Epidemiology and
Public Health Medicine

For Churchill Livingstone

Commissioning Editor: Michael Parkinson
Project Development Manager: Jim Killgore
Project Manager: Nancy Arnott
Design direction: Erik Bigland

Epidemiology and Public Health Medicine

Norman Vetter MD FFPHM
Reader and Honorary Consultant in Public Health
University of Wales College of Medicine and Bro Taf Health Authority
Cardiff, UK

Ian Matthews MSc PhD
Reader in Epidemiology
University of Wales College of Medicine
Cardiff, UK

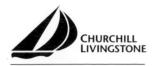
CHURCHILL
LIVINGSTONE

EDINBURGH LONDON NEW YORK PHILADELPHIA ST LOUIS
SYDNEY TORONTO 1999

CHURCHILL LIVINGSTONE
An imprint of Harcourt Publishing Limited

© Harcourt Publishing Limited 1999

is a registered trademark of Harcourt Publishing
Limited

The right of Norman Vetter and Ian Matthews to be
identified as authors of this work has been asserted by them
in accordance with the Copyright, Designs and Patents Act
1988

First published 1999

ISBN 0443-05704-4

British Library Cataloguing in Publication Data
A catalogue record for this book is available from the British
Library

Library of Congress Cataloging in Publication Data
A catalog record for this book is available from the Library of
Congress

Note
Medical knowledge is constantly changing. As new
information becomes available, changes in treatment,
procedures, equipment and the use of drugs become
necessary. The authors and the publishers have, as far as it is
possible, taken care to ensure that the information given in
this text is accurate and up-to-date. However, readers are
strongly advised to confirm that the information, especially
with regard to drug usage, complies with the latest
legislation and standards of practice.

The
publisher's
policy is to use
**paper manufactured
from sustainable forests**

Printed in China
NPCC/01

Preface

This textbook is intended to cover an undergraduate medical course in epidemiology and public health. It will also be a useful adjunct for masters degrees in public health and for post-graduate nursing courses. It is intended to be the first integrated textbook of epidemiology and public health, with the epidemiological methods leading logically into their application in public health practice.

1999   N.V.
Cardiff   I.M.

Acknowledgements

We wish to acknowledge the assistance given to us in the preparation of this book by Dr Michael Burr, Consultant in Public Health with Bro Taf health Authority, and to Ms Julia Hodgson and Ms Ann Bushell, our secretaries, in the preparation of the text.

Contents

Principles of epidemiology

The scope of epidemiology

1

This chapter discusses:

- what epidemiology is
- the information obtained in epidemiological studies
- the use of epidemiology in infectious and non-infectious diseases
- the use of epidemiology to assess population phenomena
- the use of epidemiology to assess clinical effectiveness.

Introduction

Medical epidemiologists have been described as 'doctors who don't care about a single person'. It is true that they do not often treat individuals across a desk or a bed, for they deal with illness in groups of people. Another analogy is more appealing. This suggests that doctors who treat patients individually are like people who stand beside a fast-running river, diving in and pulling out those who are being swept along by the current. This is an important and time-consuming job. Epidemiologists ignore those drowning in order to travel up-river, discover what is throwing them in and try to stop it.

Epidemiology is the study of the distribution and change in diseases. It initially developed to explain and prevent the spread of infectious diseases but in the period from the early 1960s it has acquired increasing importance in assessing risk factors for and reducing the incidence of multifactorial diseases such as heart disease. The *purpose* of epidemiology is to identify things in people and their surroundings that affect the occurrence of disease. It forms part of preventive medicine and public health. Epidemiological methods are also used to assess the effectiveness of new preventive and therapeutic treatments and the impact of different patterns of health care delivery.

Risk factors are characteristics or habits that are consistently more common in those who suffer a disease than in those people who do not. They may be suspected as a partial cause of the disease in question if that is unknown. Risk factors make people more vulnerable to the disease in some way.

Public health is defined as 'The process of promoting health, preventing disease, prolonging life and improving the quality of life through the organised efforts of society.' It is the systematic, practical application of epidemiology.

The **epidemiological approach** can be considered as occurring as a number of steps:

- definition of the disease
- the cause, aetiology
- how it spreads / occurs: risk factors:
  - in the population
  - in the environment
- how to control it
- how to prevent it
- how to eliminate it.

These aspects will appear again and again in subsequent descriptions of various diseases.

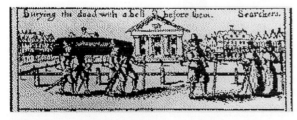

Fig. 1.1 Burying victims of the plague.

Infectious diseases

In developing countries and in the past in developed countries the main concern of epidemiologists was

The use of epidemiology

➤ To identify factors that can affect the occurrence of disease.

➤ To assess the effectiveness of preventive and therapeutic treatments.

➤ To assess the impact of health-care services.

➤ To predict future health care needs.

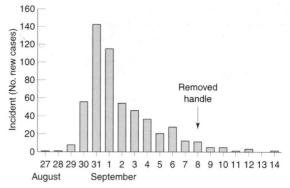

Fig. 1.2 Early attempts to find how cholera spread. The removal of the pump handle prevented access to what was a suspected source of contaminated water.

infectious diseases. The subject originated in the UK with the setting up and study of bills of mortality from infectious diseases. These were studies of deaths, which gave some warning of a severe outbreak of disease. It has been suggested that the studies were initiated and supported because the bills gave a warning for when to leave an area. Collecting data was, therefore, part of epidemiological practice from its beginnings (Fig. 1).

Early studies on cholera

One of the fathers of epidemiology, John Snow, was a clinician. He carefully studied different diseases in individuals and attempted to work out the effect of those diseases on the community at large. He suspected, before germ theory became accepted, that something in contaminated water might be responsible for the spread of cholera. In particular he suspected a water pump in Broad Street in Soho in London of being responsible for a particular cholera outbreak:

> There is a brewery in Broad Street, near to the pump, and on perceiving that no brewer's men were registered [nb] as having died of cholera, I called on Mr Huggins the proprietor. He informed me that none of them had suffered from cholera – at least in a severe form – only two having been indisposed, and that not seriously, at the time the disease prevailed. The men are allowed a certain quantity of malt liquor, and Mr Huggins believes that they do not drink water at all; and he is quite certain that the workmen never obtained water from the pump in the street …

Snow studied the progress of cases of cholera in the area then decided to act. He removed the handle of the pump in a great blaze of publicity. Figure 1.2 shows the data on deaths. We can see that he chose a good time to removal the handle in terms of publicity, but not a very persuasive time for his hypothesis that the pump contained contaminated water. Common sense suggests that the outbreak had almost stopped anyway.

As John Snow knew, there were a number of different water authorities competing for custom in the area of Soho. It was unlikely that the source of the water for both companies was contaminated if, as he suspected, the disease was in the water. The companies competed for custom by racing to dig pipes to the houses in the different streets. John Snow, therefore, had a natural experiment in which people living in otherwise similar surroundings received supplies from different water companies. In some streets, houses took water from both companies. He had data only on which street a victim came from not which house, so he could not distinguish houses in mixed-supply streets. He, therefore, divided the people who died into three groups: two groups receiving water from one company exclusively and a group where the water supply might have come from either (Fig. 1.3).

Three important principles of epidemiology are illustrated by this example:

● the crude number of affected individuals must be related to the number at risk: giving a *rate*

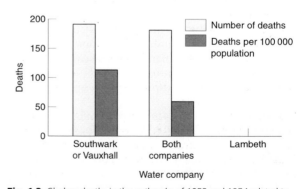

Fig. 1.3 Cholera deaths in the outbreaks of 1853 and 1854 related to the source of water.

- all the data should be used where possible
- the source and methods of limiting a disease can be identified without necessarily knowing the cause.

The first principle avoids the potential problem that the crude number, in this case deaths, may be misleading. Those people who received water solely from the Southwark or the Vauxhall Company and those who received their water from both had similar numbers of deaths. However, when Snow studied the number affected by cholera divided by the number getting water from each company, there was a much lower figure for one company. Dividing the number affected by the number at risk is a classical use of a rate.

The second principle is to use all the data whenever possible. Snow must have been tempted to ignore people in streets that received supplies from both companies and simply to compare those receiving water from one or the other. The inclusion of the mixed group, however, adds weight to the hypothesis that water from one of the companies was responsible. The death rates for people from these 'mixed' streets fall between the other two. The addition of this group, which ensured that he had used all the relevant data, increased the conclusions that could be drawn.

The use of epidemiological techniques enabled Snow to identify the source and limit the spread of a disease, cholera, without knowing its causative organism.

Cholera is virtually unknown in developed countries now but remains a scourge in developing countries. However, epidemiology has provided the necessary information to tackle the problem. It is no longer a mystery.

Smallpox

Ethiopia and Bangladesh were the last countries to suffer from epidemics of smallpox before it was eradicated from the planet in 1979. Smallpox was a major disease that killed 10 million people a year until 1968. The *International Journal of Epidemiology* wrote about the success of the eradication campaign: 'The Napoleonic conquests, World Wars I and II, the lunar landings and the space programme fade to secondary importance compared with the single achievement of eradication of smallpox'.

Figure 1.4 shows the last known sufferer of smallpox (variola major) in Bangladesh. This girl was the last naturally occurring case. The World Health Organization (WHO) workers diagnosed her disease on the 16 October 1975. The last two occurrences of smallpox on Earth were in Birmingham as a result of a tragic laboratory accident some years later.

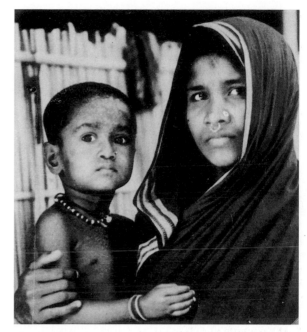

Fig. 1.4 The last known case of smallpox in Asia.

The general approach to a problem used by epidemiologists, listed above (p. 3), can be illustrated by the campaign against smallpox, where epidemiologists were largely responsible for its eradication.

In the case of smallpox the *definition* was of an infectious disease; its *cause* was the variola virus. In this instance, the disease is defined in terms of the cause, since the cause is known.

The mechanism for the way the *risk factors* increased people's vulnerability to smallpox in Bangladesh was easy to understand. Given that smallpox is an infectious disease, overcrowding, a very mobile population and disruption caused by political upheaval were obviously likely to increase the vulnerability of the population. Further factors were extreme poverty, leading to poor hygiene and poor nutrition. These are common risk factors for many infectious diseases. Epidemiologists could not reverse or eliminate the risk factors, but they could attempt to try something that they had never attempted before, to eliminate the virus, in effect to make it extinct.

One of the main breakthroughs was when to act. Figure 1.5 shows the great fluctuations in the number of outbreaks year on year in Bangladesh before its eradication. The numbers increase and decrease dramatically from year to year. They also fluctuated greatly from season to season. The epidemiologists suggested that extra people should be drafted in to vaccinate against

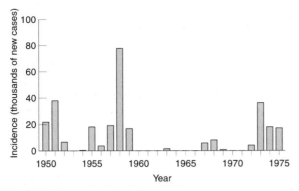

Fig. 1.5 Incidence of smallpox in Bangladesh.

smallpox when the numbers were low, rather than high. In this way the disease could be eradicated. In the past all of the effort had been concentrated on times when outbreaks were at their maximum.

Luckily, for *prevention*, there is a very effective vaccine for smallpox. The virus spreads only from close person-to-person contact. Using this knowledge, the WHO perfected a method of isolating and eliminating the virus, known as *surveillance and containment*. This consisted simply of setting up a network of workers throughout the country in question who reported on every case thought to be smallpox. To assist with this, people who reported a case received a reward. The workers then guarded the house of the infected person for a week to make sure that he or she did not leave the area. They then identified and vaccinated all people who had had contact with that person in the previous 2 weeks. The WHO originally developed this approach when workers had run short of vaccine during a mass vaccination campaign. It proved to be more successful than simply trying to find and vaccinate everyone. People knew the cause of smallpox, the variola virus, years before it was eradicated.

Control of smallpox had been possible in industrialised countries using mass vaccination since the population immunity and relative lack of personal contact stopped the spread of the disease. In developing countries, other factors closely related to poverty, overcrowding, poor nutrition and large families meant that mass vaccination did not work.

Non-infectious diseases

We can use epidemiology for any of the health problems people have. One disease that has received intense interest is myocardial infarction, sometimes known as coronary thrombosis or a heart attack. Diseases with multifactorial causes are far harder to define clearly in the way used for smallpox to give an unequivocal list of cause(s), prevention methods, etc (p. 3).

Definition of the disease

The definition of a myocardial infarction is a disruption of the blood supply to the muscle fibres of the heart causing damage to those fibres. It is normally impossible to inspect the damage directly so an indirect definition has to be used. This is said to be when characteristic new ECG changes are accompanied by an increased concentration of serum enzymes, released into the bloodstream from the damaged cardiac muscle fibres.

Aetiology

Intense efforts have been made to find the cause of myocardial infarction but so far, unlike smallpox, no single cause has been defined. Instead we know of certain characteristics that are more common in people who get myocardial infarction compared with people who do not. These are the risk factors.

Risk factors

Although certain factors do appear to be clearly associated with an increased risk of myocardial infarction, the situation is far less defined than for an infectious disease. Many people would say that the evidence against smoking is such that it is a cause beyond reasonable doubt. Despite this, people without any of the known risk factors often get myocardial infarction, suggesting that we still have a lot to learn. There are around 20 well-documented risk factors associated with coronary heart disease of which three have received the most attention, partly because they are capable of modification:

- cigarette smoking
- hypertension
- dyslipidaemia: serum cholesterol and other lipid factors.

Other population risk factors include:

- diabetes
- family history
- regional factors: identified regional variations in incidence
- relative poverty: leading to other factors such as poor diet.

Some factors can be identified but are hard to assess; for example, soft water *may* be a risk factor, hard water is certainly not.

A family history is a risk factor for any disease because families have both their genetic make-up and their environment in common. Children parted from their mother at birth still have environmental factors in common with her for they shared her body for the most formative 9 months, during gestation. Many diseases of lipid metabolism have a genetic aspect.

The environment appears to increase the risk of myocardial infarction. The classical example of this is for Japanese people who have a low risk in Japan but increase that risk when they move to the USA.

Control of myocardial infarction

Reversal of risk factors for myocardial infarction has been possible in a few experiments and the rates of myocardial infarction suffered by those people has fallen. Curiously there is a marked and virtually instantaneous fall in the rate of coronary heart disease for those who stop smoking. The disappointing part of this story has been the inability of doctors to persuade other people to stop. Doctors in the UK have persuaded themselves. They have the lowest rate for doctors in Europe. Despite this there is an increase in smoking rates among young girls in many developed countries, including the UK and USA.

Prevention of myocardial infarction

Elimination of risk factors for a disease is the ideal situation. For myocardial infarction, not all factors are known and population education, as discussed above for smoking, does not always work. In addition, in myocardial infarction there is evidence that the factors may interact in a complex manner.

Promotion of protective factors will also reduce the incidence:

● diet: increase fruit, vegetable and fatty fish content
● exercise
● aspirin for high-risk groups
● moderate alcohol intake.

We have failed to prove, on a population basis, that we can appreciably prevent or eliminate coronary heart disease by such measures. Despite this, the death rate is declining appreciably in most developed countries.

Non-disease epidemiology

Epidemiology can be applied to phenomena that are not diseases. One such is the process of ageing in humans. We can use the same subheadings to collate data as used in other epidemiological approaches although the groupings may have a different emphasis, for example ageing is not 'caused' and risk factors will be those that tilt the population to a more senescent profile.

Definition of ageing

The definition of ageing for a species is a process of accelerated senescence and death after a period of relatively low death rate. Humans in developed countries begin to age at about 70 years. Curiously not all living things age. Cox's Orange Pippens, the popular apple type, do not age. All Cox's were formed from one original tree by grafting and continue to be propagated that way. Each new generation of grafting acts like a young tree. They do not reproduce sexually. Other trees, giant redwoods and the oak, do have the possibility for sexual reproduction but they do not age. They occasionally die, through disease or woodcutters, but do not have an accelerated phase of death rate hence their great longevity.

Single-celled animals, such as the amoeba' do not age. They reach a certain degree of maturity then split into two, both being young animals again.

Aetiology

Ageing is an intrinsic feature of all mammals but its cause is difficult to define. There have been suggestions that ageing is built into the genetic make-up of some species as part of the evolutionary process to make way for the coming generations, but the evidence is slim. An aged population is much less common in countries where the environment is severe or the people have little resistance to disease, especially infectious disease. In these situations, the adverse conditions cause people to die relatively young. They, therefore, do not live long enough to enter into the ageing process. It seems unlikely that humans have, in

---

Principles of epidemiology

➤ Crude numbers of affected individuals must be related to the number at risk, giving a rate.

➤ All the data should be used wherever possible.

➤ The source of a disease and methods of limiting it can be identified without necessarily knowing the cause.

➤ Risk factors are characteristics or habits that are consistently more common in those who suffer from a disease than in those who do not.

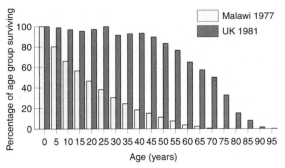

Fig. 1.6 Population structure in the UK and Malawi. (Open University Press 1984)

the past, lived long enough for evolutionary pressures to have come into play.

Figure 1.6 shows the population survival curve for Malawi and the UK. It can be seen that in the UK people survive until they reach their 70s then have a rapid death rate. In Malawi the death rate is a constant proportion of the number of people alive. The UK survival curve is typical of a country that ages, Malawi of one that does not because of the high prevalence of infectious diseases in young age groups.

We can study the possible cause or causes of ageing by looking at its associations. We think of elderly people as being likely to be handicapped and near to death. So we can see its effects in relation to deaths and morbidity even if we are not completely sure what it is. Figure 1.7 shows a group of 2000 people aged 60 and over, living at home, and their degree of disability, which causes them to be dependent upon others. As one might

expect, those with the most dependency had the greatest need for health service support. Perhaps the most interesting thing about depending is the amount it varies from person to person and place to place. In some instances, a 70-year-old may be completely dependent or in others completely independent.

Factors increasing an aged population

If ageing was a disease, the following factors would be risk factors. For a phenomenon like ageing, the epidemiological thrust is not necessarily to eliminate the process but rather to provide information to enable a society to cope with the results, for example providing more service support.

Population factors, that will affect the proportion of the population that are aged include:

- smoking (probably)
- genetic, e.g. progeria and Down's syndrome
- poverty
- excessive alcohol
- reduction in death rate: possible effect of medical services.

Generally those who age slowly, i.e. those who are *not* disabled until they are very old, and those who live a long time are those who are well off. This one factor seems to override all of the others.

Control of age span

If ageing was a disease, control would imply prevent-

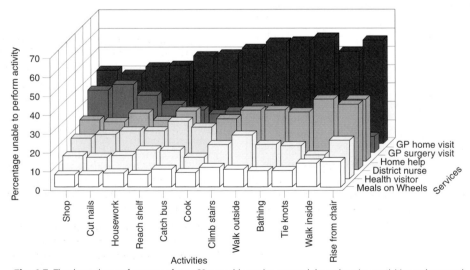

Fig. 1.7 The dependency of a group of over 60 year olds can be assessed through various activities and grouped by service use in the previous month.

ing it from occurring. For ageing, most individuals would wish to achieve a substantial age without disabilities that reduced the quality of life. In addition to avoiding the risk factors for early death, some factors may have positive effects:

- increase active life through exercise
- alter dietary pattern to more fresh fruit and vegetables.

Limitations of epidemiology

Association and causation

We should say a few things about the limitations of epidemiology. The first is that although we look for and assume that there are direct *causes* of disease. The epidemiological method can only point a finger of suspicion, indicating an *association*; we can never be certain. We can tell other people, e.g. bacteriologists or physiologists, where the cause is very likely to be but cannot actually identify it. For example, if we say 'smoking causes lung cancer' what we mean is 'in a large population, the smokers were much more likely to get lung cancer than the non-smokers'. Only an experiment can prove it beyond reasonable doubt, by exposing lung tissue to cigarette smoke and seeing the consequences over a long time.

For an epidemiologist the most persuasive experiment would be to take a cross-section of the population and persuade a randomly allocated group of people to smoke or not smoke. We could study the consequences for these people over a period. This approach is, of course, ethically and logistically very difficult. The strongly suspected risks of smoking mean that persuading people to smoke is unethical. There is, however, at least one significant experiment of persuading people to stop smoking. This showed a significant reduction in lung cancer in the group where persuasion was attempted.

Epidemiologists can point out suspected risk factors using population-based methods but these methods can only lead to associations based on statistical probability. They cannot prove that a cause leads to an effect. This is only possible in very tightly controlled laboratory experiments and even then only when the suspected causative factor always leads to the disease in question. These experiments are usually carried out in animals or in in vitro experiments.

Prevention

Prevention may be better than cure but it is certainly not cheaper. While epidemiologists may be striving to find ways of preventing or eliminating disease, there is still as much need as ever for active medicine for those suffering from the disease. So we have to pay for both at once. It is not cheaper for many years until the epidemiologist begins to succeed. Even then not even an epidemiologist would claim to be able to keep everyone alive for ever. As a result we will always have to bear the cost of the treatment of our final disease, the most expensive one for most of us.

Epidemiology applied to health care

The cause of infectious and non-infectious disease can be clarified using epidemiological methods. We are also able to make scientific statements about the natural history and outcome or prognosis of disease based upon epidemiological inquiries. These alone would be enough to emphasise the importance of the subject. However, epidemiology is also concerned with making scientific statements about the clinical effectiveness of treatments and the accuracy of diagnoses. For example observational studies have revealed the unacceptable variations in the way that many clinical treatments are carried out. Epidemiology is, therefore, needed to evaluate treatment and screening programmes and to guide us towards the best clinical approach for common and important diseases. Methods that are useful for discovering the antecedents of disease can also be used to compare the effectiveness of different treatments and be used to judge the likely outcome of disease over the long term.

> ### Wider applications of epidemiology
>
> ➤ Data on other general characteristics of populations (e.g. ageing) can be analysed using epidemiological methods.
>
> ➤ Epidemiology can indicate associations between causes and effects but cannot provide direct proof.
>
> ➤ Epidemiology is also used to assess clinical effectiveness of treatments and the accuracy of diagnoses and to evaluate screening programmes.
>
> ➤ Public health is the systematic practical application of epidemiology to promote health, prevent disease and prolong high-quality life.

Measuring health and disease

2

In this chapter the basic definitions and parameters used to describe health and disease are described, including:

- diagnosis of disease
- prevalence and incidence
- death rates and life expectancy
- morbidity.

Definitions of health and disease

Health and disease are difficult to define precisely because they are closely interwoven with the way that people view one another in a particular society. The WHO in 1948 in its original constitution proposed the most ambitious definition of health: 'Health is a state of complete physical, mental and social well-being and not merely the absence of disease or infirmity.'

People have criticised this definition because of the difficulty of defining and measuring well-being, but it remains an ideal. In 1977, the World Health Assembly resolved that the main target of governments in the WHO in the coming decades, should be 'The attainment by all citizens of the world by the year 2000, of a level of health that will permit them to lead a socially and economically productive life'.

Another suggestion for a definition of health, originally adapted from Freud, is at least a little easier to measure 'Health is the ability to love and work'.

Epidemiologists have to use working definitions that simplify these concepts in order to carry out their work. They need to have more practical definitions of health and disease and to measure the health status of large numbers of people. It is important, therefore, to concentrate on states that can be measured relatively easily. Definitions of health states used by epidemiologists tend to be simple, such as 'dead' or 'alive', or 'disease present' or 'disease absent'. Criteria for the presence or absence of a disease need to rely on definitions of normality and abnormality. Since there is considerable individual variation in most measures in humans, it is often difficult to define what is 'normal'; there is sometimes no absolute distinction between 'normal' and 'abnormal'.

Diagnosis

Diagnostic labels are often inconsistent in the way they are applied. They must be defined consistently for studies on causation, the effectiveness of treatment and prognosis to be carried out.

Reaching a diagnosis usually uses information on:

- symptoms
- signs
- test results.

For example, we can identify hepatitis by the presence of antibodies in the blood. We can detect asbestosis by symptoms and signs of lung function changes, signs of fibrosis of the lung tissue or pleural thickening on radiographs and a history of exposure to asbestos fibres.

Problems in reaching a diagnosis

In clinical practice many diagnostic criteria will consist of 'disease present', disease absent' and 'disease probably present'. Many diseases are complex and a group of *diagnostic criteria* are needed to decide whether a person with some symptoms and signs has a disease.

Table 2.1 shows the modified Jones diagnostic criteria for rheumatic fever. We describe rheumatic fever, despite its rarity these days, because it is a disease with no absolute measure of whether it is present or not. We can make a diagnosis based on several manifestations of rheumatic fever. However, some signs are more important than others. We may feel that a few

Table 2.1 Jones criteria for rheumatic fever: there is a high probability of rheumatic fever if two major or one major and two or more minor manifestations are present, plus evidence of a preceding streptococcal infection

Major signs	Minor signs
Carditis	Fever
Polyarthritis	Arthralgia
Chorea	Previous disease
Erythema marginatum	Abnormal laboratory reaction
Nodules	ECG changes (long PR interval)

people fitting the clinical criteria do not have the disease. The approach identifies people who are very likely to have rheumatic fever. It is important to be as accurate as possible in the case of rheumatic fever. People who believe that they have the disease may be afraid of the future possibility of getting rheumatic heart disease and may avoid living a full life because of this. People who have the disease need therapy and we need to follow them up to make sure that they have not developed rheumatic heart disease. For this reason it is important that we try not to miss cases or label people with the disease who have not had it.

Absence of diagnostic signs

The commonest disease in developed countries, myocardial infarction, has strict criteria for its diagnosis relating to coronary obstruction or damage to the heart muscle. However, a significant proportion of the patients thought to have myocardial infarction die suddenly. Many of these will have no significant pathological evidence of disease, but the most likely diagnosis is that they had a sudden cardiac arrhythmia, caused by an abnormality of the coronary circulation. We believe this because mobile coronary care units have effectively treated many people, notably in Seattle in the USA, who have collapsed instantaneously. The doctors in Seattle have found that many of these do not have coronary obstruction or, indeed, much damage to their heart muscle.

Simple diagnostic criteria: diagnosis in developing countries

In some situations we can justify very simple criteria. For example, the reduction of mortality caused by bacterial pneumonia in children in developing countries is dependent on rapid detection and treatment. The WHO case management guidelines recommend that pneumonia case detection is based on clinical signs alone, without listening to the heart, or making chest

X-ray or laboratory diagnostic tests. The only equipment required is a simple device for timing respiratory rate. One can justify the use of antibiotics for suspected pneumonia based only on a physical examination in places with a high likelihood of bacterial pneumonia and where treatment carries a very low risk if the diagnosis is wrong.

Changing criteria for disease

Criteria for disease may change. For example, the WHO modified its criteria for myocardial infarction in epidemiological studies by introducing an objective method for assessing electrocardiograms, called the Minnesota Code. The criteria to make a definite diagnosis of myocardial infarction are based on three things:

- the first and most important is a classical history
- the second the release of enzymes from the damaged heart muscle
- the third consists of changes to the electrical field that co-ordinates the normal heart beat, seen as abnormalities to the electrocardiogram according to Minnesota Code measures.

It is difficult to outline damage to the heart muscle using direct imaging techniques. Because of this people rarely use the method for reaching a diagnosis when patients are acutely ill.

Diagnostic criteria for epidemiology

Whatever the definitions used in epidemiology, it is essential that we state them clearly. They must also be:

- easy to use
- easy to measure in a standard manner
- easy to measure under a wide variety of circumstances
- easy to measure by different people
- highly likely to produce the same result if used twice by the same person.

Within clinical practice, definitions are often quite loosely used so that clinical judgement plays a larger part in defining whether someone has a disease. This is partly because clinicians often reach a diagnosis by eliminating other possible causes using a series of tests until they reach the final, most likely diagnosis. They also need to treat the patient. This trial and error approach is reasonable while diagnostic testing continues. Definitions need to be more rigorous if the decisions will be used, for instance, to decide on the cause of a disease.

Measures of disease frequency

Measuring disease frequency (occurrence) is an important part of epidemiology. There are several measures of disease frequency based on two important ideas, prevalence and incidence. We can measure these as raw numbers or more usefully using rates.

Use of rates

A rate is a simple idea, about which there can be much confusion. The commonest rate used in daily life is the **percentage**. This is the number in question divided by (per) one hundred (cent). Most people have a general feel that 50% is half and 25% is a quarter of the people in question.

Rates may be out of any number not just out of 100, e.g. based on per 1000, per 100 000, per million. We choose the bottom figure, the **denominator** so that the rate is a whole number that we can deal with easily. The number on top, usually the number of occurrences (for example infant deaths) is the **numerator**. Table 2.2 shows some examples of numerators, denominators and the subsequent rate.

It is obvious that the different measures of frequency depend on precise estimates of the denominators. These are the figures for the population on which the calculation is based. Ideally this population figure should include only the people who are susceptible to the disease studied. For instance, we should not include men in calculations of the occurrence of carcinoma of the cervix. Curiously the denominator is often more difficult accurately to measure than the numerator. This is often forgotten.

Population at risk

We call the part of the total population that is susceptible to the disease the population at risk. We can often define this using **demographic measures** (for example, age, sex, marital state, or where people live) or environmental factors. For instance, occupational injuries only occur among working people, in this case the population at risk is the workforce. In some countries, brucellosis occurs only among people handling infected animals. The appropriate population at risk in this instance should be farm and slaughterhouse workers.

Prevalence and incidence

A case of disease can either be an existing case, someone that has had the disease for some time, or a new case, someone that has just fallen ill. These are two ways of measuring occurrence and for specific diseases the relation between prevalence and incidence is often quite different. The definitions of these terms is important in ensuring that data are expressed in a suitable way and that the rates expressed are understood clearly by all who subsequently use them.

Incidence

Incidence measures the number of new episodes of illness arising in a population during a specified period. It can be measured as a rate.

$$\text{Incidence rate} = \frac{\text{Number of new cases over a period}}{\substack{\text{Population at risk for the time period} \\ \text{during which cases collected}}}$$

Sometimes measuring incidence is difficult because of changes in the population at risk during the time over which data was collected. This can be overcome by dividing the number of cases per year by the total number of person-years at risk. In this we add the periods during which each member of the population is at risk. In this way, people who die or move away are no longer at risk and we can take them out of the calculation.

The incidence rate should take into account the variable time periods individuals are disease-free and,

Table 2.2 Numerators, denominators and rates			
Example	Numerator	Denominator	Rate
Infant mortality in the UK, 1994	Deaths in infants aged 1 year and under	Live births during the year	5.1 infant deaths per 1000 live births
Deaths from breast cancer in the UK 1993	Deaths from breast cancer in women (rare in men)	Females of all ages at mid-point of year	24 per 100 000 female population
Patients consulting their GP for neurotic disorders 1991/92	Patients consulting their GP for neurotic disorders (first time only)	Population registered with the GPs in question	344 per 10 000 people at risk

therefore, at risk of developing the disease. Since it may not be possible to measure disease-free periods precisely, we often calculate it approximately by multiplying the average size of the study population by the length of the study period. This is reasonably accurate if the population size is stable and the incidence rate is low. For diseases that one may catch more than once it is necessary to say whether the incidence refers to the first attack only or to each separate attack.

Prevalence

Prevalence of a disease is the number of people in a population that have the disease (are cases) either at a particular time (**point prevalence**) or over a stated period (period prevalence). A 3-month prevalence will be the number of people identified with the disease or problem at any time during a 3-month period. We calculate prevalence rate by dividing the number of cases by the corresponding number of people in the population at risk.

$$\text{Prevalence rate} = \frac{\text{Number of cases in a given time}}{\text{Population at risk during that time period}}$$

$$\text{Point prevalence rate} = \frac{\text{Number of cases at a given time}}{\text{Number at risk at that time}}$$

Data concerning the ideal 'population at risk' are not always available and in many studies the total population in the study area is used as an approximation. The prevalence rate is always a proportion, but it is often expressed as 'cases per 100 population' or 'cases per 1000 population'. We refer to it as a prevalence rate or just prevalence.

Since prevalence rates are influenced by the chance of surviving with a disease, prevalence studies do not give very strong evidence when we are trying to determine the cause of a disease. Measures of prevalence rate are helpful for deciding the need for health care

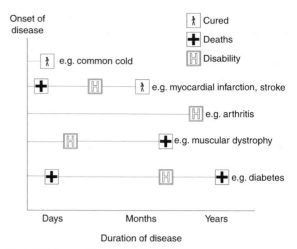

Fig. 2.1 Patterns of disease.

and the planning of health services. High rates can suggest those areas that, because of the nature of the population or the environment, are generating more cases. When deciding where to site a new health centre or hospital it may be more useful to know the actual number of cases in a year, rather than the rate.

Comparison of prevalence and incidence

Figure 2.1 shows the factors that link incidence and prevalence for different diseases. Diseases that are short-lived, because they are rapidly cured or are fatal at an early stage, will have a relatively low prevalence compared with their incidence. Diseases with a low mortality and low cure rate, leaving people with the disabling effect of the disease, will have a high prevalence compared with their incidence.

Table 2.3 shows the types of disease for which measuring prevalence or incidence will be most useful and the uses to which we can put them. It is obvious that

Table 2.3 Types of disease and measures of prevalence and incidence		
Type of disease	Use of incidence	Use of prevalence
Relatively rare severe chronic disease with fairly low early mortality, e.g. diabetes, muscular dystrophies	Estimates of numbers found by screening. Will give information about future needs, e.g. age groups in need	Estimates of numbers needing continuing care
Common dangerous disease with long-term consequences, e.g. myocardial infarction, stroke	Estimates of need for early emergency treatment	Need for rehabilitation
Short-lived non-dangerous diseases, e.g. common cold, childhood infectious diseases	Estimates of demand on GPs, especially if epidemics	
Common chronic disease with slow onset and low mortality, e.g. arthritis	Estimates of need for specific interventions in chronic conditions, e.g. hip replacements	Need for treatment and rehabilitation

diseases that are common will have higher incidence and prevalence rates than those which are rare.

Measuring prevalence and incidence involves the counting of cases in defined populations at risk. The number of new cases alone can give an impression of the overall size of a health problem or of short-term time trends within a given population, for instance during an epidemic. The WHO *Weekly Epidemiological Record* contains incidence data as case numbers. These, despite their crude nature, can give useful information about the development of epidemics of communicable diseases, for example cholera and dengue fever. In the UK, similar data are available from the Communicable Diseases Surveillance Centre at Colindale, near London.

Uses of incidence and prevalence data

Routine data on the incidence and prevalence of different diseases are often not available. Because of this, attempts have been made to work out the overall incidence or prevalence of some diseases from hospital data which are easily available. It is thought that hospital admission of people with fractured neck of femur is one disease where hospital data closely resemble the true incidence. The reason for this is that the great majority of cases are admitted to hospital. Figure 2.2 shows the estimated rates based upon admissions to hospital. It must be made clear whether the incidence refers to each attack, for patients commonly fracture their other neck of femur or re-fracture the original side.

An example of a disease where it is said that we can estimate prevalence from hospital data is schizophrenia. Here it is assumed that the severity and specialist nature of the treatment required for the disease means that virtually all cases are admitted at least once during a 5-year period. If people admitted or seen at in- or

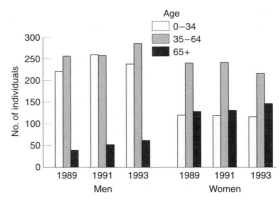

Fig. 2.3 Prevalence indicated by hospital data for schizophrenia over a 5-year period.

out-patients are counted and readmissions removed, it is said that a reasonable estimate of the true prevalence can be made. Figure 2.3 shows such data for a health authority with about 400 000 people in its population.

Uses of prevalence rate

We often use prevalence rates to measure the occurrence of conditions where the onset of disease may be gradual, such as maturity-onset diabetes or rheumatoid arthritis. The prevalence rate of non-insulin-dependent diabetes mellitus (per 100 population) in various populations using criteria proposed by the WHO varies greatly from place to place. These differences suggest the importance of environmental factors or ethnic background in causing this disease and indicate that there are markedly different needs for diabetic health services in different populations (Fig. 2.4).

Figure 2.5 shows the incidence rate of stroke in 100 000 women who were 30–55 years of age and free from coronary heart disease, stroke and cancer in 1976.

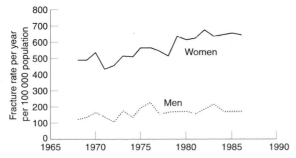

Fig. 2.2 Hospital admission rates for fractured femur as an indication of incidence. Data taken from the Oxford Record Linkage standardised by the 1981 population. (Evans, Seagroat & Goldacre 1997)

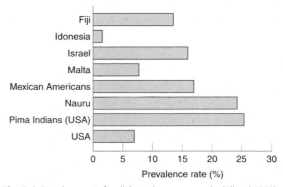

Fig. 2.4 Prevalence rate for diabetes in young people. (Alberti 1993)

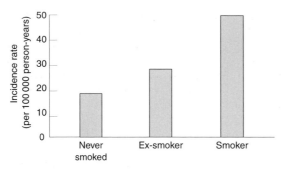

Fig. 2.5 Incidence rate of stroke in female smokers and non-smokers. (Wolf et al 1988)

The researchers identified 274 stroke cases in the 8 years of follow-up. The incidence rate was 30.2 per 100 000 person-years of observation. It was found to be higher in smokers than non-smokers; ex-smokers had rates in between the rates of non-smokers and smokers.

Inter-relationship of prevalence and incidence

Prevalence is dependent on both the *incidence* of the illness and the *duration* of the study period. Provided prevalence is low (and only then):

Prevalence = Incidence × duration

The **cumulative incidence rate** of a specific disease depends on both the incidence rate and the length of the period of interest. The incidence rate usually changes with age, so age-specific incidence rates must also be considered. Cumulative incidence is a useful approximation when the incidence rate is low or when the study period is short. New cases are collected over a period and these are simply added to the total over that period. It is used where the disease in question is chronic or, at least, continues over the collection period. An example is in the cumulative incidence of dementia, where some researchers have collected new cases over a number of years then divided the total by the number of years to give an annual incidence, about 4% for people over 65 years.

Confidence interval

Values for a whole population are calculated from values measured for a sample population. The confidence interval (CI) is the range within which we can have a certain degree of confidence that the value for the whole population will fall. For example, a parameter can be described as x (CI 95%: x_1–x_2): we can be 95% confident that the value lies between a minimum of x_1 and a maximum of x_2. The larger the size of the sample

> ### Measures of disease frequency
>
> ➤ Diagnosis depends on signs, symptoms and test results. Unambiguous diagnostic labels are needed for studies assessing causation and treatment.
> ➤ Incidence measures the number of *new* cases during a specific period.
> ➤ Prevalence is a measure of the number of cases present in a population at a particular time (point prevalence) or over a certain period (period prevalence).
> ➤ Measures of disease intensity, as prevalence and incidence, indicate the pressure of a disease on a population.
> ➤ Cumulative incidence rates are useful for diseases that extend over a reasonable period.

on which we base the calculation the smaller will be the confidence interval.

The confidence interval is taken as the value plus and minus twice its standard error where the standard error is given by

$$\sqrt{\frac{p\,(1-p)}{n}}$$

Where p is the proportion of a population (n) showing the characteristic. The proportion p and the standard error can be expressed as percentages and the 95% confidence interval is $[p - 2 \times (SE)] - [p + 2 \times (SE)]$.

Crude, specific and standardised rates

Estimations, whether of incidence, prevalence or mortality rates, are known as crude values if they refer to the population as a whole. Specific rates are used commonly to examine data for different groups, usually made on the basis of:

● age
● sex
● social class.

By narrowing the population in this way, one can compare different places that may have considerable differences in the composition of their age groups, or the proportion of males or females or their proportion of different social classes. The term **demography** is used to describe the study of populations on a national, regional or local basis in terms of age, sex or rates for more than one population.

Changes in population

For whole populations, three measures are commonly derived:

- death rate
- birth rate
- life expectancy.

Figure 2.6 shows births and deaths in England and Wales as recorded for the 100 years up to 1991. The figure shows:

- the number of births each year from 1991 back to 1891 recorded as the age of the group in 1991
- the population of England and Wales for each relevant year.

The difference between the two lines represents the number of people who have died for each age. Both lines show marked peaks and troughs. The two lines begin to diverge markedly for people aged 70 and over. Despite this, the peaks and troughs in the birth rate continue to have a marked effect upon the number of people still alive. This continues until people are in their 80s. Therefore, fluctuations in the number of births have a dramatic effect upon the numbers of people in the population, including the numbers of elderly people.

Even today the greatest age spike resulted from the rise in the number of births after the First World War. These people were 73 in 1991. As a result, in 1981 there were 50% more people aged 61 than aged 63. As time passes and people grow older, the peaks and troughs move across to the right and we can use them to understand future trends.

A useful habit epidemiologists have is to try to see themselves as being in the centre of the universe. For example, if someone says 'There is a projected increase of 60% in the over 85s in the next 25 years', an epi-

demiologist will not say, 'how awful, how will we cope?' or even, 'how wonderful that all these early 20th century babies survived'. Instead, the epidemiologist asks, 'what was it over the past 25 years?'. The answer to that question is that the over 85s increased by 120%, a considerably greater proportional change than in later years.

Deaths

Chadwick, one of the founding fathers of epidemiology, said, 'Death is certain – the rest is surmise'.

Curiously, epidemiologists often begin the investigation of the health of a population with data on deaths. In most countries, people are legally required to record the fact and the cause of death on a standard certificate that includes information such as:

- age
- sex
- birth date
- place of residence
- cause of death.

The data are open to various sources of error, but from an epidemiological perspective, routine death data often provide invaluable information on trends in the health of the population. How useful the data are depends on many things. These include the completeness of the count of the deaths and the accuracy of the diagnosis of the cause of death, especially in elderly people for whom autopsy rates, to confirm the diagnosis, are often low.

Deaths are usually accurately measured. However, people may not report deaths for cultural or religious reasons and the age at time of death may be inaccurate. In particular, people may under-report suicides in countries where there is a religious aversion to that diagnosis.

Internationally agreed classification procedures (the International Classification of Diseases prepared by the WHO) are used for coding the cause of death and the data is expressed as death rates. The coding of cause of death is quite complex and is not yet routine in all countries. Even with the International Classification there are differences in time and between countries owing to diagnostic fashion and differences in the interpretation of the classification.

The **death rate** (crude mortality rate) is calculated:

$$\text{Crude mortality rate} = \frac{\text{Number of deaths in a specified period} \times 100}{\text{Average total population during that period}}$$

The main disadvantage of a crude mortality rate is that

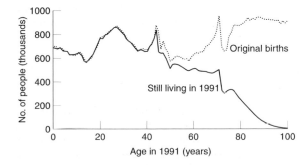

Fig. 2.6 Births and population of England and Wales in the period 1891 to 1991. The original births and population in 1991 are recorded on the basis of age in 1991. (OHE Compendium of Health Statistics 1997)

it takes no account of the fact that the chance of dying varies according to age, sex, race, socioeconomic class and other factors. It is usually not appropriate to use crude death rates for comparing different time periods or different geographic areas. For example, the death rates of people living in a new housing estate with many young families will be very much lower than that in a seaside resort where many retired people choose to live.

Life expectancy

Life expectancy is another frequently used summary measure of the health status of a population. We define it as the average number of years we expect an individual of a given age to live if current mortality trends continue.

International differences in life expectancy

It is not easy to interpret the reasons for the differences between countries in life expectancy. Different patterns among countries emerge when we use different life expectancy measures. Life expectancy at birth, as an overall measure of health status, attaches greater importance to deaths in infancy than to deaths later in life. Life expectancy at later ages may be used to examine the impact of the environment or health services on older people. Figure 2.7 shows the range for a number of countries. In the least developed countries, the life expectancy at birth may be as low as 40–50 years because of high infant mortality rates.

Other mortality-based measures of health status

People have proposed other measures of health status based on mortality data. **Years of potential life lost**

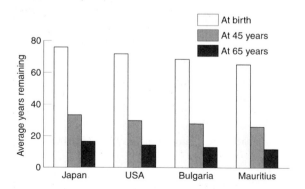

Fig. 2.7 The life expectancy at various ages in different countries. (OHE Compendium of Health Statistics 1997)

(YPLL) are based on the life lost through premature death, before some arbitrarily determined age, for example 70 years. More complex measures take into account not only the duration of life but also some analysis of its nature, e.g. **life expectancy free from disability**, or **quality-adjusted life years** (QUALY). People increasingly use the latter measures in estimates of cost effectiveness of various medical procedures.

Case fatality

Case fatality is a measure of the severity of a disease, in terms of deaths. We define it as the proportion of cases of a specified disease or condition that are fatal within a specified time.

Specific death rates

As with population rates we can express death rates more usefully for specific groups of the population. These may be age, race, sex or occupation groups. They may be in a geographic location or may have specific causes of death. For example, we define an age- and sex-specific death rate as:

$$\text{Age/sex specific death rate} = \frac{\text{No. deaths in each age/sex group in a period}}{\text{Average number of people in age/sex population in period}}$$

The measurement of death rates in communities is a very accurate measure of the size of that problem. Specific rates tell you which part of the community is most affected by this mortality.

Standardised rates or adjusted rates

Standardised rates are a way of summarising the specific rates for two or more populations. The specific rates in each population are used as if the subgroups (in, for example, each age group) were the same (standardised) for both populations. The standard structure may be based on that for the UK or the local area or we may simply add together the structure of the different populations being compared. By tradition, the standard structure is given a value of 100. This lets us compare, for instance, the death or disability rates of two or more populations while holding steady the known differences between them, usually their age structure, sex or social status. Standardisation is, therefore, useful when we try to describe the underlying differences in populations holding steady their known attributes, e.g. age, race, socioeconomic status, by the standardisation.

The classical example is the comparison of a retirement area with a new area of council housing, mentioned above. Wealthy elderly people live in the retirement area. Poor, younger people live in the council housing estate. The retirement area will have a high crude death rate because of the greater age of the population. This gives us no information about the fitness of the two populations. By standardising the mortality rate using age-specific death rates we can compare the two areas holding constant the difference in age between the two areas. In such circumstances, the best known standardised rate, the **standardised mortality rate**, sets the standard rate at 100 for both areas. Manipulation of the age-specific rates will then influence the rates for the two areas in question. A higher age-specific mortality will lead the poorer area to have a high standardised mortality (say 130), whereas the better off area will have a lower than standard rate (say 80).

Comparison of crude, specific and standardised mortality rates

The use of standardised rates allows a direct comparison to be made of the impact of a disease on mortality in different areas with different population structures. By using the age-standardised rates we can eliminate the influence of different age distributions on the mortality rates. For example, there is a great variation between countries in the reported crude mortality rates for diseases of the circulatory system (Fig. 2.8). Finland has a crude rate approximately five times higher than that of Mexico, but the standardised rate is less than twice as high: the difference between these countries is not as large as it appears from the crude rates. Developing countries have a much greater proportion of young people in their populations than the

developed countries and young people have low rates of cardiovascular disease compared with older people. Therefore, the age-standardised rates give a more accurate impression of the differences in mortality rates in different countries.

Mortality in early childhood

Mortality before and just after birth is commonly described as the **infant mortality rate**. It is often used to summarise healthiness, or lack of it, in a community. Infant mortality reflects the well-being and fitness of the mother and, therefore, of the society generally. It measures the death rate in children during the first year of life. The denominator is the number of live births in the same year. It is calculated as:

$$\text{Infant mortality rate} = \frac{\text{Number of deaths of infants less than 1 year}}{\text{Number of live births in year}}$$

The infant mortality rate is often used as a measure of overall health status when comparing different countries; it varies enormously from country to country (Fig. 2.9).

The assumption is that it is particularly sensitive to socioeconomic changes and to health care interventions. The measure does relate to the socioeconomic status of an area or country, but there is little or no evidence that it reflects the quality of the health services in the places being compared. Social elements, especially poverty, are so closely associated with infant mortality that it is difficult to imagine anything else making a significant impact upon it. Figure 2.10 shows the infant mortality rate for OECD countries compared with the gross domestic product per person (used as a measure of average wealth) for those countries. We can see the close relationship between the two measures. Infant

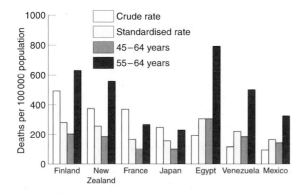

Fig. 2.8 Crude rates and age-standardised rates for deaths from circulatory disease in different countries. (OHE Compendium of Health Statistics 1997)

Population rates

➤ Crude rates based on the whole population can be narrowed to a specific group (e.g. one sex), giving specific rates.

➤ Life span can be indicated by death rates or life expectancy at a certain age and can be extended to take into account quality of life as well as duration.

➤ Standardised rates allow a direct comparison between different areas with different population structures.

➤ Infant mortality rate is often used as an indicator of the health status of a community.

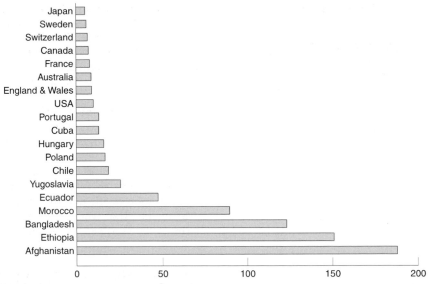

Fig. 2.9 Infant mortality rate in different countries (1989). (OHE Compendium of Health Statistics 1997)

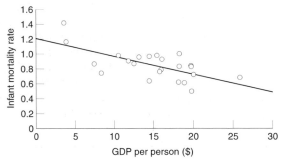

Fig. 2.10 The relationship between the infant mortality rate and the gross domestic product (GDP) for OECD countries in 1987. (World Bank 1993)

health tends to be closely correlated with the wealth of the parents and of the country as a whole.

Other measures of mortality in early childhood include:

- fetal death rate
- stillbirth rate
- perinatal mortality rate
- neonatal mortality rate
- postneonatal mortality rate.

Precise guidelines to the definition of stillbirth, fetal death and live births are given in the International Classification of Diseases.

Morbidity

Death rates are particularly useful when a disease has a high fatality. However, many diseases have a low death rate. Examples are varicose veins, rheumatoid arthritis, chickenpox and mumps. In these diseases, data on morbidity (the effect of illness) are more useful than mortality rates. Even in cases with a relatively high mortality, the effect of treatment on the morbidity of the disease may vary considerably between different treatments. Morbidity is a better measure of health status than mortality for people with diseases that are long term and disabling. In contrast to mortality, morbidity has many facets, some of which are set by the society in which the measurement is made. There is, therefore, no single, agreed measure of morbidity in health care.

We often need morbidity data to clarify the reasons for mortality trends. Changes in death rates could result from changes in morbidity rates or from changes in the severity of the disease. For example, the recent decline in cardiovascular disease mortality rates in many developed countries result either result from a fall in the number of new cases or from a reduction in how lethal it is, its case fatality. It is important to know which of these is true for it indicates the success of the preventative services in the first case and the treatment services in the second.

Classification of morbidity

Increasingly measurements in epidemiology concern not only the occurrence (for example, incidence rates, morbidity rates) but also the persistence over time or the long-term consequences of disease. These are known as the prevalence of impairments, disabilities and handicaps. The WHO has established definitions of these terms:

impairment: this is organ based, and discribes failure or loss of that organ for example in renal or cardiac failure or the loss of a limb or other organ, e.g. an eye

disability: this is person based, for example if someone is unable to walk, wash themselves or catch a bus

handicap: this is socially based, for example if someone is unable to fulfil the functions of a student, a parent or a plumber.

Impairment

We can classify impairments, once we understand the scientific basis for a disease, as present or absent, all or nothing. We can perform a function test to see if the organ is normal.

Disability

Disabilities differ from impairments in that they usually need to be described in terms of severity. For example, someone with arthritis may be able to wash him or herself but they may be slow because of pain or stiffness of their joints. Alternatively, they may require assistance or a special adaptation to the room to do so.

The severity of disability is measured in a number of ways. Some researchers have described the ability to do certain activities by the time people take. They compare this time with the expected average for healthy individuals to give the variation from the average. More usually, the classification contains three categories: the person performs the function without difficulty, with difficulty or not at all alone. We may add a further subcategory depending on whether the individual uses an aid or adaptation to perform the function.

Disabilities and their severity depend upon the immediate environment in which the person finds him or herself. This environment may be unalterable or may be changed to reduce the impact of a disability. Some work on the progression of disabilities with time showed which people were most likely to become ill over a 2-year period. They were people who were very elderly and those who were frail at the beginning. Neither of these characteristics were open to being altered for the better. However, two other important

---

Morbidity

➤ Morbidity is the state of being diseased and its measurement is important in long-term or disabling conditions.

➤ Morbidity can be classified as impairment (organ loss/failure), disability (person based, inability to do certain things) or handicap (social based, inability to fulfil a function).

➤ Disabilities can have varying severity, which will be affected by environmental factors (such as poor housing conditions).

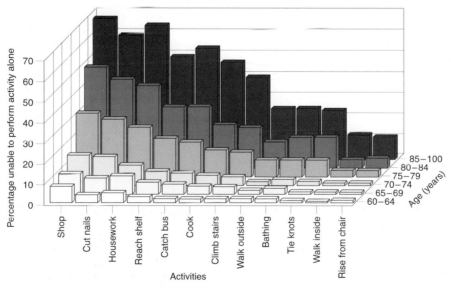

Fig. 2.11 Dependency profile for people over 60 years of age.

factors were poor housing conditions and isolation. Although these occurred in a small proportion of the people in the study, both were things that could be changed and were, therefore, important. Figure 2.11 shows data for elderly people and the proportion who were unable to perform certain tasks, such as go shopping or walk indoors. If a person is disabled to the extent that they are unable to do the task they are said to be dependent. There is a dramatic difference in the proportion of people who are dependent for different things and this rises rapidly with age.

Handicap

Handicap is more difficult to classify. It implies that an impairment or disability prevents the fulfilment of a normal *rôle* for that individual. We must, therefore, define a normal rôle for the age, sex and culture of that person. An elderly female in a remote village in Ethiopia will have a very different expected rôle from an elderly female in Sweden. The proximity of their family will have a major effect upon the degree of handicap suffered by an individual.

Causation

3

In this chapter the association between cause and effect is assessed with emphasis on:

- strength of association
- multiple and interacting causes
- confounding variables
- clinical investigation and assessment.

Cause and effect

The dictionary defines *cause* as 'Something that brings about an effect or a result'. In medicine it is sometimes very easy to work out cause and effect. This is most obvious for treatment. For example, a patient on the point of dying because of raised intracranial haemorrhage may, from being almost dead, be brought back to life by burr holes being drilled in their skull. This may even be achieved with a well-manipulated screwdriver on the street. Patients near death in extreme cardiac failure may respond amazingly to intravenous therapy. The relationship between cause and effect is so dramatic, so obvious in these cases, that there is no problem about what caused what.

The cause of disease may also be fairly obvious. A chest X-ray will show dramatically the cause of a lobar pneumonia. At operation, the cause of acute abdominal pain may be obvious as an inflamed appendix.

More often, as prevention and early treatment become more sophisticated, the relationship between cause and effect for diseases becomes more tenuous. It is difficult to work out whether an environmental hazard causes a disease or whether a treatment has caused a cure in a number of people. The days of magic bullets and miraculous cures have given way to careful statistical analysis of the treatment in large groups of patients.

Cause and effect and association

Epidemiologists have difficulties deciding that some-thing is a cause, when it may simply be associated with the disease in question. An association between two things occurs when their presence or absence appears to be linked, one increasing with changes in the other (a positive association), or one decreasing as the other increases (a negative association). The relationship is arithmetic and, therefore, may be a chance finding or may result from a third factor causing them both to alter in concert. The strength of the association can be assessed and will provide evidence of a causal relationship.

Analysing data for cause and effect

The relationship between cause and effect is not always obvious. in the ratio of exposed to non-exposed in the case group divided by the same ratio in the control group. One method of indicating the relationship is the **odds ratio**.

Betting odds are understood to be a ratio between amounts staked, e.g. a bookmaker may offer odds of 5:1 that Manchester United will win the Football League. Analogously the odds that a case is exposed divided by the odds that a control is exposed determines the odds ratio.

The fourfold table

Data on the exposure to risk factors of cases and controls can be put into a table organised in a two-by-two or fourfold table (Table 3.1). By tradition, we show the disease of interest in the columns. The patients who have the disease are counted in the left-hand column and those without in the right-hand column. Traditionally, data about the factors associated with the disease is given in the rows. The factor believed to be associated with the disease is usually in the top row. These are not hard and fast rules but they do help to reduce confusion.

Table 3.1 The distribution of cases and controls among the cells of a fourfold table

Suspected causal factor	Disease	
	Present	Absent
Present	a	b
Absent	c	d

Total with causal factor is a + b
Total without causal factor is c + d
Total with disease is a + c
Total without disease is b + d

The odds ratio in Table 3.1 is given by

$$= \frac{a/c}{b/d} = \frac{ad}{bc}$$

In other words the opposite cells are multiplied and the results divided by one another.

This analysis of data is illustrated by a study in the mid-19th century by Oliver Wendell Holmes (then Professor of Anatomy and Physiology, and later Dean of Harvard Medical School). He looked at the hand washing habits of obstetricians and the occurrence of sepsis and puerperal fever in mothers (Table 3.2)

In order to compare the effect of obstetricians not washing their hands with those washing their hands the odds ratio can be used: the odds that a case (with puerperal fever) is exposed (treated by obstetricians who did not wash their hands) is divided by the odds that a control (without puerperal fever) is exposed. In mathematical terms we have derived this as ad/bc. In numerical terms this is:

$$\frac{140 \times 620}{60 \times 180} = 8.0.$$

One can see that the chances of a patient catching puerperal fever is much higher if treated by obstetricians who did not wash their hands.

Holmes' observations led him to conclude: 'The disease known as puerperal fever is so far contagious, as to be frequently carried from patient to patient by physicians and nurses'. One response to Holmes' assertion that unwashed hands caused puerperal fever was

that the finding made no sense. 'I prefer to attribute puerperal sepsis cases to accident, or Providence, of which I can form a conception, rather than to contagion of which I cannot form any clear idea, at least as to this particular malady', wrote Professor Meigs, the Professor of Midwifery at the Harvard Medical College. The same happened in Edinburgh where Sir James Young Simpson completely ignored the advice of the young Lord Lister, his son-in-law, about keeping his hands clean when delivering babies.

The issue of *causation* confronted Simpson and Lister. Lister's data convinced him that obstetricians caused the spread of puerperal sepsis by not washing their hands between deliveries. He could not, however, say what the link was between hand washing and the disease. He did not know about bacteria causing sepsis. Simpson, therefore, remained unconvinced that anyone had established the cause of puerperal sepsis (and presumably did not bother to wash his hands).

Table 3.2 shows a number of important things. First, not all mothers, even when the obstetricians did not wash their hands, caught puerperal fever. Second, not all mothers treated by obstetricians who did wash their hands avoided it. Failing to wash hands is, therefore, not a simple cause of puerperal fever. Other things must have been involved. There is an **association** between not washing hands and getting puerperal fever.

Strength of an association

A causal relationship is indicated by the strength of an association. Patients whose obstetricians did not wash their hands are about 8 times more likely to get puerperal fever than those where the obstetrician did wash. This is a considerable difference and strongly suggests that the association is one of cause and effect. The greater the value of the odds ratio the stronger is the association between cause and effect.

Toxic shock syndrome: cause and effect relationship

An example of exploring the relationship between cause and effect occurred in the late 1970s when cases of a new and lethal disease, called toxic shock syndrome, began to appear. Patients were usually young women who suffered the onset of:

● fever
● rash and desquamation
● hypotension
● mucous membrane inflammation
● laboratory evidence of abnormalities affecting many systems.

Table 3.2 Hand washing and puerperal fever in 1843

Obstetric practice	Puerperal fever	
	Present	Absent
Do not wash hands	140 (a)	180 (b)
Do wash hands	60 (c)	620 (d)

The disease often appeared during menstruation. Scientists from the Center for Disease Control began studying the epidemic. In 1980, the researchers thought that using a new type of tampon caused many cases of the syndrome. They did not know how or, for certain, if the tampon caused the syndrome. The manufacturer voluntarily removed the tampon from the market, doing so with less evidence than Holmes gave Meigs. Upon removal of the tampon from the market, the incidence of the disease declined dramatically.

The value of identifying causes

Authors of medical textbooks usually discuss cause under such headings as 'aetiology', 'pathogenesis' or 'mechanisms'. Cause is important to practising physicians primarily in guiding their approach to three clinical tasks:

- prevention
- diagnosis
- treatment.

Less directly, the diagnostic process often depends on information about cause using the presence of **risk factors** to identify groups of patients in whom disease prevalence is likely to be high.

Analysis of causes

Single and multiple causes

In 1882 Koch wrote his postulates for determining that an infectious agent is the *cause* of a disease. These were:

- the organism must be in every case of the disease
- the organism must be isolated and grown in pure culture

Association between cause and effect

➤ The strength of an association between cause and effect reflects the likelihood that a causal relationship is involved.

➤ Odds ratios enable the linkage between cause and effect to be assessed.

➤ The fourfold table compares the proportion of people with a risk factor who later get a disease with the proportion without the factor who got the disease.

➤ Identifying causes assists in prevention, diagnosis and treatment.

- the organism must cause the specific disease when inoculated into a susceptible animal
- the organism must then be recovered from the animal and identified.

Koch's postulates contributed greatly to the theory that different bacteria cause different diseases. Using his postulates helped to clarify the causes of many diseases and allowed important scientific advances. They are still useful today; for example, Koch's postulates were the basis for the statement in 1977 that a Gram-negative bacterium causes Legionnaire's disease. However, there are many diseases where we cannot decide on the cause using Koch's postulates. His approach depended on a particular disease having one cause, and one cause resulting in a particular disease. Would that all diseases were so simple!

Smoking is so closely associated with coronary heart disease, lung cancer, chronic obstructive pulmonary disease, peptic ulcers and bladder cancer that there can be little doubt that it is causal. However, these diseases have many other associated factors that may also be causal, for coronary heart disease these include hypertension and hypercholesterolaemia. It is also possible to have coronary artery disease without any of these known risk factors being present. For example, a 55-year-old man with all five risk factors for ischaemic heart disease will have about a 6% chance of dying of ischaemic heart disease in the next 5 years. Without such risk factors, he will have about a 2% chance. His chances of dying of ischaemic heart disease are four to five times as great with all of the risk factors. These data also mean that the chances of survival of such a man are 94% if he has all risk factors, 98% if he has none. Even though the risk of disease is much greater than when there is no risk the overall chances of survival are good. We can see that avoiding the 'causes' of ischaemic heart disease for someone trying to give up smoking or taking an unpalatable diet to reduce their serum lipids may be less persuasive than the immediate enjoyment they receive from their cigarettes and chips.

There are many causes for the diseases commonly found in the developed world, most of which are, as yet, unknown. A causal factor for any one disease often results in many other diseases as well. Even in seemingly straightforward disease processes, many things act together to cause disease. This process has been called the 'web of causation'.

Interaction of causes

When several causes act together, their effects are not

necessarily simply additive. Often, the resulting risk is greater than would be expected by simply adding the effects of the separate causes. Figure 3.1 shows the probability of developing cardiovascular disease over an 8-year period among men aged 40. Those men who did not smoke cigarettes, had low serum cholesterol values and had low systolic blood pressure readings were at low risk of developing disease (12 in 1000). The risk increased to 60 in 1000, when the various factors were present individually. When all three factors were present, the risk of cardiovascular disease (317 in 1000) was almost three times greater than the sum of the individual risks.

Proximity of cause to effect

When scientists study the causes of disease, they usually search for the underlying pathological mechanism. Most clinicians accept this as the basic approach in deciding the relationship between cause and effect. These changes occur earlier in the chain of events leading to a disease. In contrast, epidemiologists look for things that occur commonly in situations where the disease in question is common, known as risk factors, then attempt to decide if the relationship is causal.

It is important to understand the contribution of these two ways of considering cause. If the pathological mechanism is not clear people may assume that we do not know the cause of a disease and, therefore, that therapy is not possible. In such situations, knowledge of risk factors may lead to very effective treatments and prevention, which can be applied without knowing the pathogenic mechanism of a disease. Tuberculosis is an example of a disease with a rich array of

causes, many of which are amenable to interventions that either prevent or reverse the disease.

Cause of tuberculosis

Originally Koch's postulates were used to establish that tuberculosis is caused by inoculation of the acid-fast bacillus *Mycobacterium tuberculosis* into susceptible hosts. From a pathological perspective, curing the disease required antibiotics or vaccines that were effective against the organism. However, the development of the disease tuberculosis is far more complex. Other important causes are the degree of susceptibility of the host and the degree of exposure. In fact, these causes determine whether invasion of the host's tissue can occur. Figure 3.2 shows some of these causal factors. Some clinicians would be hesitant to label host susceptibility and level of exposure as causes of tuberculosis, but they are very important components of cause. Control of social and economic factors influencing host susceptibility have played a much more prominent role in controlling tuberculosis than treatments developed through the biomedical–pathogenic research model. Figure 3.3 shows that the death rate from tuberculosis had dropped dramatically long before we introduced antibiotics.

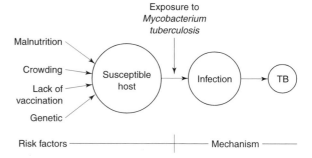

Fig. 3.2 Causes of tuberculosis.

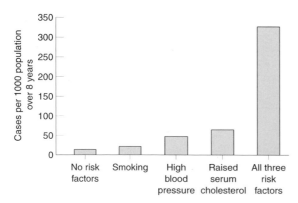

Fig. 3.1 Interaction of risk factors for diseases: in cardiovascular disease the presence of three potential 'causes' had a greater risk than simply adding the individual risks. (Stykowski 1990)

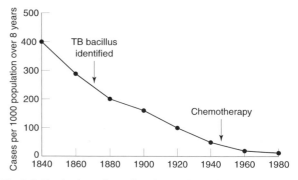

Fig. 3.3 The death rate from tuberculosis in the UK. (McKeown 1979)

Establishing cause

In clinical medicine and more so in epidemiology, it is rarely possible to *prove* causal relationships beyond reasonable doubt. However, one can mount evidence against a cause until a cause-and-effect relationship becomes implausible. This is most important and is a reason why there is often a great deal of controversy about medicine on television. Television presenters like to have things cut and dried. They like to say 'eating fat makes you die of a coronary, eating beef burgers gives you mad cow disease'. However, medicine, life indeed, is never that simple.

Association and cause

Two things must obviously be associated if they are to be considered cause-and-effect. However, not all associations are causal. Figure 3.4 outlines other kinds of association that we must exclude. Selection and measurement biases and chance are most likely to lead to apparent associations that do not exist. If these problems are unlikely, an association exists. Before deciding that the association is causal, it is necessary to know if the association occurs indirectly, through another (confounding) factor, or directly. If confounding is not found, a causal relationship is likely. However, one should always keep in mind that in the future another factor may be found that is more directly causal.

Confounding variables

Variables that are associated with both the disease and the suspected causative factor may indicate a relationship between the cause and effect when no such relationship exists. These are known as confounding variables and are often difficult to detect.

Common confounding variables include:

- time
- place
- poverty.

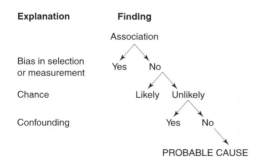

Fig. 3.4 Types of association in establishing causes.

> **Analysis of cause**
>
> ➤ Several causes affecting one disease may have a greater effect if they occur together than the simple sum of their individual effects.
>
> ➤ Associations that are not causal can occur by chance and if selection or measurement procedures are biased.
>
> ➤ Confounding variables may erroneously appear to link causes directly with disease; common confounding variables are time, place and poverty.

The commonest confounding variable is time. Many things change with time. Disease incidence often alters with time. As a result, we may assume that other factors that change with time are causing the increase or decrease in incidence.

Disease prevalence often varies greatly from place to place. Almost all disease groups are more common in the north-west of the UK than in the south-east. It is tempting to link this difference with any other similarly distributed factors. One such is the distribution of hard and soft water, which is soft in the north-west and hard in the south-east. The mechanism for any possible causative link has not been very convincing.

A further factor that is closely linked with disease prevalence is the wealth of groups of people. A close alternative to this is occupational class. Poorer people have higher rates of almost all diseases, so that any potential cause that is related to poverty may also appear to be causative.

Clinical investigations

The most important evidence establishing a cause-and-effect relationship is the research work used to establish the relationship. A number of methods are available, with varying strengths in supporting proposed relationships (Fig. 3.5). This figure is a summary of research designs used in clinical investigation.

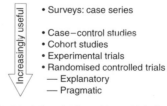

Fig. 3.5 Epidemiological methods used to establish the cause of disease.

Case series are weak studies with no defined population and no comparison group.

Case–control studies (Chapter 5) do contain a comparison (control) group but are subject to measurement confounding and selection biases, They differ from a cohort study in that they identify the cases and controls *before* the risk factor.

Cross-sectional studies are vulnerable because they provide no direct evidence of the sequence of events. True prevalence surveys are cross-sectional studies of a defined population. They guard against selection bias but are subject to measurement and confounding biases.

Cohort studies (Chapter 4) are used to analyse changes over time in a group or cohort of people who have been subjected to different risk factors but who are initially disease free. This approach helps to overcome biases in dividing the control group. They can assess the time relationship between cause and effect, can minimise bias and can examine multiple effects. They produce direct measurements that can be used to calculate risk. However, they require large groups and require adequate records or long-term follow-up.

Randomised controlled trials (Chapter 6). Well-conducted randomised controlled trials, with adequate numbers of patients, 'blinding' of therapists, patients and researchers, and carefully standardised methods of measurement and analysis are the best evidence for a cause-and-effect relationship. This is because they are best for studying the unique effects of a single factor in a complex situation. They guard against differences in the groups being compared for factors not already known to be important. Known differences can be overcome by stratifying or by methods other than a randomised controlled trial. However, randomisation is used as a means of *equally distributing unknown confounding factors that we have not yet identified*.

Examining the evidence

A cause-and-effect relationship is more likely when many lines of evidence all lead to the same conclusion. The case for a causal association is strong if an association:

- has a logical time relationship
- has a large relative risk
- demonstrates a dose–response relationship
- is reversible
- is found consistently to be present in different sites

- is consistent for various study designs
- is biologically plausible.

Time relationships

Causes should obviously precede effects. When this is clearly not so, a cause-and-effect relationship is not possible. This fundamental principle seems self-evident. However, we can overlook it when we interpret cross-sectional studies and some case–control studies, in which we measure both the supposed causes and effects at the same point. The controversy about whether better therapy for reducing high blood pressure and smoking in the USA led to a marked reduction in coronary heart disease is an example of this problem. The coronary disease rates began to fall long before anyone established a national approach to reducing blood pressure or smoking habits.

Evidence that a factor is responsible for an effect is stronger if we make observations at more than two points in time (before and after) and in more than one place. In a **time series study**, we measure the effect before and after the suspected cause has been introduced. Figure 3.6 shows an example from a study that suggested that a particular make of tampon might have caused women to fall ill with toxic shock syndrome. This natural experiment showed that the company making the tampons, the possible causative agent, introduced them before the increase in the cases of toxic shock syndrome. The number of cases fell after the withdrawal of the tampon from the market. The evidence is not completely convincing. However, the company felt that the withdrawal of the product was a small price to pay compared with the effect upon its sales of other products if it had demanded less equivocal proof. We cannot regard a

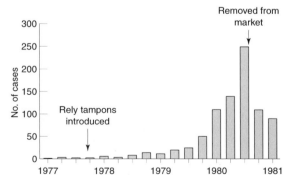

Fig. 3.6 Time series study showing the link between toxic shock syndrome and tampon use in the USA. (Rheingold et al 1982)

time series study alone as strong evidence for a cause-and-effect relationship.

Strength of the association of cause and effect

A strong association between a purported cause and an effect is better evidence for a causal relationship than a weak association. The 4-fold to 16-fold increase in lung cancer among smokers, compared with non-smokers, in eight different prospective studies is strong evidence that smoking causes lung cancer. The evidence is more convincing than the finding in the same studies that smoking is related to renal cancer because the relative risks are much smaller for renal cancer.

Dose–response relationships

A dose–response relationship is present when we find that varying amounts of the alleged cause relate to varying amounts of the effect. If we can demonstrate a dose–response relationship it strengthens the argument for cause and effect. Figure 3.7 shows the clear dose–response curve when we plot lung cancer death rates (responses) against the number of cigarettes smoked (doses).

Reversible associations

A factor is more likely to be a cause of disease if its removal results in a decreased risk of disease, that is the association between purported cause and effect is reversible. For example, people who give up smoking decrease their likelihood of getting lung cancer.

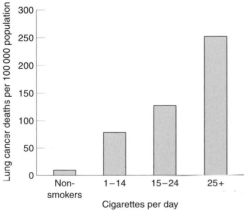

Fig. 3.7 Dose – response relationship between the number of cigarettes smoked and the lung cancer death rate. (Kabat 1998)

Consistency

There is strong evidence for a causal relationship when several studies, conducted at different times in different settings and with different patients, all come to the same conclusion. We may especially suspect cause and effect when studies using different research designs all lead to the same result. Lack of consistency does not necessarily mean the results of a particular study are invalid. One good study should outweigh several poor ones.

Biological plausibility

The biological plausibility of a suspected cause-and-effect is often given considerable weight. Biological plausibility means that the theory is in line with our knowledge of the mechanisms of the disease. It is important to remember, however, that what we consider plausible depends on the state of medical knowledge at the time. In Simpson's day, contagious diseases were biologically implausible.

Grading the evidence

The different methods used to gather evidence for cause, and the relative strength of a positive result in helping to establish or discard a theory about cause, can be divided into groups

Strong evidence derived from:

- randomised controlled trials
- cohort study.

Clinical investigations

➤ The most effective clinical method of establishing a cause-and-effect relationship is the randomised control trial.

➤ Evidence supporting cause-and-effect relationships can also come from:
  - time relationship: cause should precede effect
  - strength of the associations
  - a relationship between 'dose' of the cause and amount of the effect
  - reversible association where removal of factor results in decreased disease
  - consistency of results from several studies
  - biological plausibility: relationship fits with our knowledge of the mechanism of pathogenesis.

Less strong evidence derived from:

- large relative risk (see cohort studies)
- dose–response relationship
- reversible effect
- case control study
- time series.

Weak evidence derived from:

- cause before effect
- cross-sectional study
- small relative risk
- biologically plausible
- consistency of results.

Cohort studies

4

In this chapter the design and use of cohort studies is discussed and the values that can be obtained from this type of study:

- relative risk
- absolute risk
- attributable risk.

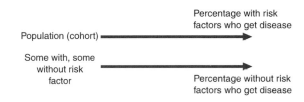

Fig. 4.1 The cohort approach.

Introduction

One tenth of a legion of Roman soldiers, about 400 men, was a cohort. Epidemiologists have adopted this terminology for the group of individuals in a cohort study. We usually set up cohort studies to look at the causes and especially the natural history of diseases. They are also useful for examining the prognosis of people who already have the disease and for tracking physiological variables like blood pressure or body mass in the population.

Use of an initially disease-free cohort — aetiological studies

In the commonest form of cohort study we choose a group of people free of the disease in question at the beginning of the study and follow them up for a time. Our aim in setting up the cohort in relation to cause is to decide, at some later time, if the incidence of the disease is greater in people exposed to a suspected cause than in those not exposed. The number of the people in the cohort must, therefore, be large so that an appreciable number of people in either group will succumb to the disease.

The suspected cause or causes, often known as 'risk factors' must be checked with all of the patients at the beginning of the study. These characteristics or risk factors may be part of the person, e.g. blood pressure or weight, or external, e.g. whether the patient smokes cigarettes or drinks alcohol. An essential feature of a

cohort study is that we can identify the data on risk factors at the same time as knowing that the cohort are disease free. In this way we can be sure that the possible cause is present before the effect. The simplest form is when we follow the whole cohort forward in time (i.e. prospectively). We must perform regular follow-ups to check on which of the people in the cohort get the disease of interest. Figure 4.1 shows the general form of the study. The relative risk is calculated as the ratio between incidence of disease in the exposed and incidence of disease in unexposed. The higher the relative risk the greater the strength of the association.

Use of a disease cohort — non-aetiological studies

In other situations, cohort studies may be used to compare the outcome of different groups of patients who have, for instance, suffered from a specific disease and are then followed over time to find out what the outcome of the disease will be. The method may be used to compare two different forms of treatment over the long term. A better method for this sort of study is to do a randomised controlled trial comparing the two forms of treatment, but sometimes randomisation into different treatment groups is not possible. This may occur when we compare different management of a disease where the approach is broadly based. An example may be where district nurses are organised to work from general practices rather than covering a geographical area. It would be extremely costly to have both approaches working at the same time in one area. It is, therefore, necessary to set up cohort studies in two areas and compare the results between the areas. In order to reduce bias, it is necessary to examine each initial cohort in detail in order to try to hold constant those differences that may be important.

Longitudinal studies

Longitudinal studies are characterised by the ascertainment of cause and effect at two different points in time. In this instance, the intention is to survey a single group of people over time. These may be patients, where the natural history of a disease in a group of patients is followed, for instance in people who have suffered a stroke, or in people who do not have a disease. A longitudinal study may also measure physiological variables such as blood pressure or body weight over time. It is probably best to keep the term cohort for studies where two or more groups are being compared.

Finding the cause of disease

It is easiest to measure precisely the effect of risk factors on disease using a cohort study. The patients may often need to be followed up over a number of years. Commonly studied risk factors include high blood pressure, heart murmurs or smoking cigarettes. Cohort studies are especially useful for studying risk factors for long-term, non-infectious diseases where the factors that put people at risk appear to be long term and cumulative. Such diseases are the main causes of death in developed countries, especially ischaemic heart disease, cerebrovascular disease and cancers.

A number of risk factors for the common chronic diseases can be studied using a cohort taken from a defined area. The make-up of the cohort may be restricted to an age and sex group. They are then examined periodically to decide on their health status. One of the best known examples of such a cohort study is the **Framingham study**. Researchers set it up as a step toward the possible prevention of coronary heart disease. They decided to work out the epidemiology of the disease before they suggested preventative measures. In 1950, the National Heart Institute of the Public Health Service in the USA set up this longitudinal prospective study in the town of Framingham, Massachusetts in the USA.

At that time there were a number of hypotheses about age, sex, occupation, race, smoking, exercise,

serum lipid levels and blood pressure as potential risk factors for ischaemic heart disease. The researchers decided to investigate how these characteristics related to people later getting ischaemic heart disease. The power of the cohort study was that it could study a number of risk factors at once and decide the relative importance of each. Another strength, which was later used with the Framingham population, was that the risk factors could also be related to other diseases, such as stroke. Framingham was selected because of the size of population. It is 'the largest town in North America', where people were reasonably easy to contact and was stable in terms of the numbers who moved in and out. As a result, the loss of people in the cohort at follow-up was minimal. Its socioeconomic and ethnic mix was near the average for the USA.

The researchers randomly chose a sample of 5000 persons in the age range 30–59 years from the total population. They estimated that approximately 1500 of this sample would develop coronary heart disease over a 20-year period. Follow-up consisted of clinical examination every 2 years and, death registration and records of illnesses and hospital admissions. As they collected the data, the researchers analysed them by comparing the incidence of disease between groups of individuals who had different measures of their initial risk factors. Using these data, they showed that raised serum cholesterol level, raised blood pressure, heavy weight and cigarette smoking were more likely to be present in people who subsequently developed coronary heart disease.

Since the Framingham study, there have been many other cohort studies examining different hypotheses. The WHO set up a study of coronary heart disease in seven countries. A cohort in Finland studied over 1400 middle-aged men free of clinically evident heart disease in 1959. These had their serum cholesterol measured and were followed up for 10 years. The point of choosing middle-aged men was that they were more likely to suffer from coronary heart disease over the following period, allowing relatively small numbers to be studied. Similarly, in the early 1980s a study of patients with possible risk factors for stroke was started in Finland to assess the longitudinal trends in incidence and the death rate.

Other researchers have set up studies to investigate experiences from birth onwards and clarify possible relationships between childhood experiences and adult disease. The 1958 National Child Development cohort study in the UK had its origins in a perinatal mortality study, which recorded birth weight for all 17 000 children born during a particular week in that year. Long-term follow-up of this cohort has investigated the association between birth weight and other factors measured at the time of the birth and later diseases and socioeconomic problems.

A prospective cohort study of health and nutritional status based on a national sample of the USA population was set up in 1971. The first follow-up between 1982 and 1984 obtained information on hospital admissions and self-reported health conditions. Further follow-up in 1986–7 suggested that a high body-mass index, a measure of fatness, was a strong predictor of risk for immobility in older women.

Researchers also devised a cohort study of infants born to HIV-infected mothers. They set this in 51 obstetric and paediatric departments in France in 1986. Data from this cohort showed that approximately one third of the infants born to seropositive mothers will have evidence of HIV-1 infection or of AIDS by the age of 18 months and 20% will have died in the first 18 months. They also showed that the rate of disease progression varied with the severity of the disease in the mother at the time of delivery. This work spurred on further research, which showed that people could reduce the rate of cross-infection between mother and baby by preventing contamination of the baby with the mother's blood during the birth.

A cohort study can provide information on other diseases, which the researchers had not considered when they designed the study. People have shown that risk factors for cardiovascular disease also predispose to atrial fibrillation. This was discovered in a recent investigation based on 38 years of follow-up of the original cohort of the Framingham study. Cohorts that are already set up can also be used for further work as they age. Subjects in the Framingham study cohort who were free of dementia in 1976 were followed and the incidence of dementia and probable Alzheimer's disease obtained after 10 more years.

Cohort studies can show the importance of physiological measures as risk factors for disease. In addition, they allow us to make estimates of the risk of exposure to toxins. Researchers used a longitudinal study of recipients of blood from donors later found to be infected with HIV to estimate the risk of HIV infection from transfusion of HIV-infected blood. Most patients who received HIV-infected blood became seropositive and about half developed AIDS within 7 years. This was an example of a retrospectively gathered cohort of people. In 1976, the Nurses Health Study cohort of over 110 000 nurses aged 30 to 55 with no history of cancer was set up in the USA. The nurses completed a questionnaire regarding possible risk factors for breast cancer. Over 7000 reported that they were using oral contraceptives. Over the next 10 years use of oral contraceptives was not associated with a substantial risk of breast cancer. This is an example of one of the many large cohort studies made on the effect of the contraceptive pill.

Cohort studies are, by their nature, often long-lived so that some continue to provide data for many years and become quite famous in their own right.

Choice of comparison groups

Comparison groups in cohort studies can be chosen in three ways.

A single study group chosen from, for example, an area in which some people have been exposed, others not exposed, to the suspected risk factors in question.

Two groups specifically chosen because one of the cohorts has been exposed. The rate at which the two cohorts get the disease being studied is compared between them. The two cohorts can be matched in some way to make them more comparable, for instance, by age groups or by sex. This approach can be used when the risk factor is relatively uncommon, such as exposure to unusual toxins or ionising radiation.

A single exposed group form the cohort. Results are compared, for the proportion of people who get the disease, with the general population. The average exposure of the population to the suspected risk factor must be known or it must be virtually absent in the general population. The cohort will need to be similar to the general population in other respects that may affect the incidence of the disease.

Comparison of cohort studies with case-control studies

The essential features to remember, when comparing cohort studies with case-control studies are that:

- cohorts are initially disease free
- exposure to the suspected risk factor is analysed at the initial stage and if possible over time but before the disease status of the population is known.

Loss of people in the cohort

A long-term cohort study must take into account the ageing of the population being studied over time. Some people in the cohort will have a greater exposure than others, both in terms of the degree and the time over which exposure occurs. Cigarette smokers, for instance, may smoke few cigarettes a day but continue to smoke over a long period, or may give up smoking after some time. In order to get around this problem, the exposure may be measured by **person-years** of exposure.

Sir Richard Doll and Dr Bradford Hill first suggested this classical way to compare disease incidence for different groups of people exposed to differing risk factors. They did this in a very large cohort study of all the medical doctors in the UK. Doctors were chosen because they are relatively easy to keep in contact with over time, for their names and addresses are registered with the General Medical Council. They contacted all of the doctors and asked them how many cigarettes they smoked. Over the following years they calculated the incidence rates of death from lung cancer for doctors with different smoking patterns. They studied the death rates at specific ages and compared people smoking different numbers of cigarettes. They had to take into account some that had started smoking during the study and some who had given up.

The researchers calculated the death rates from lung cancer per 1000 population per annum for men aged 35 or more. The figures were

- 0.07 in non-smokers
- 0.93 in cigarette smokers
- 2.23 in smokers of 25 or more cigarettes a day.

This increase in the rate with increasing exposure to the suspected risk factor is an example of the

---

Cohort studies

➤ A cohort is a group of individuals followed over a period of time to examine the cause or progress of a disease (or physiological variable) or to chart its long-term effects.

➤ The Framington study was a large cohort study designed to assess risk factors for ischaemic heart disease.

➤ Cohort studies provide data that can be used in ways not originally envisaged, e.g. assessing linkages of collected data (e.g. toxin exposure) with different diseases.

➤ Comparison groups can be a single group from a population that may or may not be exposed to a risk factor, a single group who have all been exposed (and are compared with an otherwise matched general population) or two groups chosen because one has been exposed.

➤ Exposure measured in person-years allows for variable degrees of exposure to a risk factor over time.

---

dose–response effect, mentioned in Chapter 3. It is powerful evidence to suggest that smoking is closely related to getting lung cancer.

Parameters obtained from cohort studies

Cohort studies have a number of strengths:

- they can assess cause–effect relationships
- they can provide information on diseases other than those for which the original design intended
- they can indicate the importance of physiological variables
- they can estimate the outcome of rare exposures
- they can assess relative, absolute and attributable risks.

Relative risk

One of the most useful attributes of a cohort study is that it can be used to measure relative risk. This measures the extent to which someone with a risk factor is likely to get the disease in question compared with someone who has no such risk factor. A relative risk of 32 means that the person with the risk factor is 32 times more likely to suffer the disease than someone without the risk factor over the period measured.

Comparison of the incidence rates of the disease in the exposed and non-exposed groups indicates how strong the association is between exposure to a risk factor and a disease. This ratio of incidence rates is the relative risk. If exposure is related to the disease, the incidence is higher in the exposed group of people. The greater the impact of the risk factor on the disease the greater the difference in incidence and, therefore, the higher the relative risk. (In the fourfold table method of laying out data (Table 3.1, p. 24), the relative risk would be $a/(a+b)$ divided by $c/(c+d)$.)

In the Doll and Hill study of cigarette smoking, the relative risk for lung cancer mortality in smokers of 25 or more cigarettes a day compared with non-smokers was 2.23 for smokers, 0.07 for non-smokers. Dividing one by the other gives the relative risk of 32:1. We have mentioned the evidence of a dose–response relationship since the relative risk for *all* smokers compared with non-smokers is 0.93:0.07 or 13:1, less than that for heavy smokers. The relative risk data mean that a smoker has a 13 times greater chance of dying of lung cancer than a non-smoker, someone smoking 25 a day or more has 32 times the chance of getting lung cancer.

Absolute and attributable risk

Absolute risk, is the incidence rate for a group exposed to a risk factor. This is not very useful because it assumes that there is no risk of disease in people who are not exposed. This is virtually never the case, mostly because common diseases in developed countries have many causes, some of them unidentified. The **attributable risk** is the *difference* in incidence rates between exposed and non-exposed groups. It describes the number of people who will succumb to disease specifically because of their exposure. This information is useful to health-policy makers for it gives the likely effect on the disease of reducing the exposure.

For example, the data derived by Doll and Hill can be used to show that the excess mortality rate for cancer of the lung in cigarette smokers over non-smokers is 0.93 − 0.07, or 0.86, deaths per 1000 population. If 20% of smokers stopped smoking the impact that this would have on lung cancer rates can be calculated. If the risk factor cannot be changed but there is an effective treatment for the disease, people known to be at risk can be preferentially offered regular screening. This might alleviate the effects of the disease by catching it at an early stage.

Cohort design

The design of a cohort study needs to be carefully planned to ensure that the data collected is fully useful.

Selection bias

Selection bias is when the group of people in the study is very different from the general population, so that the results of the study cannot be *generalised* to the whole population. Cohort studies tend not to have

---

Assessment of risk

➤ Relative risk is a measure of the extent to which those exposed to a risk factor are likely to get a disease compared with the non-exposed group.

➤ Absolute risk is the incidence rate for a group exposed to a risk factor.

➤ Attributable risk is the difference in the incidence of a disease between the exposed and the non-exposed groups.

---

problems with selection bias if the cohort is taken from a large number of people.

There may be problems with people being lost during the cohort study, either because they move away or because they refuse to take further part. These are likely to be different from those who remain in the study. As a result biases, may arise if we cannot obtain information about every subject or if the information is of better quality in one group compared with another. In general, the longer the cohort is followed the more difficult it will be to get a complete follow-up. For this reason, studies often use groups such as doctors or civil servants who are relatively easily found if they move.

The need for accuracy

Cohort studies must be designed to ensure that certain essential parts are accurately assessed.

Exposure to the risk factor

Exposure must be accurately assessed if effects are to be linked to causes. We can sometimes find objective measures of exposure. Patient doses during radiotherapy, for instance, will be documented in hospital notes. It is more usual to get information from the individuals themselves. In this case they may be biased when they report their measures of exposure. Individuals who are ill, or who have preconceived notions about the possible risk, may give a biased reply. This is especially so when they are questioned about the number of cigarettes they smoke or the quantity of alcohol they consume.

Criteria for the diagnosis of the disease

Criteria must be standardised accurately preferably using objective criteria. It is especially valuable if we can confirm the diagnosis using someone unaware of the previous history of each patient. This **blinded** approach ensures that the person making the diagnosis is not biased.

Surveillance system

An accurate system for assessing if patients have had the disease or have died should be equally applied to those exposed and those not exposed. If patients are aware of the potential risks, for example of smoking, they may go to their doctors more often and, therefore, be diagnosed earlier than those who do not. It is possible to take a note of how often each person contacts medical care to check this.

Change in the cohort with time

There is a further problem for cohorts where the

population is followed for a long time, with the regular routine checks that such a study requires, in that the people in the study become different from the general population, thus making the findings less generalisable. This was a potential problem in the Framingham study where the effect of risk factors for coronary heart disease was followed for an extended period.

Special approaches: retrospective design

Retrospective cohort design is a particularly efficient method when the disease takes a long time to develop after the exposure. In this instance the risk data are gathered from notes or records taken in the past. For example, a computerised search of the hospital discharge register in Denmark from 1979 to 1989 identified 73 000 men who had had a vasectomy. The Danish cancer registry identified cases of testicular cancer in those men. Cancer rates were found to be no different from that in the Danish population generally. A similar linkage between patients admitted to hospital with diabetes and the Swedish cancer registry found a higher number than expected of cases of pancreatic cancer in these people.

Retrospective cohort studies usually evaluate exposures that occurred many years previously so they may need to depend on risk factor data that may be inaccurate or incomplete. In a prospective investigation, the investigator can usually assess the exposure directly or through questioning the participants and can also obtain data about potential confounders.

Strengths and limitations of cohort studies

Cohort studies have the following strengths and weaknesses.

Strengths

- allow direct measurement of the incidence of disease in the exposed and non-exposed groups
- can account for the relationship between the exposure and disease, in particular they can confirm that the exposure occurred before the onset of the disease
- when prospective, they can minimise bias in estimating the degree of exposure
- can examine multiple effects of a single exposure

- can enable calculation of attributable risk
- can enable calculation of the outcome for rare exposures
- Can indicate the natural history of disease (longitudinal studies).

Limitations

- are inefficient for studying rare diseases. Unless the attributable risk is high, huge numbers of people are needed in the study group
- if prospective, they can be expensive and time consuming
- if retrospective they require adequate records to be available
- the validity of their results can be seriously affected by losses to follow-up.

Is the cohort study a good one?

Tests for whether a cohort study is a good one or not are:

- was the initial cohort complete?
- were the risk factors well defined?
- was a high proportion followed up?
- were objective diagnostic or outcome criteria used?
- was the assessment for the final diagnoses made in a blinded fashion with regard to whether the patient had been exposed to the risk in question?

Cohort design

- ➤ Selection bias is minimised by using a large cohort.
- ➤ Accuracy is essential in estimating exposure to a risk factor, in establishing criteria for diagnosis of a disease and in surveillance of both exposed and non-exposed groups.
- ➤ Retrospective design is effective for diseases with a long development time. Health records enable groups of people with a common history to be assessed for development of a disease.
- ➤ Prospective design allows exposure to risk factors to be assessed directly and confounding variables to be considered.

Case–control studies

5

A noticed link between a risk factor and a disease can be initially examined using matched cases and controls. This chapter discusses:

- how to design case–control studies
- how to analyse the results
- how to minimise confounding factors.

Introduction

The purpose of a case–control study is to determine whether or not an association exists between a disease and a particular risk factor. It may be considered as a first step in testing an hypothesis. If positive, the hypothesis may then be tested using a cohort study. The methods used are different for reasons that should become obvious during the chapter.

New ideas about the possible cause of a disease usually come from people working with patients, often because of a chance cluster of a particular disease in a group of people. It may be that a doctor working in a particular industry notices many people with a particular unusual disease. On occasion, an epidemiologist working on, for example, cancer registration data may notice an especially high prevalence in one area or one industry. Sometimes the concerns may come from the public, when they may complain about a large number of cases of asthma in an area and blame an especially noxious factory effluent, because it is unpleasant to sight or smell. We may follow up this initial curiosity by testing whether there is an association between the possible cause, the risk factor and the disease.

The disease is, therefore, the important trigger in a case–control study. Case–control studies, which start with a group of people suffering from disease, are often the first formal approach to deciding whether a possible risk factor may be the cause. For instance a cluster of cases of a rare disease, scrotal cancer, in men working in a factory made people suspect that expo-

sure to the oil used by them for sharpening their tools and that regularly soaked their clothing may have been the cause. It is possible to discount this relationship by formal testing, in other words we can overturn the idea by showing no association between the risk factor and the disease. We cannot prove it, only disprove it. We describe the idea or hypothesis of a relationship between a suspected cause and a disease. In order to test whether this idea is true we develop the **null hypothesis**. In this the idea is reversed, we assume that there is no relationship and then use statistical tests to try to disprove the null hypothesis. This odd double-negative approach can show that the idea had some foundation but does not prove it.

General approach

The method used for this kind of study is first to identify the cases, those people with the disease. A comparison group of people are then chosen who are as similar as possible to the first group, *except* that they do not have the disease. We compare these two groups for how frequently the cases and controls were exposed to a suspected risk factor in the past. An example would be the proportion of the cases and controls that were exposed to ionising radiation in the past 20 years.

If the possible risk factor can come in different doses, rather than being present or absent, we can compare its does at the initial stage in the two groups. An example of a numerical measure is blood pressure, where we can compare the average blood pressure in each group. An example of an all-or-nothing exposure would be having blue eyes or being of a particular race. Figure 5.1 shows a general outline of a case–control study.

Identifying cases

It can be seen that the cases are identified first. It is important to set exact criteria for the diagnosis and

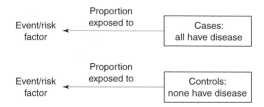

Fig. 5.1 Typical case – control study.

inclusion of cases. It is sometimes not possible to decide if the patient was exposed to the event or risk factor before the disease process began because it may be difficult to get people to remember past events, especially if the suspected risk factor occurred in the distant past. In Figure 5.1, the study is retrospective since the investigator is trying to measure past events in people already diseased. The central difference between such a study and a cohort study is that in a case–control study the cases and controls are identified before the risk factors.

The criteria for the disease being present in the cases must be both *sensitive*, able to detect the disease if present, and *specific*, able to separate those with disease from those without. The degree of specificity required of a diagnosis may be defined by some generally accepted standard. The International Classification of Diseases, produced by the WHO, is often used to define the diagnosis. This is also a way of specifying the amount of precision one needs for a particular study. For example, stroke not specified as haemorrhage or infarction has the three-character code (ICD) 164. The required diagnostic specificity can then be chosen from any of 48 subclassifications within ICD 160–169, Cerebrovascular Disease.

Patients can be chosen from those with the disease in an area (prevalent cases) or from those who are new cases (incident). If we choose prevalent cases, it may be difficult to decide whether the suspected risk factor is a cause or an effect. An accurate diagnosis is more important than trying to identify all the patients in an area with the disease. The reason for this is that the main concern is to find any association between exposure and the disease. If less exactly diagnosed cases are accepted there is the the risk of diluting the cases with some non-cases. This lessens the chance of finding a difference in exposure to the suspected risk factor between the cases and the control group and reduces the chance of finding an association between the exposure and the disease.

Cases can be selected from the general population, as has been done in a national case–control study of oral contraceptive use and breast cancer. Researchers identified cases from local cancer registries and hospital discharge data. These women had to have a positive biopsy between 1982 and 1985 and be less than 36 years of age. Patients can also be selected for a particular medical care setting. For example, a study was set up based on patients with hepatocellular carcinoma admitted to a department of medicine over a 3-year period. These were compared with a control group hospitalised in the same period. This study showed that patients exposed to hepatitis B virus were at significantly greater risk of developing carcinoma. Selection bias may occur, for example, researchers found in one study that multiple sclerosis patients referred for treatment had less severe illness than patients from the same community but not referred.

Identifying controls

Once the disease to be investigated has been defined, controls are sought that are similar to the cases except that they do not have the disease being studied. Biases often occur during the process to identify controls. Controls can be selected to match the characteristics of the neighbourhood by taking next-door neighbours. This is a way to control for unknown risk factors relating to socioeconomic state and access to medical care.

It is also important to make sure that the control group is exposed to the suspected risk factor at a similar rate to the general population. This can be a particular problem when hospital patients are the control group. When, for example, comparing people with heart disease and analysing their diet as a possible cause, it is important to avoid controls that are diabetic since their diets are unusual. It is especially difficult to avoid bias in hospital controls for it is often impossible to know whether the disease, which was the cause of the patients' admission, is truly independent of the suspected risk factor. For instance, people have found associations between smoking and being overweight for many diseases. Because of this, control patients with diseases not related to smoking or being overweight may be difficult to find. Selection of a different number of diseases into the control group reduces this potential bias to some extent. Despite these considerations hospital controls are convenient and can reduce the bias of selective recall between cases and controls.

Selection of the control group usually involves taking a sample. If there are limited resources, the control group will usually be about equal in size to the case group. In other situations, there may be more controls, often two or three times more than the number of cases. These greater numbers help to reduce the sampling variation in the control group. Controls and cases are often chosen in pairs, that is, for each case one or more controls are picked according to preset criteria. For example, in the national breast cancer study, the researchers chose a control whose birth date matched that of the case to within 6 months. They decided this by studying the lists held by GPs. Researchers often choose hospital controls by selecting the next patient after the case admitted to a particular out-patient clinic that is of the same sex and approximately the same age.

Identifying possible risk factors

Having obtained groups of cases and controls, we analyse whether the suspected event or risk factor is present in each of the two groups. A person who is unaware of whether the person being examined is a case or a control best carries this out (known as blind assessment). The suspected risk factor may have a direct bearing on the presence of the disease, for instance a type of operation. In this case, it may be impossible to 'blind' the person assessing the presence or absence or the extent of that risk factor.

Objective measures that do not need interpretation by either the clinician or the patients are ideal. It is especially useful if someone has reported on them before either the cases or the controls were identified. Examples could be lung function tests or other investigations taken some time before. Measures that need interpretation by a doctor, for example radiography and electrocardiography, after the cases and controls have been chosen are less ideal. If possible, the person interpreting the results should not know to which

---

Case–control studies

➤ Identification of suitable controls is a major problem; controls must have as similar a background as possible to the cases except that they do not have the disease in question.

➤ Identification of cases can be made from the general population using health registers and data, or from a particular medical setting.

➤ The diagnostic criteria for disease presence must be sensitive and specific.

➤ Objective measures of the presence of risk factors are best, ideally carried out in a 'blind' assessment or before the cases and controls are identified.

---

group patients belong. It is especially unsatisfactory, if we ask for patients' symptoms in retrospect. Reporting of symptoms of depression or angina, for example, may be biased if the patient already suspects that there is a link between the risk factor or symptom and the final disease.

There should be no major difference between the people in the case group and the control group with respect to the quantity or quality of the information collected. There is no better evidence of a poor study than differences in the amount of missing data between the cases and controls.

Analysis of the study

Analysis consists of a comparison between cases and controls to discover the frequency of occurrence of factors that might be responsible for the disease in question. Traditionally data from case–control studies is set out in a two-by-two or **fourfold table**. This is discussed in Table 3.1 (p. 24). Data are entered into the table according to the exposure to risk factors for the cases and the controls.

The parameters that can be derived from case–control studies differ from those of a cohort study because of the study design. A cohort study, in contrast with a case – control study, begins with a population who do not have the disease being studied, so an incidence rate can be calculated for the disease as people are affected. The population in the study group is used as the denominator for measuring these incidence rates. We can also calculate a relative risk index. In a case–control study there is no such population-based denominator, only groups of cases and controls. However, one would expect that if exposure to a risk factor were a cause of the disease there would be more exposure amongst the cases than the controls. A good index for deciding whether this has occurred is the **odds ratio**.

Odds ratio and relative risk

The odds ratio is defined as the ratio of exposed to non-exposed in the case group divided by the same ratio in the control group. In Table 3.1 (p. 24) this was given as ad/cb for the entries in the fourfold table. This is sometimes called the cross odds ratio because the numbers to be multiplied are found diagonally across the table. The relative risk of a factor, usually derived from a cohort study, gives a population-based estimate of its risk. Odds ratios in a case–control study give only the difference in odds between the cases and controls in that particular study. These two groups are not often representative of the wider population so that it is difficult to draw general conclusions for the population at large. However, it can be shown that when the number of persons with the disease is small compared with the number unaffected, then the odds ratio is not dissimilar in number to the relative risk measure. This is the case in most studies.

An example of a case–control study

Table 5.1 shows data from the case–control study by Doll and Hill; this examined the aetiology of carcinoma of the lung, which was suspected to be related to cigarette smoking. The extension of this study into a cohort study was discussed in Chapter 4.

If the suspected risk factor is quantitative, as in this case for cigarette smoking, then the odds ratios can be calculated for different categories of exposure compared with no exposure. In Table 5.1 the odds ratios increase with exposure, giving a clear indication of a dose–response relationship.

The equivalent measure to an odds ratio that is derived in a cohort study is relative risk. Using the fourfold table method of ordering data (Table 3.1, p. 24), the odds ratio is ad/cb and the relative risk is $a/(a + b) \div c/(c + d)$. In other words, the incidence in the exposed is divided by the incidence in the unexposed.

Confounding variables

A confounding variable is any variable which is associated with both the disease and the risk factor being tested. If such variables exist there is no way for the researcher to know whether the difference in the risk factor or the confounding variable is the one that is truly causing the disease in question.

The association of a disease and a suspected risk factor with this third variable may lead us to believe that there is a relationship between the risk factor and the disease when no such relationship exists.

The problem is to identify such confounding variables. This involves searching the data from the cases and controls to work out the ways in which they differ. For each factor where there is an important difference between the cases and controls one must decide if that factor is also related to the possible cause being studied. For example, the data in Table 5.1 show a difference in the smoking habits of cases and controls. However, male sex is associated with both smoking and lung cancer. Because of this, differences noted between the smoking habits of cases and controls might be because more smokers are males (Fig. 5.2). It could, therefore, be male sex rather than smoking which is of most significance in the aetiology of lung cancer. To get around this problem we have to make sure that cases and controls need to have similar numbers of men and women. One can examine the results separately for men and women to be sure that the effect is independent of sex. Sometimes this may be difficult, for instance if there are small numbers of women.

Confounding variables are very important. The possibility of unknown confounding variables means that we cannot state categorically that any factor is the *cause* of the disease with which it is associated. The commonest confounding variable is age. Many diseases that are common in the UK increase rapidly with age, notably most forms of ischaemic heart disease, cerebrovascular disease and most cancers. Any other factor that is related to age can, therefore, be related to the prevalence of these diseases unless the data are measured age-specifically, i.e. comparisons are made for the different age groups. Other important possible confounding variables are sex and occupational class, a substitute measure for poverty. Most diseases are more prevalent in men compared with women, though there are a few exceptions such as rheumatoid arthritis and thyroid disease. Most diseases are more common in poor than in rich people.

Table 5.1 Carcinoma of the lung and smoking (Benhamou et al 1989)

Average daily cigarettes	Lung cancer cases	Controls	Odds ratio
0	7	61	1
1–4	55	129	3.7
5–14	489	570	7.4
15–24	475	431	9.6
25–49	293	154	16.3
50+	38	12	27.7
Total	1357	1357	

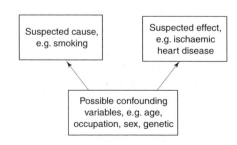

Fig. 5.2 An example of the effect of confounding variables.

Examples of confounding variables

In a case–control study to test the hypothesis that juvenile-onset schizophrenia may be predated by motor and language problems in infancy, researchers tried to decide which factors might confound the association. They decided that possible confounding variables included social class, the position in the family (i.e. first, second or third child) and race. To make sure that these factors did not confound the original hypothesis they needed to ensure that the cases and controls were comparable for all of these confounders.

If we have not controlled for confounding at the beginning of a study it is still possible to stratify the cases and controls later. This means taking each subgroup and comparing the two groups. One can then compare the differences between the original groups within different subsets, for instance in the schizophrenia example examining first children only. The difficulty with this is that some subgroups can be very small or even non-existent. For example, with age groups the smaller the age band, e.g. 5-year age groups, the more comparable will be the patients. However, it may be difficult to find sufficient cases within each. Another good reason for selecting more controls than cases is that this helps to ensure that there will be controls for cases at all relevant levels of a confounding variable. This means that we can make better comparisons.

Matching and overmatching cases and controls

Controls need to be generally similar to the cases except that the disease is absent. Matching for a particular characteristic eliminates it as a reason for the difference between the cases and controls. Matching tries to eliminate differences between the cases and controls for factors that often have an important impact on other diseases. For example, if the suspected cause of a disease is hypertension we may match cases and controls by age because age is related to changes in blood pressure. This matching then eliminates age as an the explanation of the blood pressure difference.

The study should not match factors that are related to the suspected cause but not to the disease. For example, social class may be a suspected risk factor. If the investigator matched cases and controls by educational background it would seriously undermine social class comparisons since this is closely related to education. In addition, variables should not be matched if they are likely to be intermediate in the causal pathway between a risk factor being considered and the disease. For example, if smoking altered blood cholesterol, which in turn was causally associated with cardiovascular disease, then smoking would be considered a cause of cardiovascular disease. However, matching for blood cholesterol would mask the association between the disease and smoking. When controls are chosen to be similar to the cases for a characteristic and when this tends to mask a disease's associations with another characteristic of interest, the cases and controls are said to be overmatched.

Bias

Bias is a systematic error that results in over- or underestimation of the strength of the association, that is the odds ratio. The accuracy of any study depends upon the accuracy with which we assign subjects to the four categories of the fourfold table: exposed cases, unexposed cases, exposed controls, unexposed controls. Misclassification may occur because of over- or underdiagnosis. The disease may be difficult to diagnose and criteria for diagnosis may not be uniform. Misclassification is much less in a disease entity if it is:

- well defined
- has a diagnosis that is uniform and established
- the majority of cases come to medical attention
- there is little selectivity by physicians in putting the patient into hospital.

Some diseases (e.g., thromboembolic phenomena) are difficult to diagnose, they may present as complications of another medical or surgical condition and criteria for their existence are not uniform. Even if objective clinical diagnostic tests were available, clinicians might not interpret them uniformly. Exposure to the possible risk factor under study may be difficult to define and measure. For example, the value used for the total number exposed to a risk factor may over- or underrepresent the exposure in the sample. Information about exposure to risk factors may be obtained by interviewing patients or by sending them a questionnaire. Their recall of past events may be inaccurate or the information supplied may be biased, particularly among the patient group as they know they have a disease and may already associate it with exposure. It is an advantage, in this case, to employ hospital controls since they too have been ill and will supply similar quality of information as the patient group.

When the interviewer is seeking an association, bias can be introduced unconsciously by probing the patients in the case group for more information than the controls. To minimise bias from this source, ideally the interviewer should be unaware of which participant is a case or a control, but this is difficult to achieve in practice. The proportions of the case group and the control group supplying information should be equal. If the response rate differs between the two groups, it is evidence of lack of comparability. At the patient level, the quality of information obtained from the cases and the controls should be similar. They should not differ as a result of differences, for example, in educational status, knowledge of the disease, or psychological state.

A good example is the accuracy of self-reporting of alcohol use and smoking during pregnancy. This is poor when the outcome of pregnancy is adverse. Different results for alcohol intake are obtained depending on whether the information comes from obstetric records or personal interviews by researchers. This offers a plausible explanation for the disagreement between reports about the link between prematurity and alcohol use during pregnancy.

Use of case–control studies

Adenocarcinoma of the vagina

An historical example of the use of the case–control method was the investigation of the unusual occurrence of a small number of the rare disease adenocarcinoma of the vagina. These were treated at the Vincent Memorial Hospital, Boston between 1966 and 1969. The doctors there saw seven girls aged 15 to 20 years of age. The correct diagnosis was delayed since prolonged bleeding was mistaken for anovulatory bleeding, vaginal cytology was often negative and the tumour was not palpated on rectal examination. The correct diagnosis was only achieved after a vaginal examination. The researchers intended to use four matched controls for each patient with vaginal carcinoma. They were to select these by examination of the birth records at the hospital in which each patient was born. They identified females born within 5 days of the cases on the same type of ward. However, they could not locate 25% of this control group, which could have led to selection bias. Therefore, since the families of the patients were still living in the community where the patients were born, the researchers decided to choose controls from the community.

A trained interviewer questioned all the mothers of the girls to uncover factors that might be related to the sudden appearance of these tumours. They collected information retrospectively on:

- the mother's age at the birth of the child
- the mother's smoking habits
- bleeding during pregnancy

- prior pregnancy loss
- maternal oestrogen therapy
- X-ray exposure.

The researchers found a highly significant association between the treatment of the mothers with the oestrogen diethylstilboestrol during pregnancy and the subsequent development of adenocarcinoma of the vagina in their daughters. At a lower level of significance, maternal bleeding during pregnancy and prior pregnancy loss were also different between cases and controls. The mothers of patients had both more frequent prior pregnancy loss and more frequent bleeding than controls, which is why they were given the oestrogen diethylstilboestrol. The authors concluded that it is unwise to administer the drug to women early in pregnancy.

Thalidomide

Another case of iatrogenic (doctor-caused) illness that

Analysis of results

➤ Because there are no population-based data in case–control studies, results are best expressed as an odds ratio, the ratio of exposed to non-exposed in the case group divided by the same ratio for the control group.

➤ When the number with disease is small compared with the number unaffected, the odds ratio is closer in value to the relative risk, which is a population-based estimate derived from cohort studies.

➤ Confounding variables are variables other than the risk factor for which case and control groups differ; age is the most common example. The possibility of unknown confounding variables makes it difficult to state categorically that a factor is a cause.

➤ Matching of cases and controls can eliminate the matched parameter as a cause of difference. Overmatching occurs if a variable matched could, in fact, be an intermediate on a causal pathway; this would mask a disease association.

➤ Bias is a systematic error in the estimate of an association between cause and effect; it may result from poor diagnosis, poor case choice or variation in the way risk exposure is assessed in cases and controls.

was investigated using a case–control study was the thalidomide tragedy. In 1960 and 1961 at 13 departments of obstetrics in Hamburg medical staff noticed that there had been 27 infants born with types of malformation that they had not observed between 1930 and 1958. Retrospective case–control analysis of 112 mothers of malformed infants and 188 control mothers of healthy infants implicated thalidomide as the risk factor. The mothers had taken this to prevent sickness during a critical period between the 27th and the 40th day after conception.

HIV infection

Another famous case–control study matched cases of Kaposi's sarcoma and *Pneumocystis carini* pneumonia (PCP) in homosexual men. The researchers used four different male homosexual controls matched by age, race and residence. The study found striking differences in the number of sexual partners reported by cases and controls. This enabled preventive measures to be publicised for these diseases before identification of the causative agent, subsequently shown to be HIV.

Randomised controlled trials

In this chapter important aspects of randomised trials are described:

- trial types and assessment
- sampling and randomisation
- compliance
- interpretation and ethics.

Introduction

The idea of randomisation in trials is traditionally credited to R.A. Fisher's work *The Design of Experiments* in 1935. He developed this interest trying to improve the yield of grain in agriculture. Austin Bradford Hill, a statistician, carried out the first practical randomised clinical trial of recognised significance for the Medical Research Council in 1946. He designed the trial to decide the effectiveness of streptomycin in the treatment of tuberculosis, published in 1948. Hill used random numbers to decide which patients should be given which treatment. The details of this allocation were unknown to the investigators administering the trial to eliminate bias. Shortly before this another pioneer, Archie Cochrane, later to achieve fame through his work and by publication of a book, *Effectiveness and Efficiency*, was conducting what he described as his 'first, worst and only successful randomised trial'. He carried this out on British soldiers with nutritional deficiencies in a prisoner-of-war camp during the Second World War. In this study, he gave a random group of soldiers gruel made up by boiling the husks of rice, thought to contain essential vitamins. He claimed that this reduced the nutritional deficiencies suffered by the men.

Trials

We use cohort and case–control studies to analyse the relationships between risk factors or characteristics of patients and their likelihood of getting a particular disease. In these the researcher is passive and the patients are only observed. We do not subject patients to any intervention. In an experimental trial, the researcher allocates the patients or other subjects to different groups and each group will be given a different exposure to the factor, often a treatment, in question. The researcher controls the level of this exposure. We must not put patients at known risk any more than they would have been if they had not taken part in the trial. For this reason, this approach is most often used for comparing a standard treatment with a new one that appears to show promise.

Trial types

Experimental trials can be divided into:

- therapeutic trials: people with disease are given a therapeutic treatment to prevent death or improve health
- preventive trials for healthy individuals: individuals from the general population are subjected to a prophylactic agent or procedure and the efficacy of such prophylaxis is determined by following them up over time
- preventive trials for at-risk groups: people with characteristics thought to increase their risk of disease, for example a genetic abnormality, are subjected to some intervention (e.g. drugs, diet or behaviour modification) to prevent the development of disease.

Design of trials

Certain experimental design features improve the quality of the results that can be obtained from a trial:

- sampling: chosing a suitable population
- randomisation: dividing participants between groups in a random fashion

- stratification: grouping participants according to a characteristic before randomisation
- controls: chosing a good control 'treatment'
- crossover: switching treatment and control groups after a period of time
- placebos: using a placebo to mask what treatment is being received
- blinding: assessment by those unaware of the treatment group.

Sampling the population

The aim of a trial is to apply the conclusions of the experiment to people in the general population. For example, a preventive trial, concerned with cardiovascular disease or cancer, might aim to give results that will apply to the whole population aged over 40 years of age who are free of these diseases. The people included in a trial should, therefore, be representative of the population.

Before a trial begins, we need to estimate the sample size needed to provide a level of confidence in the hypothesis that the intervention gives benefit. Reviews of many trials published in journals have shown that researchers often design and conduct trials with a sample size that is too small. This is not only stupid in that the researchers waste considerable effort but it is also unethical, for patients will have been included in a trial that was of no benefit to them or others. Part of the art of setting up a trial is to choose a group of patients in which one can reasonably foresee the result. We need to prejudge whether the group will experience enough outcomes, either deaths or new disease, to let us compare the treatment groups. The data for making these decisions may often be scanty and much will depend upon the experience of the researcher in choosing the right study group.

In therapeutic trials even for common diseases a single hospital would not see enough patients to test with confidence an idea or hypothesis that the treatment would give moderate benefit over a reasonable time scale. Much research is funded for a 3-year period; therefore, most experiments have to fit into that period. In addition, the characteristics of disease and, even more, the range of therapies available change over time so that if trials are to have an impact they need to be completed reasonably quickly. People design multicentre trials, often internationally, to collect enough cases within a reasonable time span.

Setting up a trial

Figure 6.1 shows the general outline of a randomised

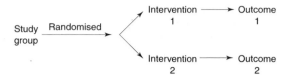

Fig. 6.1 Scheme for a randomised control trial.

controlled trial. The researchers invite people from the population of interest to take part in the proposed trial. The informed consent of patients must be obtained. This consent will include letting patients know about the aim of the trial, the likely benefits and risks and that they may be randomly allocated to a group receiving a new or no treatment. Some people will not wish to participate in the trial. It is well recognised that these non-participants are likely to differ from those who do take part in many ways that may affect the outcomes under investigation. This will not affect the accuracy of the result of the trial but it will affect whether the results will be useful when applied to the general population.

Some people may be excluded from trials, which makes the trial less generalisable. In a preventive trial for men with primary hypercholesterolaemia, the criteria for eligibility were men aged between 35 and 59 years, with plasma cholesterol concentrations of at least 6.85 mmol/l. People with high plasma triglyceride levels, with hyperlipoproteinaemia and with conditions associated with secondary hyperlipoproteinaemia were excluded from the trial. The researchers also excluded people with clinical coronary heart disease. Such a wide range of exclusions obviously limits the applicability of the findings for the general population. Critics of this highly selective approach to trials have said that virtually no patients with diabetes have been entered into trials of therapy for coronary heart disease. This makes it difficult to know the best treatment for people with diabetes who suffer from coronary heart disease.

Randomisation

The central point of randomised controlled trials, the most effective experimental model, is one in which patients or other subjects are divided into groups by random allocation. The chance of an individual being included in one or other group is, therefore, independent of anything that might influence the result. Random allocation has the further advantage of eliminating selection bias.

We can randomly allocate patients to different treatment groups using tables of random numbers. This is the most effective way of making sure that the groups receiving the different interventions are comparable. In non-random assignment, e.g. alternate assignment of patients to different treatment groups, we find that the, often subconcious, views of the researchers may introduce bias. No amount of matching in non-random studies can balance the treatment groups concerning unknown characteristics or those not understood to be of significance.

The larger the sample size the more successful will be the randomisation in equally distributing known and unknown factors that may bias the outcome. Having said this, it is usual to check the basic differences between the treatment groups (e.g. age and sex characteristics) at the end of the trial. This ensures that randomisation has resulted in a reasonably comparable split of the study group for factors we know about. For example, in the trial of cholestyramine and placebo groups for hypercholesterolaemia, there was no statistically significant difference between the two groups for any of the coronary heart disease risk factors (e.g. weight, blood pressure, cigarette smoking) following randomisation.

Explanatory randomised controlled trials

Explanatory randomised controlled trials are intended to answer the question, 'In optimal circumstances does this treatment work?' Such a trial will, therefore, take a study group that is as homogeneous as possible and test the treatment with close supervision to make sure that patients take the treatment in an optimal dose for as long as is needed. The study group is typically of one sex and a fairly narrow age range. This study group is randomly allocated to an intervention or control group.

Pragmatic randomised controlled trials

In a pragmatic trial the question asked is, 'In normal day-to-day circumstances does the treatment work?' In this situation, the treatment is given to a wide range of people, as it would normally be given in practice. The trial should also be set up in the situation where it is likely to be used in practice. For instance, if it is a treatment likely to be useful in general practices the trial should be held in general practice.

Comparison of explanatory and pragmatic trials

The essential difference between an explanatory and pragmatic trial is the degree of homogeneity of the study group before it is randomised into subgroups. A

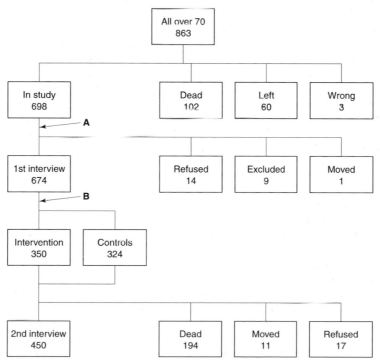

Fig. 6.2 The structure of a randomised trial. In a pragmatic trial randomisation occurs at B after those that do not fit the criteria have been eliminated. In an explanatory trial, randomisation occurs at A when those who would not participate have been excluded.

pragmatic trial provides a more conservative estimate of the benefit of a treatment. In both explanatory and pragmatic trials, once we have randomly allocated patients to a particular treatment group we must analyse them along with the others in that group regardless of whether or not they remain in the study or comply with their treatment. The **intention-to-treat principle** requires analysis of a trial according to allocation at randomisation not according to whether patients received or completed treatment. The use of this principle removes the bias that may occur if patients experience poor outcomes or side effects and are selectively taken out of the analysis. At the point of randomisation the two (or more) groups are identical. Therefore, if patients are lost or taken out of the study after randomisation the study, will no longer be as accurate. In other words all randomised controlled trials should use the intention-to-treat approach for greatest accuracy.

Figure 6.2 shows the structure of a randomised trial. In this, a large group of patients aged 70 years and over were identified in a general practice, from the age, sex register. The register was inaccurate in that a number of patients had died, moved away or were not, in fact, over 70. These are identified in the second row. In an exploratory trial the randomisation will occur at B, once those who do not fit the criteria have been eliminated. However, during the course of the trial some patients refused to take part; the GP refused to let them be visited and one moved away. These would be randomly allocated and included in the trial in a pragmatic model at point B.

A pragmatic trial is weakened in its ability to find a difference between the two groups. The strength of a pragmatic trial is that it more truly mimics real life and gives realistic estimates of the benefit patients are likely to receive.

Random stratification

If we know that a characteristic is strongly related to the outcome we are studying, we may first group the patients according to this characteristic, then randomise to treatment or control within each group. This is a form of stratification. For example, if we know that age or sex has an important effect on the outcome of the disease, the study group may first be split into subgroups for different ages or for men and women. We then carry out the randomisation within these subgroups. This makes sure that we have equally distributed the characteristic between the different treatment groups. This is most important when the sample size is relatively small since in larger samples randomisation

---

Design of randomised trials

➤ Trials may be of therapeutic treatments, of preventative measures or for preventative measures in at-risk groups.

➤ Sample size and composition is important; multicentre trials often occur to obtain a large number of patients in a reasonable time period.

➤ Randomisation removes selection bias and ensures that unknown factors that might affect the trial are, as far as possible, equally distributed between the two groups.

➤ Stratification is the grouping of patients according to a known characteristic affecting outcome before randomisation to groups. This ensures equal representation of the characteristic in each group.

➤ Intention-to-treat analysis uses patient's data according to their allocation at randomisation not according to whether they received or completed treatment. It removes bias that can arise from patients leaving trials through poor outcomes or side effects.

➤ A placebo group is useful in assessing side effects and subjective treatment outcomes.

➤ Blinding ensures that patients and, if possible, assessors are unaware of the treatment group.

---

is more likely to achieve comparability between the subgroups.

Use of placebos

The placebo effect is the name given to the tendency for individuals to report favourably on the effect of treatments regardless of their actual efficacy. A placebo is an inert substance that appears, to the patient and the doctor, to be identical to the active treatment. They can be very useful for assessing the effectiveness of a new treatment where no treatment at all is a reasonable option. Placebos can be especially useful for working out whether side effects of active medicines are truly caused by the drug or not. It is common to find a number of supposed side effects in patients receiving the inert preparation. At the other end of the spectrum, if we do not use a placebo control it may be impossible to tell whether subjective outcomes result from the treatment. They may be caused by the patient's belief that the treatment will help.

Blinding: measuring outcome

All comparative studies, whether cohort, case–control or randomised controlled trials can be improved if the outcome variables are measured by someone unaware of the group to which individuals belonged. Ideally, studies are designed so that patients are unaware of their treatment category. This means that their compliance with their regime and their reporting of symptoms is not biased (single blind). Doctors should also be unaware so that their management is unchanged between treatment and control groups (double blind). This is sometimes not possible. Both patients and surgeons would be aware of, for instance, the treatment they had received in a comparison of traditional and keyhole surgery for cholecystectomy. It might be possible to have a blind assessment to monitor pain control methods.

It is frighteningly easy for investigators to be biased towards a positive result of a research study if they know which patients are on the new or active therapy. For this reason, different specialties have attempted to define standardised outcome measures. For example, health-related quality-of-life questionnaires have been developed and tested for outcome measurement in randomised controlled trials of inflammatory bowel disease and rheumatoid arthritis. A double-blind trial is the ideal.

Examples of randomised trials

Trials in coronary heart disease

Coronary heart disease is a major cause of mortality in the developed countries and there have been many therapeutic trials to test the effectiveness of different treatments. For example, large-scale trials of thrombolytic therapy in patients with acute myocardial infarction have shown marked improvements in survival. Researchers have shown that these advantages are confined to patients presenting to hospital within 6 hours of the onset of their symptoms. Also, it has been shown that coronary artery bypass surgery reduces mortality in the long term in patients with a previous myocardial infarction.

A large number of trials have also been set up to examine preventive measures aimed at reducing the incidence of coronary heart disease. The Multiple Risk Factor Intervention Trial (MRFIT) randomly allocated men who were at high risk of developing coronary heart disease to one of two groups. They intervened with one group to reduce their smoking, blood pressure and blood cholesterol concentrations. At follow-

up there was no significant difference between the groups in coronary heart disease mortality. However, they found that the un-targeted group had also reduced their risk factors, no doubt through their knowledge of health promotional material. This pinpoints the difficulty of intervening in large community-based prevention trials.

Trials in infectious diseases

There are many historical landmarks of randomised experimental trials used to examine the prevention of infectious diseases. These include the prevention of tuberculosis by means of BCG, of poliomyelitis by means of Salk vaccine and of malaria by various drugs.

Preventive trials for infectious disease involve larger numbers of people compared with therapeutic trials. The reason for this is that when we try to prevent disease the proportion of healthy people who succumb to infectious disease is relatively small. As a result, many people have to be given protection who would not normally be affected. In treatment trials, in our experience, at least 10% of the patients need to be affected by the treatment. If less than this are likely to benefit, the trial can be very difficult to control, often needing many centres to collect enough patients.

Continuation within a trial

Compliance

The effect of non-compliance, or refusal to take part in the study, is to make the experience of the intervention and placebo groups more similar. This decreases our ability to detect true differences between the groups if any exist. Subjects who are aware of having a high risk are more likely to agree to take part in a trial. A general technique for improving compliance during a trial is to screen participants regarding their potential to comply. For example, the Physicians Health Study in 1985 tried to assess the effects of aspirin on cardiovascular deaths and of beta-carotene on cancer incidence. Over 33 000 male physicians aged over 40 years who were willing and eligible were enrolled in the run-in phase of the trial. This lasted 1–6 months, in which they were assigned to active aspirin and beta-carotene placebo. The purpose of the run-in phase was to improve compliance. The researchers randomised into the trial only those physicians who tolerated aspirin and complied with medication at least two thirds of the time. These techniques gave in a more powerful result than would have been obtained if a larger mixed group of compliers and non-compliers had been randomised.

Non-compliance can occur as a result of:

● therapy becoming contraindicated for a particular patient
● the patient withdrawing consent
● the patient choosing an alternative treatment instead of or in addition to therapy (co-intervention).

For example, if we set up a therapeutic trial comparing surgery with high dietary fibre in the treatment of haemorrhoids, it is possible that surgical patients, learning that dietary fibre may be important, might eat a high fibre diet. Their intervention would decrease the ability (power) of the trial to detect a difference in outcome, if present, between the two groups.

Since non-compliance can decrease the power of a trial it is important to monitor compliance throughout the trial. Patients can be questioned directly or by postal questionnaire but this is obviously open to bias. For some drug trials, metabolites or markers in their blood or urine can be assayed but this is time consuming and expensive. Ideally patients should be unaware of their treatment category to avoid bias in their compliance or symptom reports.

The ethics of stopping a trial

If a therapy obviously gives immediate and significant improvements in mortality or morbidity, as for example when penicillin was introduced, it is unethical to withhold its use to test its effectiveness. Surprisingly few treatments are as effective as penicillin. In modern clinical practice, clinicians are usually looking for small improvements in the treatment of disease. Even small improvements may be worthwhile to the patients and, if the disease is common, can be considerable for the health of the public, for instance in cardiovascular or respiratory disease.

It is also unethical to adopt a new treatment before conducting an experimental trial. It is not only unethical to subject patients to treatments that confer no benefit and may cause some risk but there are also wasted costs incurred in the worthless treatment. As a result, other patients with treatable disease will lose out, for there may well not be enough money left to treat them.

Unfortunately in many situations, the untested beliefs of either doctors or the public may make it difficult or even impossible to carry out a trial. This is especially the case for treatments that have been accepted for many years. Sometimes this may happen for a relatively new treatment, because a logical but untested argument seems to be overwhelming. An example of this was the untested belief of the medical profession that radical mastectomy for breast cancer was more effective than lumpectomy. The central problem here was that treatment of all types is ineffective if the cancer has progressed beyond its earliest stages. Surgeons, therefore, felt under pressure to operate more and more widely in the hope of eradicating the disease. Eventually Fisher performed a randomised trial in 1985. This showed no appreciable difference in 5-year survival between the two treatments. The staging (i.e. severity) of the disease was the overwhelming factor that made a difference to survival.

Ideally, the decision about when to stop a trial should be included in the protocol at the design phase. The data should be reviewed periodically and if a treatment is showing clear benefit or obvious harm then it is ethical to stop the trial. It is, of course, important not to stop the trial prematurely because of a trend that may disappear as the trial progresses. Data monitoring committees, which are independent of the study investigators, examine the data and make recommendations about whether trials should continue. There are concerns, however, that stopping early because an effect is present results in a serious loss of accuracy in estimating the size of the benefit. This leads to inaccurate claims that then form the basis for future practice. It is possible to use statistical tests of the significance of data accumulated up to that point in the decision-making process. For example, in the MRC preventive trial of folate supplements and neural tube defect, the trial was terminated before the scheduled end on the recommendation of the data monitoring board.

Assessment of trial results

Trial results may be presented in different ways. If the primary outcome measure is a continuous clinical variable, e.g. blood pressure, then the mean value in each separate treatment group is measured. The null hypothesis may then be tested by calculating the statistical significance of the difference between the two means, or a confidence interval determined for the measured difference (Fig. 6.3).

If the primary outcome measure relates to the proportion of people showing some improvement in each separate treatment group then similarly the proportions may be compared. The approach adopted sometimes refers to proportions adversely affected rather than improved, in which case a relative risk of adverse outcome is presented (Table 6.1, 1 and 2).

Trial results tend to be presented as relative risk (RR) when the numbers enrolled are large but as an odds ratio (OR) when numbers are small. In this case the definition of odds ratio differs from that used for a case control study and is defined:

$$\text{Odds ratio} = \frac{\text{Ratio of improved to not improved for new treatment}}{\text{Ratio of improved to not improved for old treatment}}$$

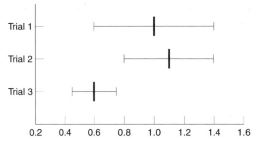

Fig. 6.3 Mean (dark bar) and confidence intervals (horizontal range) of relative risk in three trials.

Table 6.1

	No. of patients improved or cared	No of patients not improved or not cared
Number of patients receiving intervention A	a	b
No of patients receiving intervention B	c	d

Results of trials are reported as either:

1. Relative risk, i.e. of adverse outcome

$$\frac{b}{a+b} \div \frac{d}{c+d}$$

and if treatment A B more effective than treatment B then the value of the RR will be < 1.

2. Odds ratio for improvement between treatments, i.e.

$$\frac{ad}{bc}$$

where if treatment A is more effective than treatment B then OR > 1. The interpretation of RR and OR in terms of statistical significance and clinical importance is detailed on pp. 39–40 in Chapter 5.

3. The difference between mean values of a continuous clinical variable in each separate treatment group.

Continuation within a trial

➤ Non-compliance makes the difference between intervention and control groups less marked. It can occur because of withdrawn consent, contraindications or patient choice of a different or additional therapy.

➤ Early termination of trials can occur if there are clear benefits or harm indicated by the data accumulating.

➤ Assessment of progress of a trial requires statistical analysis of the relative risk (adverse outcome in new versus old/placebo treatment). An effective therapy has a relative risk of less than 1.

Applying epidemiology in clinical practice

Measurement

7

The aims of this first of the applied chapters (7 to 12) are that you should be able to:

- define the reproducibility and validity (accuracy) of measurements and distinguish between the two concepts
- identify sources of variability in measurements and distinguish between *intra-* and *inter-* observer variability.
- distinguish between random (non-systematic) and biased (systematic) observer error and know their importance in clinical medicine
- describe at least three techniques for reducing measurement variability.

Definitions and techniques

Fourfold table

An important aspect of assessing results is the degree of *agreement* achieved by one observer over time (**intraobserver variation**) or by several observers (**interobserver variation**). This can be shown clearly in a comparison of agreement table (Table 7.1) set out in the manner of a fourfold table (p. 39).

Definitions

The following definitions form aspects of measurement

Validity is the extent to which a measurement represents a true value.

Reproducibility is the degree to which results can be repeated to give the same value.

Random errors suggest a lack of competence at carrying out a test or function. The difference between the gold standard and the actual reading is haphazard. Random errors can be overcome by repeated measurements.

Biased errors are also inaccurate compared with the gold standard but the inaccuracy tends to be in one direction. It suggests that the person is using an instrument that has a consistent error or is using the machine consistently in the wrong way. This suggests poor training, rather than lack of it.

Problems

PROBLEM 1

Nurses in a postoperative recovery ward are being assessed on their abilities at measuring blood pressure. They are tested against electronic blood pressure-measuring equipment that accurately records the true blood pressure. The nurse and the instrument measure the diastolic pressure simultaneously. The nurse is not aware of the reading on the instrument. Figure 7.1a–d represents the results obtained for four nurses, on several patients. These results show two types of error being made by the four nurses. Assess their relative importance in each case and how the errors could be rectified.

PROBLEM 2

A 21-year-old woman is making her first visit to an antenatal clinic. She is 18 weeks into her first pregnancy. Three workers measure her blood pressure and the results are:

medical student	150/90
midwife	140/88
obstetrician	120/80.

Table 7.1 Comparison of agreement

Observation 2	Observation 1	
	Positive	Negative
Positive	Agreement	
Negative		Agreement

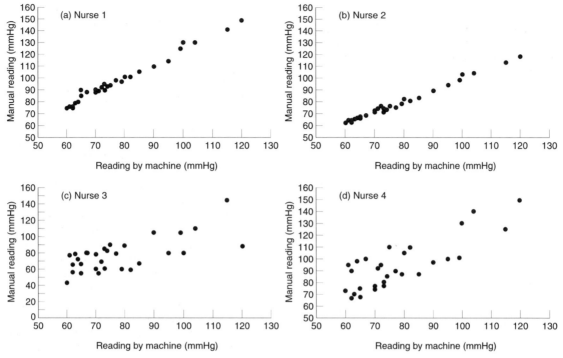

Fig. 7.1 Manual diastolic blood pressure readings taken by four nurses (a–d) compared with the simultaneous machine reading.

Discuss why these results differ. Suggest methods for preventing these discrepancies. The difference is important because it is between a blood pressure possibly suggesting a complicated pregnancy and one progressing normally.

PROBLEM 3

Get together with a group of colleagues or family. Do not tell anyone your height. Each one of you should use a tape measure to measure the height of a member of the group. Repeat the exercise after discussion of how to reduce the variation in measurement.

PROBLEM 4

Foot length is sometimes used as a rough guide for assessing height. For a group of people measure height (in inches) and foot size (in inches). Take three measures and average them. Plot foot length on the *y* axis, height on the *x* axis. Comment on the results.

PROBLEM 5

A study is performed on two physicians, A and B, each giving their opinions on the same 100 ECGs. The physicians

are asked simply to state if they think each is normal or abnormal. The results are shown in two forms Tables 7.2 and 7.3.

» Do you think that Table 7.2 demonstrates reasonable agreement between the two physicians?

» Complete Table 7.3 and consider again.

Table 7.2 Observations by the two physicians

	Physicians	
Observation	A	B
Normal	65	73
Abnormal	35	27
	100	100

Table 7.3 Correlation of agreement between physicians

	Physician B	
Physician A	Normal	Abnormal
Normal	50	
Abnormal		12

PROBLEM 6

The physicians were shown another 100 ECGs. These are in fact the same 100 as before but they are unaware of this. The results of the first and second viewing for each ECG are given in Tables 7.4 and 7.5.

The overall normal:abnormal ratios *remain the same* as in problem 5.

>> Which of the two physicians demonstrates the smaller *intraobserver* variation?

>> What does this imply for problem 4?

Table 7.4 Correlation of agreement between two viewings for physician A

First view	Second view	
	Normal	Abnormal
Normal	62	3
Abnormal	3	32

Table 7.5 Correlation of agreement between two viewings for physician B

First view	Second view	
	Normal	Abnormal
Normal	52	21
Abnormal	21	6

Answers

PROBLEM 1

A line can be drawn on each figure representing perfect agreement, i.e. passing through the zeros and the same numbers on the *x* and *y* axes. In Figure 7.1a the readings are reproducible, i.e. the scatter is small, but they are not valid as, they all lie above and away from the line. This is an example of **systematic error**. The nurse systematically obtains a higher reading than the machine but for any given pressure she will obtain nearly the same error. Repeated measurements of the same blood pressure would show little variation. The readings in Figure 7.1b are the best. The nurse's readings at any one value are tightly distributed around the actual value (represented by the diagonal line). The results are, therefore, both valid and reproducible. The third nurse (Fig. 7.1c) does not achieve reproducible results. The scatter is great. This is **random**, better described as haphazard, **error**. The readings are spread evenly around the line so there is no systematic error. The values obtained by the fourth nurse (Fig. 7.1d) are the worst. There is **systematic** and **random error**

present. The results are neither valid nor reproducible. Random errors can be overcome by repeated measurements, systematic errors cannot.

PROBLEM 2

A number of reasons may be responsible for the differences in blood pressure.

Subject variability. As the patient relaxes then blood pressure falls. This is a physiological response. Patients are less tense with people who appear less threatening and more expert. Their blood pressure will be lower.

Possible instrument bias or errors. The calibration of the instrument may be faulty. The cuff size used needs to be adjusted for patients with large arms. The cuff may be badly applied. The cuff may not be sufficiently inflated.

Observer bias. There must be an agreed definition of systolic (first sound heard – phase I) and diastolic (choose the point either at which the sound is muffled (phase IV) or when it vanishes (phase V)). Doctors will be more aware than others of the consequences of finding an abnormal blood pressure. They may, therefore, be biased towards a lower reading. This bias is usually quite involuntary and can be very potent, particularly at 2.00 am, when the doctor may not wish to face a serious hypertensive crisis, or in other situations, a diabetic going out of control or an abnormal fundus.

Variability in measurement. There are many examples in the literature of variability in measurement, covering such areas as the reading of X-ray films, palpation of pedal pulses, the interpretation of heart sounds, or eliciting a history of chest pain. *All* measurements, histories, examinations and opinions are subject to error and variation.

PROBLEM 3

Methods for reducing variability can be classified in several ways. The following are useful techniques:

- defining standards: e.g. size of BP cuff to use, type of assay for cardiac enzymes, the actual number of millimetres of ST-depression in an ECG to be called abnormal, etc.
- define instrument standards: operating technique, control samples
- training observers: use standards to assess performance
- multiple independent observers: reduces bias in particular systematic bias.

In the case of the height measurement exercise, it is usual to specify that the subject stands against a wall with a ruler or other straight edge on the top of his or her head at right angles to the wall. Measurement is then made up the wall. It is worth checking if the measurement tape is complete and accurate and compare the techniques of observers.

PROBLEM 4

In the case of foot length it is useful to draw around the foot on a piece of paper and take the maximum length. This is defining a standard method of measurement. It may affect the result if the observer doing the drawing is different to the ones measuring height (blinding the observers to the owner's of the feet).

PROBLEM 5

The rates of 65% and 73% as normal ECGs for the two physicians in Table 7.2 are comparable. Table 7.6 is the completed Table 7.3.

Table 7.3 shows the number of ECGs for which the physicians are in agreement. So both A and B think 50 are normal. This leaves 15 that A thinks are normal and B thinks are abnormal and 23 that B thinks are normal and A thinks are abnormal. As a result they are in agreement on only 12 as abnormal. A further derivation gives the other values in the table.

The comparison of the two physicians is interesting. Table 7.2 simply gives the overall ratios of normal to abnormal. This does not, however, tell us of the degree of agreement between the physicians as to which individual ECGs are normal or not. Table 7.6 shows the ECGs for

Table 7.6 Correlation of agreement between physicians

Physician A	Physician B	
	Normal	Abnormal
Normal	50	15
Abnormal	23	12

which both physicians, are in agreement (whether normal or abnormal). This is only 50 + 12 ECGs, which out of the 100 is 62%.

There is, therefore, marked **interobserver variation**, that is a difference between different observers.

PROBLEM 6

Physician A agrees with his original finding for 62 + 32, so for 100 ECGs there is 94% agreement between the two viewings. Physician B agrees for 52 + 6, so for 100 ECGs there is 58% agreement. The physician demonstrates marked intraobserver variation, that is given the same problem the physician changes the decision.

By giving the physicians the same ECG twice it is possible to assess *intraobserver* variability. Physician A does well, giving the same opinion on 94% of the ECGs. Physician B is poor at 58%. With this degree of variation, physician B's judgement is brought into question. Note, however, that physician A may be making considerable systematic errors, i.e. his opinion in the strict sense is reproducible but may not be valid against some gold standard.

Measurement

➤ A good measuring system must represent a true value (valid) and be reproducible.

➤ Errors can be random, which is overcome by multiple measurements, or biased (systematic), tend to vary in one direction owing to systematic errors of an instrument or observer.

➤ The degree of variation between multiple observations is known as intraobserver when one observer takes several measurements and interobserver when several observers measure the same parameter.

Clinical diagnosis

8

By the end of this chapter you should be able to:

- define the sensitivity and specificity of a clinical finding or diagnostic test
- discuss the role of disease prevalence in predicting the presence of disease
- understand the numerical and clinical significance of false positives and negatives
- appreciate the potential pitfalls in the indiscriminate use of diagnostic tests.

Definitions and techniques

The fourfold table

The fourfold table is used to compare two groups of findings, e.g. presence and absence of disease and positive and negative diagnostic tests (Table 8.1).

Definitions

The following definitions are used in assessing clinical diagnosis.

Sensitivity is the ability *correctly* to identify those with the disease. It is the proportion of patients with the disease in whom the test finding is positive. It is also called the **true positive rate**. In Table 8.1 its numerical value is $a/(a + c)$.

Specificity is the ability correctly to identify those without the disease. It is the proportion of those without disease in which the test finding is negative. It is also called the **true negative rate**. In Table 8.1 its numerical value is $d/(b + d)$.

Positive predictive value of a test is the proportion of those with a positive test result that have the disease. In Table 8.1 it is equal to $a/(a + b)$.

Negative predictive value of a test is the proportion of those with a negative test result that do not have the disease. In Table 8.1 it is equal to $d/(c + d)$.

The **false positive rate** is the rate of positive results occurring in those without the disease. In Table 8.1 it is $b/(b + d)$. It can also be expressed as the false positive rate of the test, i.e. $b/(a + b)$. The numbers of people who are falsely positive, i.e. who have a positive test but not the disease, are those in cell b. False positive cases are important if the outcome of the test is to have an unpleasant or dangerous treatment. This is especially so in prenatal testing where a normal fetus may be aborted if a false positive test occurs.

The **false negative rate** is the rate of negative results occurring in those with the disease. In Table 8.1 it is $c/(a + c)$. It can also be expressed as the false negative rate of the test, i.e. $c/(c + d)$. The number of people who are falsely negative, i.e. who have a negative test but who who have the disease are those in cell c. False negatives can be a problem if the test delays the accurate diagnosis of the disease.

Prevalence is the proportion of those in the base population who have the disease. In Table 8.1 it is

$$\frac{a + c}{a + b + c + d}$$

Pre-test probability is an estimate of the likelihood of a patient having the disease, given the information already available. It may depend on research data about the likelihood of the presence of disease given certain symptoms, or on the investigations performed so far.

Post-test probability is an estimate of the likeli-

Table 8.1 Fourfold table for comparison between two groups of data, for example disease and diagnostic finding

Finding	Disease		
	Present	Absent	Totals
Positive	a	b	a + b
Negative	c	d	c + d
Totals	a + c	b + d	a + b + c + d

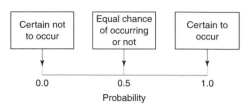

Fig. 8.1 The probability that an event will occur.

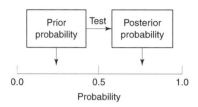

Fig. 8.2 Prior and posterior probability.

hood of a patient having the disease as a result of a new piece of information: a symptom, sign or investigation. This estimate will be different depending upon whether the test is positive or negative.

Interpreting results from tests

The straight line in Figure 8.1 represents the continuum of probability (p from 0, a state or position where an event is certain *not* to occur, to a state where $p = 1$ and an event is certain to occur. Maximum uncertainty occurs around $p = 0.5$. The purpose of carrying out a test, or series of tests, is to try and reduce some of the uncertainty in managing individual patients. The *interpretation of new information* (the result of the test) *depends on what is already known about the patient.* In Problem 2, three patients with chest pain, this **pre-test probability** is the prevalence of ischaemic heart disease in the three subgroups these patients are drawn from. The value of the test (an ECG in Problem 2) is the degree to which it reduces uncertainty. This is dependent on its sensitivity and specificity and the type of population in which it is used, the prevalence of the

underlying condition in question, and hence its predictive value. Figure 8.2 shows how a test can alter the pre-test probability to a different value, the **post-test probability**.

Sometimes test results are negative, in which case the post-test probability of disease being present is less than the pre-test probability.

Do not be muddled by mathematics. A test may have a very high sensitivity and specificity but at a *low* enough prevalence the **false positives** will become unacceptably high and eventually outnumber the **true positives**. At a *high* enough prevalence the **false negatives** will become unacceptably high and eventually outnumber the **true negatives**. The interpretation of the result of a test or clinical finding depends crucially upon the **prevalence** of the disease being sought, in the base population.

Note that populations are often pre-selected.

General population → GP → A & E → Ward → Specialist

In general the prevalence of diseases rises from left to right and findings increase in significance. Life in a GP's surgery is very different from that as a house person in a hospital. All headaches with photophobia are not meningitis. Figure 8.3 shows the actual data for the number of patients with mental illness in the population, in general practice and in hospital.

Problems

PROBLEM 1:

Exercise ECGS

The exercise ECG is positive in 60% of patients with obstructive coronary artery disease. It is also positive in 10% of normals The 'gold standard' is coronary angiography for patients admitted to hospital.

» What is the sensitivity of the test?

» What is its specificity?

» Is it a good test?

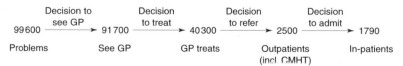

Fig. 8.3 Mentally ill people in different parts of the health service (CMHT, community mental health team).

PROBLEM 2:

Importance of the prevalence of the disease

Consider the three patients described who were seen in out-patients complaining of chest pain:

1. What is the likelihood of each patient having coronary heart disease (CHD) before the test?
2. On clinical grounds, how useful would an exercise ECG be?

Patient A. A 55-year-old man with exertional chest pain, like a heavy weight, radiating down the left arm and associated with some dyspnoea. A fourth heart sound is present. He has a family history of coronary heart disease. An exercise ECG is suggested to clinch the diagnosis.

Patient B. A 31-year-old man who is otherwise well, with no risk factors, and a 6-week history of heartburn-like pain. He is asking for an exercise ECG to be on the safe side.

Patient C. A 45-year-old man who smokes 25 cigarettes per day, with 3 weeks of pre-cordial pain, inconsistently related to exercise. It is sometimes like a heavy weight on his chest. There is slight tenderness over a costochondral junction. Will an exercise ECG be helpful?

What is the diagnosis for each patient on the basis of their symptoms?

PROBLEM 3

Using the figures for prevalence of CHD and the sensitivity (60%) and specificity (90%) associated with an exercise ECG test, construct the fourfold tables for the three patient types in Problem 2 (assuming a base of 1000 patients to ease calculation). The columns will be presence and absence of CHD and the rows will be positive and negative exercise ECGs. The pre-test probabilities are

Patient A 0.9
Patient B 0.05
Patient C 0.5

Calculate the post-test probabilities, which refers to the probability of the patient having CHD if the test is positive and if it is negative, and comment on the usefulness of the test on the basis of these results.

PROBLEM 4

In a city of 1 million people, there are 1000 people who have contracted gout. A test for gout is positive in 95% of people with the disease and is negative in 95% of people without the disease. The test is given to all the people in the city. For this city, draw a fourfold table to show what is the probability that a person with a positive test had gout:

- 1 to 3%
- 10 to 20%
- 50 to 60%
- 80 to 95%
- Over 95%

PROBLEM 5

Combined tests

In the differential diagnosis of non-specific abdominal pain (NSAP) and acute appendicitis (AA), several clinical signs and symptoms have been studied to determine their usefulness in distinguishing the two conditions. Table 8.2 gives a summary of some of their frequencies (After de Dombal, a Leeds surgeon). Assuming the diagnosis is one of either NSAP or AA.

1. Calculate the sensitivity and specificity for RIF pain
2. In an A&E population with abdominal pain where patients have either NSAP or AA, the prevalence of AA is 16%; construct the fourfold table for RIF pain for 1000 patients
3. What is the predictive value for RIF pain in this situation?

Table 8.2 Signs and symptoms in appendicitis and NSAP (de Dombal 1995)

Symptom	Percentage occurrence in	
	Appendicitis	NSAP
Bowel change	20	30
Nausea	73	58
Vomiting	72	50
Anorexia	80	54
Pain shifting to RIF	75	25
RIF pain	75	25
RIF tenderness	65	25
Rectal tenderness	43	16
Rebound	80	22
Guarding	80	10

RIF, right iliac fossa.

PROBLEM 6

Extend the data given in Problem 5 to assume that RIF pain is present and assess the value of a second symptom, guarding, as a combined analysis. The *positives* from the fourfold analysis of RIF pain and AA (Table 8.8) then become the totals for this analysis: positive RIF pain with AA = 120, without AA = 210.

1. Make a fourfold table for guarding when RIF pain is present in AA
2. What proportion of patients with both findings actually have acute appendicitis?

3. What has the use of the combined findings done for the predictive value?

The example of RIF pain and guarding in acute appendicitis and non-specific abdominal pain is an example of combining two pieces of information. Intuitively, the combination of RIF and guarding is more likely to identify those with AA than using RIF alone.

Thus for the first stage, the pre-test probability is the prevalence of AA in an A and E population = 0.16 or 16%. The post-test probability using the presence of RIF is 0.36. This post-test probability forms the (new) pre-test probability for the second stage where the use of guarding as a sign in those with RIF is now used as the 'test'.

Answers

PROBLEM 1

The sensitivity and specificity can be worked out using the fourfold table (Table 8.3). In each case the term 'per cent' means out of 100.

The test is not very sensitive: there are many false negatives, i.e. cell c. Although the definitive test is coronary angiography, it is quite dangerous and not to be undertaken lightly.

PROBLEM 2

1. From the symptoms of coronary heart disease, patient A will be likely to have had a coronary, patient B not and patient C is uncertain. Investigations should only be used where they will make a difference to the management of the patient.
2. To assess how an exercise ECG will perform in each of these situations it is necessary to know the likely prevalence of CHD in the group to which each patient belongs before the investigation is performed. This is the pre-test likelihood of the patient having the disease in question.

A clinical opinion of the likelihood of patients having CHD would be based upon experiential or research knowledge of the prevalence of CHD for sub-groups with defined groups, e.g.

Patient A 90%
Patient B 5%
Patient C 50%.

These are pre-test probabilities.

PROBLEM 3

Table 8.4–8.5 give the figures for the three patients.

Patient A. The diagnosis of CHD would be 98% likely if the test was positive, 80% if it was negative. The patient would be treated as if he had had CHD no matter what the outcome of the test. There was, therefore, no point in doing the test.

Patient B. The chance of this patient having CHD is only 24% if the test is positive, 2% if it is negative. In either case the diagnosis is not likely to be CHD whatever the outcome of test

Patient C. In this case, the diagnosis is confirmed if the test is positive (86%) and is shown not to be likely if the test is negative. The diagnosis, therefore, depends on the test result, showing that the test was useful.

Table 8.3 The sensitivity and specificity of exercise ECGs

Exercise ECG	Coronary heart disease		Totals
	Present	Absent	
Positive	60	10	70
Negative	40	90	130
Totals	100	100	200

The sensitivity of the test is 60% the specificity of the test is 90%.

Table 8.4 Patient A

Exercise ECG	Coronary heart disease		Totals
	Present	Absent	
Positive	540	10	550
Negative	360	90	450
Totals	900	100	1000

Pre-test probability = 0.9
Post-test probabilities:
Test positive = 540/550 = 0.98
Test negative = 360/450 = 0.80

Table 8.5 Patient B

Exercise ECG	Coronary heart disease		Totals
	Present	Absent	
Positive	30	95	125
Negative	20	855	875
Totals	50	950	1000

Pre-test probability = 0.05
Post-test probabilities:
Positive = 30/125 = 0.24
Negative = 20/875 = 0.02

Table 8.6 Patient C

| Exercise ECG | Coronary heart disease | | |
	Present	Absent	Totals
Positive	300	50	350
Negative	200	450	650
Totals	500	500	1000

Pre-test probability = 0.50
Post-test probabilities:
Positive = 300/350 = 0.86
Negative = 200/650 = 0.31

The usefulness of exercise ECG. In each patient, the post-test probability refers to the probability of the patient having CHD if the test is positive or negative. The following conclusions can be drawn:

- Patient A was a certainty to begin with and the test adds little to the overall diagnosis
- Patient B was a very unlikely candidate for CHD and the test cannot make the diagnosis of CHD
- Patient C benefits the most in that the diagnosis will move usefully away from 50% depending on the result of the test.

It could be argued that A and B should not have the test. This problem highlights two important features of tests.

Usefulness of tests, especially investigations. Unless there is real doubt about the diagnosis or the best next course of action to take there is no point in doing further tests. What is more, unnecessary tests cause confusion, may be dangerous and are certainly expensive.

False positives and negatives. Always give careful consideration to false positives and negatives. Consider patient B. If the test is negative then he is reassured, which could be done anyway. If it is positive, what are the consequences? It is probably a false positive and a normal young man can be labelled as a heart patient with all that implies for his job, insurance, mortgage and peace of mind. This has to be weighted against the lesser chance of missing the diagnosis. For patient A, the converse is true and a negative test is most likely to be a false one and a patient with CHD would be incorrectly diagnosed.

PROBLEM 4

This example changes the clinical details but again emphasises the importance of the prevalence in influencing the positive predictive values. With a low prevalence (as in this example), the false positives markedly outweigh the true positives, resulting in a very low positive predictive value (PPV) (Table 8.7).

Table 8.7 Testing a population for gout

| Test | Gout | | |
	Present	Absent	Totals
Positive	950	49 950	50 900
Negative	50	949 050	949 100
Totals	1000	999 000	1 000 000

The positive predictive value = 950/50 900 = 0.0187 = 1.87%, i.e. 1–3%.

This problem is a common one with screening when a large population is being approached, a test with high sensitivity and specificity will still generate a large number of false positives. This is especially problematical when cancer screening is involved because the false positives suffer considerable anxiety and have to be followed up with more definitive diagnostic testing very quickly to allay that anxiety.

PROBLEM 5

1. RIF pain sensitivity is 75%, specificity is 75%. This is because RIF pain was present in 75 out of 100 cases of AA, was not present in 75% of those without AA. It must be remembered that NSAP is simply not appendicitis in this example.
2. In this population, the choice is only between AA and NSAP. Table 8.8 gives the fourfold analysis for AA at a prevalence of 16% in this A&E department.

The positive predictive value is 120/330 = 0.36
Although RIF pain is much more common in AA than in NSAP, the prevalence results in a low positive predictive value. The likely value of the finding in a GP surgery at a prevalence of AA of say 5% would be, in this case, a PPV of 0.13 showing that the finding is even less useful in this setting.

PROBLEM 6

1. Table 8.9 shows the results for guarding as a sign of AA in those patients who had a positive result for RIF pain.

Table 8.8 RIF pain and AA where AA prevalence is 16%

| RIF pain | Acute appendicitis | | |
	Present	Absent	Totals
Positive	120	210	330
Negative	40	630	670
Totals	160	840	1000

2. The proportion with both findings who actually have appendicitis is, therefore, 96/120 = 0.8 or 80%.
3. The predictive value for both findings is 96/117 = 0.82 or 82%, considerably better than for RIF pain alone. The diagnostic yield can, therefore, be greatly increased by combining findings and tests. (No mention has been made of potential correlations between findings.)

Combined tests give greater accuracy for those testing positive to each test, but some people are lost at each stage. Positive tests apply to an increasingly lower proportion of the population as more tests are added. In addition, a large number of tests (usually investigation where the likely diagnosis is already reasonably certain) are a waste of resources; one needs to think about the actions that will be taken if the result is positive or negative. False positives and negatives may present a problem if a large number of tests are carried out. A good clinician will use his or her experience to estimate the prevalence of the disease in the population to which the patient belongs, and will interpret findings and the likely effects of a new test in that light.

Table 8.9 Guarding as a symptom of AA in patients with RIF pain

Guarding	Acute appendicitis		
	Present	Absent	Totals
Positive	96	21	117
Negative	24	189	213
Totals	120	210	330

Clinical diagnosis

➤ Tests used in clinical diagnosis should ideally be sensitive and specific.

➤ False positives and negatives can result in costly/dangerous treatment that is unnecessary or in delaying accurate diagnosis and treatment.

➤ Tests should only be used where there is doubt about the diagnosis or the next best course of action to take.

➤ Combined tests give greater accuracy for those testing positive to each test but at each test some people (negative results) fail to pass on to the next test.

Clinical importance

9

By the end of this chapter the student should have an understanding of:

- the problem of definition of the disease entity, i.e. defining a case
- the process by which a clinician judges the borderline between health and sickness and upon what basis such judgements are made
- the possible clinical significance of results and their interpretation
- statistical definitions of normal and abnormal ranges.

Definitions

Normality and abnormality

The first priority in any clinical encounter is to find out whether the patient's symptoms, signs or diagnostic test results are normal or abnormal. This decision is necessary before further action can be taken, whether this is more investigations, treatment or observation. It would be easy if there was always a clear distinction between the frequency distribution of observations on normal and abnormal people. Regrettably, this is rarely found, except in genetic disorders determined by a single dominant gene; modern knowledge about genetics is showing this to be increasingly unusual. Occasionally the frequency distributions overlap, but more often there is only one distribution and the so-called abnormal people are the tail end of the distribution of a bell-shaped curve. In this situation three types of criteria have been used to help clinicians make practical decisions:

- normal as common
- abnormal associated with disease
- abnormal as treatable.

Normal as common

In our experience, students coming upon the Gaussian or normal distribution (often known as the bell-shaped curve) for the first time are prone to a misconception. Frequently occurring values are considered normal and infrequently occurring values are considered abnormal. An arbitrary cut-off point is specified on the population frequency distribution. This is assumed to be the limit of normal (often two standard deviations from the mean). All values beyond this point are considered abnormal. This is an operational definition of abnormality. If the distribution is in fact normal then this cut-off point would identify 2.5% of the population as 'abnormal'. An alternative approach that does not assume a bell-shaped curve is to use percentiles. This often involves considering the 95th percentile point as the dividing line between normal and abnormal, thus identifying 5% of the population as 'abnormal'.

Because of this, if a patient has 14 tests (not uncommon with modern biochemistry equipment) he has over 50% chance of one of them being 'abnormal' – if each test is independent. The chance of each test being normal is 0.95. For 14 tests the chance of all 14 being normal is $(0.95) \times (0.95) \times (0.95)$ for 14 times. This is 0.48. Thus the chance of at least one abnormal test is $1 - 0.48 = 0.52 = 52\%$. This definition of the normal range has no necessary link with risk to health or a notion of illness as determined by symptoms and signs. Labels such as anaemia can quickly metamorphose into diseases and explanations for symptoms.

Epidemiological and clinical evidence are required to establish links between diseases and findings.

A major limitation of this criterion for normality – normal as common – is that for most variables there is no biological basis for using an arbitrary cut-off point as a basis of abnormality. For serum cholesterol or blood pressure, for example, there is an increasing risk of cardiovascular disease with increasing levels. Even within the 'normal' ranges, as determined statistically, there is an increased risk of disease compared with the lowest population levels. A majority of the excess coronary heart disease deaths occurs at levels of blood pressure that are usual, only a small proportion of cases occurs at extremely high values.

Abnormality associated with disease

This criterion suggests two populations, one healthy and one diseased. For an objective measure of health or disease many of the measures, especially investigations, may give data on the distribution of observations for both healthy and diseased. This may, for continuous variables, approximate to two bell-shaped curves overlapping to some degree. We may make attempts to define an appropriate cut-off point, which clearly separates the two groups. However such a cut-off point, which neatly separates cases from non-cases, is usually impossible. There will always be some healthy people on the abnormal side of the cut-off point who will be called abnormal and there will be some true cases that will be considered normal.

Figure 9.1 shows data for serum cholesterol in a longitudinal study of men aged 50–62 years who later developed or did not develop coronary heart disease. It can be seen that the two distributions largely overlapped apart from a bulge at the upper end of the distribution, where there were more men who had coronary heart disease, representing the 'abnormal' bell-shaped curve. The number of people who had coronary heart disease was, of course, much smaller than the number who did not. Nevertheless clearly no cut-off point will totally separate those at risk of coronary heart disease from those not at risk. One can move the dividing line along the x-axis but the more 'abnormals' are classified correctly the less 'normals' there will be.

Abnormal as treatable

The difficulties in distinguishing between normal and abnormal using the above two criteria have led to the use of measures determined by evidence from randomised controlled trials. These indicate the level at which treatment does more good than harm.

The treatment of diastolic blood pressure provides a good example of both the advantage and the limitations of this type of criteria. Early clinical trials provided firm evidence that treating very high sustained diastolic blood pressure (120 mmHg) was beneficial. Subsequent trials have indicated that the benefits of treatment outweigh the problems at lower levels, perhaps as low as 95 mmHg and this is now the recommended level of treatment in many countries. However, this approach does not take into account the economic and other costs of treatment and is, therefore, still a rather simplistic approach to determining treatment levels. With the development and application of sophisticated cost-effectiveness analyses, it may be possible to add the cost dimension to these clinical decisions. It is likely, for example, that it will be soon feasible to determine the blood pressure levels for specific age and sex groups at which treatment makes reasonable economic as well as medical sense. For example, a young woman with a diastolic blood pressure level of 90 mmHg is at low risk of cardiovascular diseases. It will be much less cost-effective to treat her than an older man with a diastolic blood pressure of 150 mmHg, who has a much greater risk of cardiovascular disease.

In addition, the level at which people are considered treatable changes with time. This is illustrated for the changing definition of treatable levels of blood pressure (Fig. 9.2). As new evidence accumulates from well-conducted clinical trials, the levels recommended for treatment will continue to change. Each new cut-off point proposed has, however, important logistic and cost implications that require consideration. The

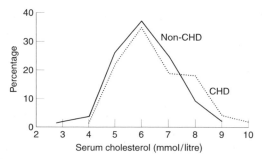

Fig. 9.1 Distribution of serum cholesterol levels in men who did or did not develop coronary heart disease. (Khow & Rose 1989)

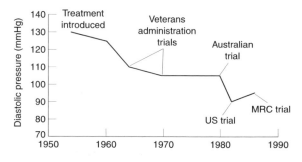

Fig. 9.2 Changing treatment definitions for hypertension over time. (Mosser 1989)

results of the most recent Medical Research Council trials have suggested that over-treatment might be occurring at least in the UK. There is therefore a tendency to move the treatment level upwards.

Statistical significance and clinical importance are not the same

A difference is regarded as *statistically significant* when the *p*-value calculated from the data is less than some pre-determined threshold value α. Usually this is equivalent to the 1–α confidence interval for the difference excluding zero. Whether statistical significance is achieved depends heavily on the sample size used.

A *clinically important* difference is one that is large enough to actually matter in clinical or public health practice. What is to be regarded as clinically important is to be judged from our understanding of the context, not from the set of data that we have collected. Thus a difference in blood pressure lowering activity of 25 mmHg between two treatments would be regarded as clinically important, a difference of 2 mmHg would not be. However, a very large study might demonstrate the latter difference to be statistically significant, with a 95% CI from 1 to 3 mmHg – clearly to be interpreted as negligible. Conversely, a very small study might produce a 95% CI for the former from –5 to 55 mmHg, and fail to show even a difference as large as 25 mmHg as statistically significant.

You will encounter references to clinical *significance*; the expression clinical *importance* is preferable, being less prone to confuse.

A single study, however extreme a *p*-value it yields, should not usually be regarded as an adequate basis for a change of policy; independent confirmation is desirable, with corroboration from studies of pathophysiology and pharmacology.

A confidence interval for a difference enables us to appraise both its statistical significance and its clinical importance. Figure 9.3 shows the possible outcomes. In small studies, the confidence interval for the difference is wide; it may (A, B) or may not (C, D) exclude 0, but it is unlikely to demonstrate that even at a conservative estimate the difference is clinically important (E).

Note that intervals A to E have been drawn with equal widths here; they merely correspond to different values for the point estimate. The effect of increasing the sample size is to reduce the width of the interval, bringing the inference into sharper focus.

A: *Statistically significant difference (H$_0$ rejected)*. The point estimate and the majority of the confidence interval lie below the threshold of clinical importance, but as some of the interval is above it, this result is compatible with there being a clinically worthwhile difference.

B: *Statistically significant difference (H$_0$ rejected)*. The point estimate and the majority of the confidence interval lie above the threshold of clinical importance. The result is, however, still compatible with the actual difference in the population being less than the threshold of clinical importance.

C: *Insufficient evidence to reject H$_0$ – 'not statistically significant'*. The confidence interval includes the null value and it also includes an area above the threshold of clinical importance. The result is thus classically not proven being compatible both with the null hypothesis being true and with there being an effect larger than the threshold of clinical importance.

D: *Not statistically significant (H$_0$ not rejected)*. The confidence interval excludes any clinically important difference so this is a substantial negative finding, i.e. any difference that exists is trivially small.

E: *Statistically highly significant (H$_0$ rejected)*. This study excludes there being a difference that is below the threshold of clinical importance.

F: *Statistically significant (H$_0$ rejected)*. This unusual type of result is both incompatible with the null hypothesis being true and with the true difference being of clinical importance.

Note that however large the sample size, A or B will sometimes occur: we cannot guarantee to be able to decide whether the true difference is greater or less than δ. C is the classical indeterminate outcome that is sometimes mis-reported as having shown that there is no difference. D is the classical firm negative outcome – compare with C. E is the ideal positive outcome, but it is relatively rare. F is a rare outcome.

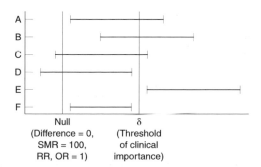

Fig. 9.3 Interpreting confidence intervals: the distinction between clinical importance and statistical significance in comparative studies (in approximate order of frequency of occurrence in published paper).

Problems

PROBLEM 1

Think of as many diagnostic labels (diagnoses) as you can. Write them down then categorise them in a table with the categories:

- symptom
- sign
- investigation
- general statement
- pathological finding
- extreme of a physiological range
- extreme range of an investigation
- mixed.

PROBLEM 2

Rheumatic fever is an acute inflammatory complication of streptococcal infection that may involve the joints (arthritis), brain (chorea), heart (carditis and valve disease), subcutaneous tissue (nodules) and the skin (rash). The disease rarely affects all five body systems and typically involves only one or two. A streptococcal throat may be involved in the initial stages of the disease. Other non-specific findings include acute fever, elevated white blood cell count and an increased red blood cell sedimentation rate.

What criteria would you use to define a case of rheumatic fever?

PROBLEM 3

Figure 9.4 shows the overlapping complex relationships of patients with sore throats and patients with positive tests for streptococcal infections. Streptococcal infections are identified by a positive laboratory test, either from a throat swab culture or in a serological rise of antibody titre, or in both. Sore throats are identified as a symptom reported by the patient. The inter-relationships of the Venn diagram show the connection between symptoms and investigations.

What are the possible situations that can occur between sore throats and these investigations?

PROBLEM 4

The epidemiological data demonstrate that rheumatic fever is a subset of streptococcal infections with high antibody titres.

What can be inferred from the diagrammatic representation of the situation shown in Figure 9.5?

PROBLEM 5

Rheumatic fever is a complication of streptococcal infection. It is a clinical entity for which signs, symptoms and investigations are arbitrarily defined by the criteria set out originally by Jones (Table 2.1, p. 12). The relationship between the symptoms of arthritis, chorea and carditis is shown in Figure 9.6 including one for patients who have severe carditis. Two other 'major' features of rheumatic fever – erythaema marginatum and subcutaneous nodules – seldom occur alone and have no prognostic or therapeutic significance. Hence they have been omitted from the main diagram.

1. When chorea occurs alone, is it an aberrant variety or form of rheumatic fever?
2. It is possible for carditis to occur alone. When the acute carditis subsides in such patients, leaving residual scars found at some later date, rheumatic heart disease is said to have developed 'without a history of rheumatic fever'.

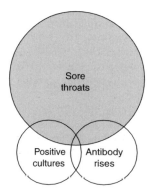

Fig. 9.4 The inter-relationship between sore throats and investigations (Venn diagram).

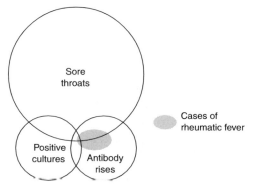

Fig. 9.5 Venn diagram showing the relationship of cases of rheumatic fever with sore throats and streptococcal infection.

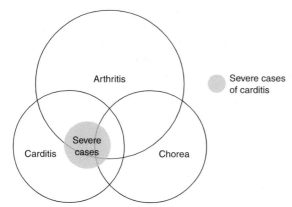

Fig. 9.6 The inter-relationship between the major symptoms of rheumatic fever.

The heart disease found in these circumstances is often called insidious. What would be a more correct description of the natural history of disease in such individuals?

PROBLEM 6

A 48-year-old man with a typical history of angina pectoris is seen in the out-patient clinic. As part of his work-up blood pressure is measured. The result is reported as 160/105. Figure 9.7 gives the distribution of diastolic blood pressure for an appropriate population.

● Is the patient's blood pressure normal?
● How have you defined normal?
● Does he require attention and will he benefit?
● What other information do you seek?

PROBLEM 7

Figure 9.8 shows the relationship between blood pressure and risk of death from heart disease.

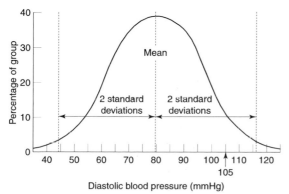

Fig. 9.7 The distribution of diastolic blood pressure in men aged 40–49 years.

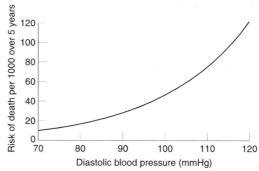

Fig. 9.8 The relationship between risk of death from heart disease and diastolic blood pressure in middle-aged men. (Kannel 1990)

1. Is the blood pressure now normal, is it clinically significant, does the patient need treating?
2. How does your definition of normal affect the potential number of cases of hypertension?
3. What other information should be sought?
4. Is age a significant confounder?
5. What is the relationship between blood pressure and total mortality?

PROBLEM 8

A 40-year old woman presents feeling tired, listless and irritable. Following the history and examination you request a full blood count. Her haemoglobin is reported as 11.0 g/dl (normal range for the laboratory is 11.5–16.4).

● Is she anaemic?
● Does her haemoglobin explain her symptoms?
● What may happen if when her haemoglobin is remeasured?

Answers

PROBLEM 1

Table 9.1 shows some examples of diagnostic labels commonly used and the categories to which they belong. The term 'diagnosis' can mean a whole range of different things. In particular' patients and doctors often misunderstand each other when talking about a label. The term 'heart attack' means sudden death to some patients, but not to doctors. A diagnosis is only useful if it helps the physician to act on it in the patient's interest.

PROBLEM 2

The diagnosis of rheumatic fever is complicated. Because

Table 9.1 Categories and diagnostic labels

Category	Diagnostic label
Symptom	Cough, sore throat, indigestion
Sign	Heart murmur
Investigation	Coronary thrombosis
General statement	Cold, heart attack, stroke
Pathological finding	Myocardial infarction, cancer, rheumatoid arthritis, Alzheimer's disease
Extreme of a physiological range	Hypertension, fever
Extreme range of an investigation	Anaemia
Mixed	Rheumatic fever, schizophrenia, measles

the disease may take many forms and affect different organ systems, the diagnosis requires the physician to have a high degree of suspicion. Diagnosis depends upon the presence of at least one and preferably two or more 'major manifestations' of the disease, which include carditis, chorea, arthritis, erythaema marginatum (a skin rash) and subcutaneous nodules. In addition to the 'major' manifestations, there should be recent evidence of a group A streptococcal infection and the presence of 'minor' manifestations of the disease (Table 2.1, p. 12). These include fever and elevation of the sedimentation rate and white blood cell count.

Rheumatic fever is related to previous infection with group A beta-haemolytic streptococci. Its boundaries are indefinite, and its differentiation from other diseases is sometimes impossible. There is no specific laboratory diagnostic test. Diagnosis must, therefore, be arbitrary and empirical. Because of the potential to develop rheumatic heart disease, diagnosis is important both to avoid missing cases and to avoid labelling those without the disease but with some indications of it.

PROBLEM 3

With reference to the Venn diagram (Fig. 9.4), streptococcal infections need not produce sore throats and sore throats need not be streptococcal. Sore throats are, of course, immensely more common than the prevalence of the positive investigations. Clinical epidemiological studies of large numbers of patients in these different situations have demonstrated that rheumatic complications emerge from only a small proportion of such people. The epidemiological data have shown that rheumatic fever can develop in patients with or without a sore throat and with or without a positive throat culture. The critical feature that makes a streptococcal infection potentially rheumatogenic is a rise in antibody titre.

The clinical significance of a variate of a particular disease can only be discovered by working out the extent to which it is present or absent in other members of the population of the same age, sex, etc. This requires us to survey populations of both well and ill people to measure of the strength of the association between the variate and independent clinical confirmation of the presence of sickness.

PROBLEM 4

From Figure 9.5 it can be inferred that the shaded area differentiates those patients with rheumatic fever from those with sore throats and streptococcal infections. This helps to explain several pertinent clinical features of the occurrence of rheumatic fever. Typical pharyngitis, with a sore throat, often fails to appear in many patients who have serologically positive streptococcal infection. In such patients, the infection can produce rheumatic fever insidiously, without previous symptomatic warning. Conversely, when the serological evidence is negative, a positive throat culture in a patient with sore throat denotes that the event is streptococcal, or the carrier state, but it cannot cause rheumatic fever.

PROBLEM 5

1. When chorea occurs alone it is not an aberrant variety of rheumatic fever but a distinct entity in the post-streptococcal spectrum.
2. When carditis occurs alone, the patient has no chorea or joint pains and may also lack fever or congestive heart failure. If they have none of these symptoms, the patient may not seek medical aid. Actually, the period of acute inflammation may have been no more than a few months. The truly insidious aspect of the disease was the absence of symptoms that would have enabled the patient to complain and be medically examined to detect disease during the acute phase of the carditis.

PROBLEM 6

Figure 9.7 is a Gaussian or bell-shaped distribution with a mean and two standard deviations from that mean in either direction. This covers 95% of the population. Using the distribution and the use of two standard deviations to define a 'normal' range, would put a pressure of 160/105 well within this range. This is a statistical concept, not a medical one. A person with a disease or at high risk from disease is not the same as someone who is near the average measure of a distribution. One has only to think about the relative importance of blood pressure well above the mean and compare it with blood pressure well below the mean. The latter are not generally considered at risk. Clinically, the blood pressure may be important, even if it is statistically similar to that of the majority of people.

PROBLEM 7

Figure 9.8 relates the risk of increased blood pressure and heart disease mortality. This introduces another view of normal, as related to risk of, or association with, disease.

1. On these grounds, a level of 105 may be undesirable. There is, however, no cut-off value where the risk suddenly rises or falls. The demonstration of a risk factor does not necessarily imply that attempted control, i.e. giving hypotensive agents, will provide benefit. In addition, treatment itself has risks, whether of side effects, the cost of using medicines over the long term or the psychological effect of labelling someone who feels well as having a disease. These risks have to be balanced.
2. As the level of blood pressure considered abnormal is reduced so the number of people requiring treatment rises very rapidly, as one moves up the bell-shaped curve.
3. In a patient who is on the margin of needing treatment, information on other risk factors that affect the patient will help to decide whether or not to treat.
4. Older people have higher average blood pressure measurements than younger in the UK. A decision has to be made about whether one point, say 90 mmHg, is regarded as abnormal for people of all ages or whether abnormal should be a defined deviation from the average, in which case the point for treatment would be higher. Most clinicians allow as normal in old people a degree of blood pressure that they would treat in younger people.
5. Total mortality is not as clearly related to blood pressure. However, because heart disease is so common there still is a relationship, though less clear, with total mortality.

Clinical and statistical significance. Problems 6 and 7 are examples of the problem in distinguishing clinical and statistical significance. A clinically significant change in a measure such as blood pressure means that, in the judgement of expert clinical opinion, the change will have an impact on the length of life or quality of life of a patient. The impact will take into account any risks or other problems, such as side effects from treatment, that the patient may be exposed to. Statistical significance simply means that the difference in the measure is such that it would not be expected to occur by chance. Treatment which caused a mean fall in blood pressure of 1 mmHg

might, in a large enough sample reach statistical significance (at, say, the 5% level) but would have no noticeable effect on the well-being of the patients.

PROBLEM 8

This question highlights the inappropriate use of statistical definitions rather than clinical ones where the problem is essentially clinical. The symptoms described have been shown not to be specific to anaemia by Elwood in a comparison between women with haemoglobins within and outside two standard deviations. Minor differences in haemoglobin concentration do not cause symptoms. If any finding outside the two standard deviation range is repeated it is most likely to be nearer to normal the next time. This is known as **regression towards the mean**. This is a statistical concept that simply means that an unusual finding, within the variation inherent in any method of measurement, is, by chance, more likely to be near the mean the next time. In addition, high or low readings are likely to have been caused by a variety of factors. These may have been:

- methodological; the machine may have been reading low or high that day
- in the taking of the sample, which may, by coincidence, have worked in the same direction as any methodological variation.

This is unlikely to recur.

> ### Clinical significance
>
> ➤ Test results can be assessed using different criteria of normal: abnormal as uncommon, as associated with disease and as treatable.
>
> ➤ Diagnoses can be defined in many different ways. The label is only important if it helps the physician to act on the diagnosis in the patient's interest.
>
> ➤ Clinical significance is changes in a measure that expert clinical opinion considers will have an impact on life quality or extent in a patient. The assessment of impact will take into account any risks, side effects or other problems treatment might cause.
>
> ➤ Statistical significance means that the difference in the measure is such that it could not occur by chance.

Treatment effectiveness

10

By the end of this chapter you should understand:

- the variability in natural history of diseases and treatment outcome
- the need to control for the inadequacies of personal clinical impressions in evaluating treatments
- the use of controls in evaluating treatment
- historical controls
- comparability of controls
- selection bias
- comparability of treatments
- 'Blinding' in trials
- double-blind randomised controlled trials
- explanatory and pragmatic (intention-to-treat) trials.

Problems

PROBLEM 1

Figure 10.1 shows data extracted from an advertisement for Vibramycin (doxycycline), a tetracycline antibiotic. The data is derived from winter studies of doxycycline in respiratory tract infections. The total number of patients involved was 1747, a substantial study. The advertisement described Vibramycin as the adult antibiotic. Discuss the following points:

- is Vibramycin effective in treating respiratory tract infections?
- which symptom is it best at relieving?

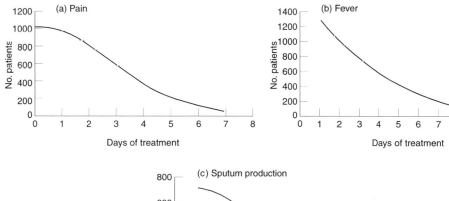

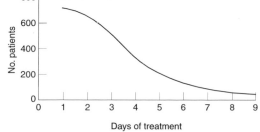

Fig. 10.1 Vibramycin treatment of upper respiratory infection: number of patients experiencing. (Hartnett & Marlin 1976)

PROBLEM 2

Following the opening of a new, highly specialised and well-equipped coronary care unit (CCU) in Australia, the paper stated 'We believe that the mortality from myocardial infarction has indeed been lowered by the new facilities we have been able to offer'.

Table 10.1 is taken from a table in the paper. The comparison is with a 2-year period prior to the opening of the new unit. Discuss the following points:

- is the new unit effective at treating acute myocardial infarction?
- the data in Table 10.2, which were taken from the text of the paper?
- possible explanations for the difference between the two periods in Table 10.2.

Table 10.1 Deaths in patients with definite myocardial infarction admitted directly to the coronary care unit

	Before CCU (1967–9)		After CCU (1973–5)	
	N	%	N	%
Total patients	196		522	
Total deaths	48	24.5%	50	9.6%

Table 10.2 Coronary care unit data taken from the text

	Before CCU (1967–9)	After CCU (1973–5)
Total admissions	Not known	1364
Total deaths	Not known	100 (7.3%)
Total definite infarcts	Not known	620
Deaths in definite infarcts	Not known (26%)	88 (14.2%)

PROBLEM 3

Childhood leukaemia data is presented in Figure 10.2 for two trials. The data come from the National Cancer Registry (96% complete in registrations and better than 99% complete in recording deaths). The study group was treated by experts, the others by non-experts. Comment was made that the experts were probably also referred the more difficult cases:

- do the experts do a better job – is survival better?
- Comment on the comparability of the groups.

This sort of problem has become more important recently for there have been reports suggesting that specialist centres have better results than non-specialist. This has resulted in a policy of conducting some forms of cancer surgery only in specialist centres.

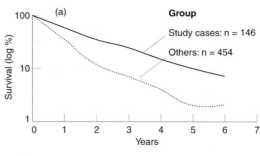

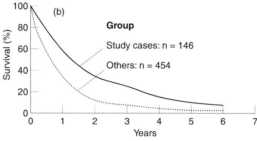

Fig. 10.2 Survival in childhood leukaemia: data displayed in two ways from a trial in which the study group was treated by experts and the others by non-experts. Numbers treated: study 146, others 454. (Gale 1984)

PROBLEM 4

Two treatment of gastric cancer are compared in Figure 10.3, radical surgery versus other modalities.

- Which is the better of the two treatments?
- Comment on the numbers in the two groups and their mode of selection.

Problems 5–7 explore experimental versus observational studies and, in particular, randomisation and the double-blind controlled trial.

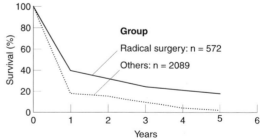

Fig. 10.3 Survival in gastric cancer with radical surgery and other treatments. (McCulloch 1996)

PROBLEM 5

During the pioneering days of surgery for ischaemic heart disease, an operation was developed aimed at improving the coronary circulation and thereby relieving angina. In this

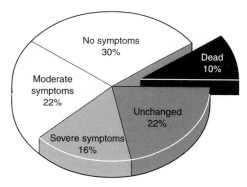

Fig. 10.4 A study of outcome at 6 months after surgery for bilateral ligature of the internal mammary arteries as a treatment for angina in ischaemic heart disease. (Orszulak et al 1986)

procedure both internal mammary arteries were ligated to increase the coronary perfusion pressure. The results of a study of this procedure are given in Figure 10.4.

● How effective is the procedure at relieving or abolishing angina?
● Given these figures would you recommend surgery for your patients?

PROBLEM 6

Further data on the procedure described in Problem 5 are given in Figure 10.5.

● What type of study is this?
● What further basic information about the study design do you want to know?
● What does it show?

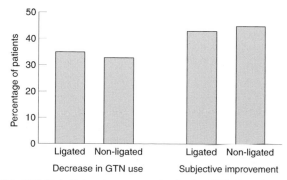

Fig. 10.5 Trial of internal mammary artery ligation. GTN, glyceryl trinitrite. (Orszulak et al 1986)

PROBLEM 7

Figure 10.6 is a proposed plan for a trial of a thrombolytic drug in the treatment of acute myocardial infarction. After

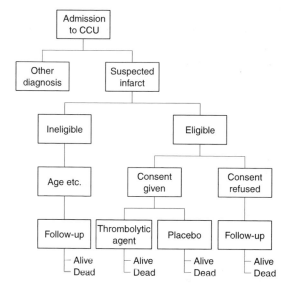

Fig. 10.6 Trial of thrombolysis in acute myocardial infarction (CCU, coronary care unit).

consent has been obtained, the patient is allocated to placebo or active agent.

● Make suggestions as to how this allocation may be done
● What should be the primary aim of this allocation?
● For the other branch points in the tree, make suggestions about how the decision required may be arrived at, and how it may affect the result.

PROBLEM 8

Figure 10.7 represents a trial of conservative versus surgical management of haemorrhoids. The allocation of patients

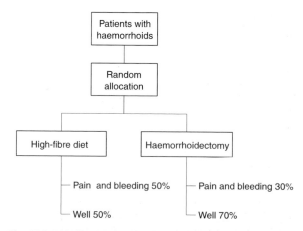

Fig. 10.7 Trial of haemorrhoid treatment assessed at 6 months. (Keighley et al 1979)

produced two identical groups. Treatment was then given and the outcome at 6 months recorded.

● Given the random allocation of patients are the results, therefore, reliable?
● What may have biased the results: list as many suggestions as possible?
● Ideally how should treatment be given as regards patient and observer?

Answers

PROBLEM 1

This is an **uncontrolled study**. There is no allowance made for the natural history of the condition. When fever is established it does not persist forever. It is not possible to comment on the success or failure of the therapy as a whole or with regard to a particular symptom. It is even possible that the treatment made things worse, and the study is unable to detect this.

PROBLEM 2

This is an example of the use of **historical controls**. A number of changes may have occurred in the intervening period that will affect the validity of historical controls. In this example, changes that may have been very important include:

● changes in the natural history of the disease
● the two groups of patients are probably not comparable on important factors such as age, sex, severity of infarction, etc.: much larger numbers were admitted into the new unit.
● treatment has improved with time irrespective of location of delivery
● the historical control and the present group may not be easily compared: Table 10.1 shows the unit in a good light, but data enabling a better comparison are not available in the table (Table 10.2). Note the total death rate from all definite infarcts is 14.2%
● other studies may affect the interpretation of the data: there have been several studies questioning the value of coronary care units on both clinical and economic grounds.

PROBLEM 3

The groups in this study are contemporary but are they comparable? Note first of all that Figure 10.2a uses a logarithmic scale, as presented in the original. Figure 10.5 is linear and removes the exaggerating effect of tail-end survivors. It is quite possible that the 'experts' were not

referred children considered to be untreatable. This **referral bias** could improve their survival figures. It should be said that since these data were produced the outlook for children with leukaemia has improved greatly. The researchers were probably right, that specialist units were better. They presented their case so badly, however, that it was not very convincing.

PROBLEM 4

Problems 1–3 concentrated on **observational studies**. The observers compared groups that happened to have received different treatments. Such studies are fraught with problems with the comparability of the two groups. In a good **experimental trial**, the aim should be to study groups that are identical except for the study treatment they receive. This treatment should also be correctly completed.

In Problem 4 survival is compared for two types of treatment. To be an effective comparison, patients need to be randomly allocated to a treatment. Figure 10.3 almost certainly represents **treatment selection bias**. Gastric cancer is often inoperable or widely disseminated at the time of presentation and such patients do not (usually) undergo radical surgery. Patients are, therefore, allocated to a treatment in a way linked to their chances of survival and it is unlikely that the comparison is a fair one.

The above does not mean that such studies are all worthless. If a disease is uniformly and rapidly fatal, then a treatment that is very effective in curing it would not require a rigid trial to demonstrate it. It could even, indeed, be unethical to perform such a trial. Such situations, however, are rare.

PROBLEM 5

The data are from an uncontrolled study. The operation was originally considered to be effective and was increasing in popularity. There has been no allowance made for the placebo effect and angina is particularly susceptible to suggestion. Given the data the procedure does not appear to be effective at relieving or abolishing angina and thus surgery would not be recommended.

PROBLEM 6

Figure 10.5 is from a controlled trial. This was a randomised trial in which the 'placebo' group of patients had a chest incision but no ligation. This study would be extremely unlikely to pass an ethics committee in the 1990s. It showed that there was very little difference between the group in which the ligation was performed compared with those where there was no ligation.

PROBLEM 7

Patients will be allocated to two or sometimes more groups. The following have been suggested as methods:

- patients on one ward and patients on another
- one consultant versus another
- day of week or odd/even date
- patient's initial or date of birth
- tossing a coin.

Most of the above introduce **bias** into the groups. Even seemingly 'random' methods such as the day of the week are vulnerable. Such methods are *systematic* and allocation can, therefore be predicted in advance. A physician may then 'play the system' to favour his preferences.

In the **explanatory** model of randomised controlled trial patients form a homogeneous sample satisfying rigorous selection criteria.

A **pragmatic trial** attempts to decide upon the effectiveness of the drug in real life. Patients who do not wish to take part are excluded at the initial stage and the rest of the patients randomised without further subdivision of the patients. This usually means taking both sexes, all ages and patients who have other complicating diseases. As a result more patients may not actually receive the drug in question than in an exploratory trial because they find the side effects intolerable or the regime too difficult to follow, but they are still retained in the drug group. This type of trial is useful for checking if a new management regime is likely to be effective at improving patient well-being. It contrasts with the explanatory trial where the question is simply whether the drug has an effect in optimal conditions. Pragmatic trials should follow successful explanatory ones. It may be, for instance, that an effective treatment has such severe side effects that most of the patients refuse to continue their medication. This will be picked up by the pragmatic trial. More detail on these trials was given in Chapter 6.

Cards in sealed envelopes are commonly used for either form of randomisation. These cards are prepared by the trial co-ordinators and an individual patient's allocation cannot be predicted before a decision to enter him into the trial. They also allow the numbers in each group to be controlled.

In trials comparing one drug with another, or placebo, the randomisation is often achieved by having numbered treatment packs, used sequentially. This means that the treatment is also **blind**, where the patient does not know what he or she is receiving, or **double-blind** where the attending doctor does not know which preparation is being given. Having said that, it is not uncommon for the medical staff to quickly learn to recognise those patients receiving the real thing. In thrombolytic trials, the bruises, nose bleeds and dysrhythmias often point the way.

It is important clearly to state the inclusion and exclusion criteria at each stage in the decision tree, of which figure 10.6 is an example. The selection of patients before randomisation can significantly affect the representativeness of the results when applied to a more general population. It can also serve to diminish or exaggerate differences in outcome between the two groups. For example, the death rate in the active treatment group would presumably rise if patients with recent gastrointestinal haemorrhage were not excluded. Note that it is proposed to follow-up all suspected infarctions.

PROBLEM 8

Figure 10.7 assumes correctly formed groups but explores possible biases in controlling treatment and assessing outcome. Problems arise in several ways such as:

- compliance with therapy especially the high-fibre group, who may not follow their instructions
- co-interventions: the surgery patients may also adopt a high-fibre diet after reading of its benefits in the media
- doctor's preference may affect his or her assessment of the outcome
- patient's preference may affect his or her assessment of the outcome.

Blinding is obviously not possible in this study. Even with a blind or double-blind trial it is possible for the 'code' to be broken either deliberately (and this does occur) or because of problems such as those outlined above with thrombolytic agents. Despite the difficulties, the double-blind randomised controlled trial remains the ideal. There can be serious difficulties with the ethics of such trials, especially if placebo controlled. The internal mammary artery example, however, demonstrates the ethical failure of not carrying out a trial.

Treatment effectiveness

➤ The quality of the data derived from trials is dependent upon the quality of the controls. Conclusions cannot be drawn from uncontrolled or poorly controlled trials.

➤ Historical controls derived from data gathered in the past may be flawed because the natural history of the disease may have altered and controls may not be available that match on important factors.

➤ The gold standard is a double-blind randomised controlled trial: effectively randomised, well-selected controls, and treatment blind for both patients *and* doctors.

Double-blind randomised controlled trials. These are the gold standard for measuring the effects of new therapy. There are some occasions where blinding or even randomisation is impossible, not usually on ethical grounds, but because of the nature of the treatment or management. Operation versus non-operative treatment can obviously not be kept from patients or attending staff. Management of patients that requires major organisational change cannot easily be hidden, indeed sometimes cannot be randomised if costs prohibit, e.g. two different types of management team working in parallel.

Clinical risk: adverse reactions to medicines

11

The aims of this chapter are:

- to outline some of the basic theory of risk perceptions
- to underline that all medicines and drugs are potentially harmful as well as beneficial
- to understand and use the concept of attributable risk
- to understand and use the concept of relative risk.

Risk perception

The probability of adverse outcomes following certain activities can be determined by recording outcomes and relating these to the base population 'at risk'. However, assessment of these risks depends upon judgements, which may be conditioned by individual psychology or anthropological considerations. Individual perceptions of the risks of an activity are affected by its familiarity, controllability or whether it is voluntary or involuntary. Perceptions of lay people correspond quite well to the rank ordering obtained from statistical estimates.

In a world where more and more people are coming to see themselves as the victims rather than the beneficiaries of technology, it is not surprising that the control of hazards has become a major concern of society and a growing responsibility of government. At the same time, manufacturers of pharmaceutical medicines are also concerned about what appears to be a changing social and political environment. Public debate about the risks, benefits and safety associated with drugs has intensified and disputes over risks are brought to court when individuals seek compensation for health problems attributed to a pharmaceutical product.

Drug-surveillance activities and reporting systems to identify drug safety problems have been strengthened. The understanding and management of drug safety is, nonetheless, beset by doubts, disagreements, and disputes. Conflict occurs over the:

- significance of risk
- adequacy of evidence
- methods used to evaluate and measure risk
- standards that guide regulation
- optimal means of communicating risk information to the public.

Types of risk

In medicine, perceptions of drug risks are likely to influence patients' treatment choices, their compliance with treatment, their acceptance of adverse reactions and their attitudes towards the regulation of drugs. Studies of risk perception of drugs have examined the attitudes of the public. People have an extreme aversion to some hazards but are indifferent to others. The discrepancies between these reactions and experts' opinions are important. Studies have shown that the risk perceived by the public is quantifiable and predictable. Figure 11.1 shows the order of ranking of risks and shows that the concept of 'risk' means different things to different people.

	Women	Students	Experts
Nuclear power	1	1	8
Motor vehicles	2	3	1
Smoking	3	2	2
Alcohol	4	4	3
Surgery	5	6	4
Mountain climbing	6	10	12
Contraceptives	7	5	6
X-rays	8	7	5
Railways	9	11	7
Food colouring	10	8	9
Antibiotics	11	9	10
Vaccination	12	12	11

Fig. 11.1 Perception of risk by different groups (ranked in order). (Paling & Paling 1993)

When experts judge risk, their responses correlate highly with annual fatalities. Lay people can assess fatalities if they are asked to and produce estimates somewhat like the technical estimates. However, their judgements of 'risk' are sensitive to other factors as well, for example catastrophic potential and the threat to future generations. As a result they tend to see risk differently from their own, and experts' estimates of fatalities.

People tend to view current risk levels as unacceptably high for most activities. The gap between perceived and desired risk levels suggests that people are not satisfied with the mechanisms to balance risk and benefits. Studies also show that people are willing to tolerate higher risks from activities seen as beneficial. People are willing to accept risks that are

- voluntary
- controllable
- familiar
- non-catastrophic
- fair in the way that risks and benefits are distributed across individuals.

Many of the risk characteristics are highly correlated with each other across a wide range of hazards. For example, hazards rated as 'voluntary' tend also to be rated as 'controllable' and 'well-known'. Hazards that appear to threaten future generations tend also to be seen as having catastrophic potential, and so on. An approach to describing these ideas is shown in Figure 11.2. One type of risk perception approach divides risks into dread risks and unknown risks.

Dread risk is defined as:

- perceived lack of control
- dread
- catastrophic potential
- fatal consequences
- inequitable distribution of risks and benefits.

Nuclear weapons and nuclear power scored highest on the characteristics that make up this factor.

Risks can also be analysed on a scale of known–unknown.

Unknown risk is defined as hazards judged to be

- unobservable
- unknown
- new
- delayed before they cause harm.

Chemical technologies scored particularly highly as unknown risks. Medical procedures and pharmaceutical products also scored high on unknown risk but they were perceived to be low on the dread-risk scale, therefore, they appear in the upper left quadrant of the space diagram (Fig. 11.2). In other words, they were seen as controllable, not fatal, not dreaded, equitable (the person who benefits also bears the risk), and individual rather than catastrophic. They also tended to be rated low in risk and high in benefit.

Research has shown that lay people feel 'dread risk'

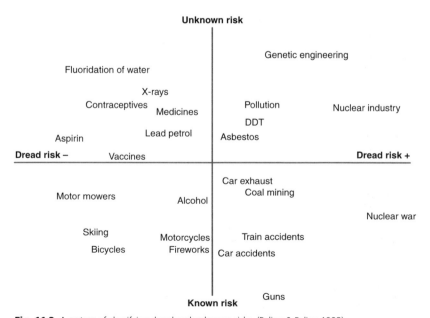

Fig. 11.2 A system of classifying dread and unknown risks. (Paling & Paling 1993)

to be the most important. The higher a hazard's score on this factor (i.e. the further to the right it appears in the space in Figure 11.2), the higher its perceived risk. For this type of risk a high proportion of people want to see its current risks reduced and want strict regulation to achieve this.

An accident that takes many lives may produce relatively little social disturbance, beyond that caused to the victims' families and friends, if it occurs as part of a familiar and well-understood system, for example a train crash. However, a small accident in an unfamiliar setup, or one poorly understood, such as a nuclear reactor, a DNA laboratory or even a prescribed drug may have immense social consequences if it is thought to be a precursor of further and possible catastrophic mishaps.

The media and risk

The media are important in risk perception. Medicine is of great interest to the media. Stories involving adverse drug reactions and their victims are generally classified as being stories about quackery, which basically means false medical claims and exploitation of the sick for profit. Given this general approach, it is hardly surprising that the starting point for a journalist investigating a story about adverse reactions to drugs is that innocent people have been harmed when they thought they were being helped. The view of the media is that the providers of the treatment must have been either less than honest in their claims or negligent in the way that they conducted their experiments. There is a belief that doctors and authorities were duped or bribed. The task of a journalist is, therefore, to prove that any or all of these assumptions are true.

Risk and benefit

Figure 11.3 shows the results of a study of perceived risk and benefit. The high level of concern about sleeping pills and antidepressant drugs may have resulted from extensive media publicity regarding the risks of addiction and overdose. Those who claimed to have experienced any sort of side effect from a prescription drug showed slightly higher perceptions of risk than did those without side effects. Perceptions of risk seemed unaffected by having experienced significant benefits from taking drugs.

It is obvious that perceived risks and benefits are not positively related. Appendicectomy, insulin, vaccines and antibiotics stood out as being quite high in perceived benefit and low in perceived risk. Other

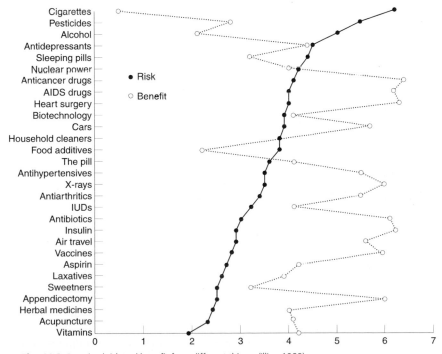

Fig. 11.3 Perceived risk and benefit from different things. (Illing 1989)

drug items, with the notable exception of antidepressants and sleeping pills, showed a similar, though less extreme, pattern. Four non-drug chemical hazards, cigarettes, alcohol, pesticides, and food additives, were judged extremely high in risk and low in benefit.

Although the scales are not strictly comparable, it is interesting to create a net benefit score by subtracting the judgement of risk from the judgement of benefit for each. In this case, the perceived net benefits for antidepressants, birth control pills, sleeping pills and antihypertensives were higher for those persons claiming to be comfortable taking medicine than for those who are not comfortable doing so. However, these two groups of people did not differ in their net benefit ratings for such high-benefit drugs as vaccines, antibiotics and insulin. Older respondents (ages 60–74 years) showed higher net benefit ratings than younger for antihypertensives, cancer drugs, antidepressants and artificial sweeteners. There was a greater variation depending on whether the risk was new, for example from AIDS and biotechnology drugs, or old, for example from cigarettes and alcohol. Most pharmaceutical products are seen as new and, therefore, a risk but with a considerable difference in perception for different drugs.

A survey on this subject was administered to members of the general public who were chronically ill with ankylosing spondylitis, a chronic rheumatic disease. About 70% of these individuals were currently taking medication. As might be expected, a higher percentage of these patients reported experiencing a serious drug reaction (47%) than did normal respondents (5%). Those patients who had experienced a serious reaction judged the incidence of reactions in general as more frequent than did persons without such an experience. Those who had experienced serious reactions were more likely than others to attribute the cause of the reaction to the patient's having:

● inadequate information about the drug
● inadequate testing by the manufacturer
● inadequate monitoring by the doctor.

Those who had experienced serious reactions were less likely than others to blame the patient for a side effect.

Almost two thirds of patients who had had adverse reactions suggested that a suspected drug should be taken off the market. These patients, in response to a question asking about comparisons between risks today and 20 years ago, said that risks were the same as 20 years ago. Unaffected samples of people were more likely to say that risks are greater now than 20 years ago.

Risk management through provision of warnings

There have been numerous surveys to show that patients around the world strongly desire warning information on prescription drugs. People have argued that extensive, frank warnings and precautions are desirable because it gives patients informed choice. It also helps the patient to use the drug safely and effectively. The idea of informed choice is a powerful idea that could revolutionise warning information in the marketing and use of prescription drugs. The idea is being implemented in studies in marketing of some intra-uterine devices and in marketing the antiacne drug Accutane.

The results from such tests of informed choice can be very useful. However, additional information is needed to discover which types of medical product best suit this approach. Warnings may deter some patients from taking essential medicines.

Measuring the risk of therapeutic agents

Modern drugs have conferred great benefits on humanity, yet by their nature it is inevitable that serious adverse reactions may occur. A past chairman of the Committee on the Safety of Medicine has said: 'Either a substance is biologically inactive, in which case it may be safe but is certainly not a medicine, or it is active, in which case it may be a medicine but it is certainly not safe'.

There is increasing concern about the possible harmful effects of treatment, both immediate and delayed. Drug overdose is now the second commonest cause of emergency admission to hospital, and some studies suggest that as many as 5% of all hospital in-patients are there for treatment of the side effects of earlier therapy. If this is true, then there is obviously justification for the idea that the effectiveness of a treatment should first be compared with no action before it is made generally available.

One of the first scientific attempts to measure the safety of a therapeutic procedure was undertaken in 1828 by Louis at the Charité Hospital in Paris, where he examined the safety (note the similarity with effectiveness) of taking blood from patients with pneumonia. He found, by prospective epidemiological investigation, that the longer the bleeding was delayed the better the outcome for the patient (Table 11.1) and he suggested that outcome might be improved further if no blood was let at all.

Table 11.1 The effect of taking blood from patients with pneumonia

Day bled after onset of pneumonia	Died	Lived
1–3	12 (50%)	12
4–6	12 (35%)	22
7–9	3 (33%)	6

At that time, blood letting was so firmly established as a necessary therapeutic procedure that failure to do this in a serious illness constituted professional negligence. In the UK in the 1950s, failure to use anticoagulants in coronary disease constituted negligence. In the 1990s, failure to put a patient with acute myocardial infarction in hospital may be similarly viewed. This, in spite of recent evidence suggesting that intensive care therapy only confers significant benefit above care at home for the first 12 hours.

Consistent figures on the incidence of adverse drug reactions are not collected nationally so it is easy to underestimate the size of this public health problem. We know that 560 million prescriptions were issued in the UK in 1994 and that, on average, there are two drugs on each prescription. If we make the modest assumption that the frequency of mild and serious reactions are 1 and 0.1%, respectively, this gives an estimate of 5 million mild and 500 000 serious drug reactions a year.

Adverse reactions

A growing number of modern treatments and investigations carry a small but definite risk of adverse reactions, for example

- antibiotics (allergy)
- surgical operations (bleeding)
- bronchodilators (cardiac arrest)
- diagnostic procedures (ionising irradiation)
- amniocentesis (spontaneous abortion).

Clinicians are well aware that adverse reactions and even deaths occur in these procedures but they believe that the likelihood of harm coming to an individual patient is less than the likely benefit arising as a result of the action. If the choice of an action is to be a rational one it follows that a decision to prescribe should be based as much upon knowledge of dangers as of effectiveness.

Unlike the universally harmful effects of blood-letting, adverse effects of therapy are usually relatively infrequent and may appear some time after treatment was prescribed. In these circumstances, even if the doctor suspects a harmful effect, he or she does not see enough similar cases to judge whether the effect is caused by the therapy. A single case can be put down to coincidence. Many doctors are in no position to set up a comparative study of safety, because they see too few cases. They are dependent upon information that they receive when they exchange views with their colleagues at conferences or by publishing their suspicions, and from reading the comments of their colleagues in the correspondence columns of medical journals.

As an example, in 1923 a physician in London described severe jaundice in a patient who had been treated for gout with cincophen, a drug that had been in wide use since 1908. A number of letters reporting similar occurrences, some of which were fatal, were published over the next few years. Despite this, cincophen remained a drug that could be purchased by the public without prescription. At an inquest at Birmingham in 1934 several doctors denied, to the surprise of the coroner, that they had ever heard of cincophen causing jaundice.

Measuring the risks of therapy

The situation in measuring risk is analogous to judging the effectiveness of therapy. One requires to understand the difficulties of collecting information about drug safety and the problems and pitfalls that surround its interpretation. Information must be collated from large numbers of patients who have received the treatment and, ideally, an equally large number who have not, as the comparison group. This will allow an estimate of the risks of the suspected adverse effect in the treated and non-treated groups. The rarer the expected adverse reaction, the larger the groups will need to be.

Safety is an idea, like effectiveness, that is best expressed in a numerical form. Very few therapies are completely safe. Surgical procedures such as cholecystectomy carry a definite risk of death. The size of this risk would be unacceptable if the same procedure were therapy for a less severe disease, say dermatitis or migraine. The term 'safe' when applied to any therapy only has meaning if the likelihood of harm is weighed against the dangers of the disease and other treatments for that disease. The safety, and the effectiveness, of a given therapeutic procedure are measured in exactly the same way: safety is merely a mirror image of effectiveness.

Toxicity testing

The effect of a toxin usually depends critically upon the dose. In clinical practice, other factors such as age, sex and susceptibility must also be considered. Toxicological testing is done first in in vitro and animal experiments. These are limited for several reasons. Effects of drugs in humans may only become apparent after a long time. Animals obviously differ in many ways from humans, especially in their biochemical reactions. The genetic variability of humans and their variations in health status also make extrapolation from animal to humans open to many possible errors.

For medicines the dose is decided by taking account of the adverse effects observed in the tissues of animals. Researchers try to assess the dose that produces no adverse effects. A major limitation in practice is estimating the 'no observed effect level' by fitting the results of the experiments to a mathematical model or dose–response curve. High doses of drugs are given to observe some useful effects while keeping the number of animals experimented on at a small number. The problem is to estimate the effect of lower doses by extrapolating the data. A number of mathematical formulae may 'fit' the data equally well in the high doses tested on the animals, but these may give very different estimates low-dose therapeutic range.

To reduce this uncertainty it would be necessary to test large numbers of animals in the relatively low doses. This is only done where the risks are of potential significance to the public health, for example with ionising radiation. Even for ionising radiation, the actual effects in the low doses are hypothetical extrapolations of effects at higher doses. These limitations of toxicity testing mean that epidemiological methods are needed to assess the risks of clinical procedures and agents in practice.

Problems

PROBLEM 1

The data of Table 11.2 are taken from a case control study of oral contraceptive use and breast cancer conducted in London, Oxford and Edinburgh between 1980 and 1984.

1. Calculate the odds ratios for the different categories of OC use before first term pregnancy
2. What inferences can be drawn from the values obtained?
3. What factors might confound this observed relationship?

PROBLEM 2

Assume that the data given in Table 11.2 is judged not to have occurred by chance then:

Table 11.2 Retrospective case – control study of oral contraceptive (OC) use and breast cancer in women under 45 years of age (Vessy, Doll & Sutton 1972)

OC use before first term pregnancy (months)	Cases	Controls
No use	235	273
1–12	27	26
13–48	43	29
48+	46	23

1. Do the findings confirm that taking the pill and subsequent breast cancer co-existed more frequently than would be expected by chance?
2. Is the risk of breast cancer doubled for women who used OC for more than a year before first term pregnancy compared with those who did not?

PROBLEM 3

The data of Table 11.3 are taken from a case–control study of fatal venous thromboembolism and oral contraceptive use in women aged between 16 and 39.

1. What is the odds ratio for current users compared with non-users?
2. What other factors may have confounded the relationship between OC use and fatal venous thromboembolism?
3. Can it be inferred from the odds ratios for fatal venous thromboembolism that the odds ratio for non-fatal venous thromboembolism would be greater than one?

Table 11.3 Case–control study of fatal venous thromboembolism in women taking OC (Anonymous 1973)

OC	Cases	Controls
Non-users	20	39
Previous users	11	31
Current users	29	45

PROBLEM 4

Relative risk provides an index for the significance of the drug or procedure being investigated and the occurrence of a disease or other effect. Table 11.4 gives data on infants born to women living in Cardiff between 1965 and 1971.

1. What is the absolute risk of a non-epileptic mother having a malformed child?
2. What is the relative risk of an epileptic mother on anticonvulsant therapy producing a malformed child

Table 11.4 Malformations in babies born of mothers with epilepsy (Lowe 1973)

	Total No.	No. malformed
All infants born to non-epileptic women in Cardiff 1965–71	31 262	893 (2.8%)
Infants born to women with a history of epilepsy:		
On anticonvulsants during first trimester	134	9 (6.7%)
Not taking anticonvulsants	111	3 (2.7%)

compared with an epileptic mother not on anticonvulsant therapy?

3. What is the relative risk of babies born to epileptic mothers not on anticonvulsants compared with that for non-epileptic mothers.

PROBLEM 5

For the management of a patient or the development of health policy, **attributable risk** is the important measure. For example, if an intervention is considered to confer benefit upon a patient by improving a condition with a risk of mortality that is very low (e.g. 1 in 50 000) then both the patient and doctor may be comfortable even if the relative risk was high (e.g. 5). However, if the background risk is not low then any extra risk from the procedure may be considered unacceptable.

In 1976, nurses aged 30–55 years with no history of cancer were enrolled into a prospective cohort study of OC use and risk of breast cancer in women. Data for a subgroup aged 50–54 in 1986 are shown in Table 11.5.

1. What is the risk of breast cancer attributable to the use of OCs?
2. How would you explain to a woman wishing to be prescribed oral OCs what were her chances/probability of subsequently suffering breast cancer?
3. In a population of ten million females aged 30–55 years, how many breast cancer cases would you expect to record over a 10-year period as a direct consequence of OC use? Assume that their characteristics and behaviour are similar to the women in the study reported.

Table 11.5 Data from a cohort study of OC use and breast cancer in women aged 50–54 years (Vessy, Doll & Sutton 1972)

OC use	No. with breast cancer	No. of person-years
Past use	133	61 657
Never used	310	158 433

PROBLEM 6

What would you estimate to be the probability of death per year from:

1. Vaccinations, England and Wales
2. Anaesthesia in surgery 1986
3. Childbirth 1987–89 England and Wales
4. Accidental death for coal miners UK 1987–90
5. Cancer in males 65–74 years of age
6. Coronary heart disease males 65–74 years of age
7. Diabetes in females 65–74 years of age
8. Asthma in males 15–24 years of age.

PROBLEM 7

By comparison with the data in Problem 6, what would you estimate to be the probability of death from:

1. Skiing per million hours in France (1974–76)
2. Travel in a car in the UK (1983) per million hours
3. Living 5 years at the boundary of a nuclear power plant
4. Murder in England and Wales 1990.

Answers

PROBLEM 1

1. Using the definition of odds ratio (Chapter 5) the odds ratios for the different durations of OC use before first term pregnancy compared with no use are:

   1–12 months: OR = 1.21
   13–48 months: OR = 1.72
   over 48 months: OR = 2.32.

2. The odds ratios suggest an association between OC use and breast cancer, with evidence of a dose–response relationship, i.e. as the dose of OC increases the odds ratio increases.
3. Parity, smoking status and alcohol consumption could have confounded the relationship, but the investigators found on analysis that these did not confound the comparison. The most important confounding variable was age at first term pregnancy. Family history of breast cancer was also shown to be a confounder. When these variables were allowed for in the analysis the odds ratios were reduced.

PROBLEM 2

1. Yes, especially the dose–response changes. The risk is not great.
2. No. The odds ratio can only compare cases and controls.

The number of women taking the pill is not known, i.e. there is no denominator. Therefore, the number affected per 100 000 pill takers was not known so the risk of OC use is not known.

PROBLEM 3

1. The Odds ratio is $(29 \times 39) \div (20 \times 45) = 1.26$.
2. The findings of the study confirmed two previously known risk factors for fatal venous thromboembolism: an increase in risk associated with a history of previous thrombotic disease and an increase in risk associated with an operation or accident.
3. No, one can only make inferences about the outcome of interest.

PROBLEM 4

1. The absolute risk for a non-epileptic mother having a malformed child is $893/31\,262 = 2.86\%$.
2. As detailed in Chapter 5, relative risk can only be determined by measuring the absolute risk in each subgroup. This requires a cohort study in which the base population at risk (i.e. the denominator) is known for the various groups concerned. The relative risk for an epileptic mother taking anticonvulsant therapy compared with one not taking anticonvulsants is $(9/134): (3/111) = 2.5:1$.
3. In a similar way the relative risk for babies born to epileptic mothers not on anticonvulsants compared with non-epileptic mothers is $(3/111):(893/31\,262) = 0.95:1$

PROBLEM 5

1. The risk of breast cancer without use of OC is $310/158\,433 = 19.6$ per 10 000 person-years. The risk of breast cancer with use of OC is $133/161\,657 = 21.6$ per 10 000 person-years. Therefore, the attributable risk is $21.6 - 19.6 = 2$ per 10 000 person-years.
2. For each year that she takes the pill, her chances of getting breast cancer over and above the natural background chance, as a direct consequence of taking it, is 2 in 10 000 or over a 10-year period 2 in 1000. Her absolute risk of getting breast cancer in the same 10-year period even if she does not take the pill is $310/158\,433$ or 196 in 10 000. Therefore, the attributable risk is about one tenth of the absolute risk, but, of course, it would be additional to the absolute risk.
3. Ten million females over 10 years is 100 million person-years. Attributable risk is 2 per 10 000 years. The Number of expected cases, therefore, would be 20 000 cases.

Personal risk compared with the impact on the country at large. For individuals the risk of the contraceptive pill is very small, but because it is used by a large number of people the impact of a small adverse effect can be considerable nationally.

PROBLEM 6

1. Vaccinations, England and Wales: 1 in 10^6
2. Anaesthesia in surgery 1986: 5 in 10^6
3. Childbirth 1987–89 England and Wales: 7 in 100 000 or 7 in 10^5
4. Accidental death for coal miners UK 1987–90: 145 per 10^6
5. Cancer in males 65–74 years of age: 12.3 in 1000
6. Coronary heart disease in males 65–74 years of age: 12.3 in 1000
7. Diabetes in females 65–74 years of age: 2.9 in 10 000
8. Asthma in males 15–24 years of age: 8 in 10^6.

By comparison, the National Childhood Encephalopathy Study estimated the risk of permanent neurological damage attributable to a completed course of vaccination against pertussis to be 1 in 10^5.

PROBLEM 7

1. Skiing per million hours France (1974–76): 1.3 per million
2. Travel in a car in the UK (1983) per million hours: 0.3 per million
3. Living 5 years at a site boundary of a typical, nuclear power plant: 4 in 100 000
4. Murder in England and Wales 1990: 12 per million per annum.

Risk and adverse reactions

➤ Public perception of risk can be divided into two groups: known–unknown risk and a severity assessment 'dread risk'.

➤ Measuring the risks of therapy requires collecting information from large numbers of patients (the rarer the event the larger the group will need to be) and then interpreting this information correctly.

➤ Assessment of a treatment must balance the size of the risk against the dangers of the disease and the other possible treatments: safety and effectiveness are two opposing aspects.

➤ An adverse effect can constitute a small personal risk but can have a large impact in a population if many people take the risk. This has implications for health service provision.

Prognosis

12

The aims of this chapter are:

- to indicate the limitation of personal clinical experience in making a prognosis
- to describe three ways of expressing the natural history/clinical course of a disease
- to describe how estimates of prognosis can be affected by sample selection (referral pattern) and disease severities, definitions of outcome, incomplete follow-up and early diagnosis.

Personal clinical experience

This section deals with personal clinical experience and seeks to show the difficulty in basing accurate prognoses on such experience. What number of patients should be seen with a condition before the clinician is experienced in the course of that condition? Consider the 'incubation period' of an outcome, the variable outcomes for any given disease, the ability of a clinician to remember the details of the clinical courses of previous patients, and the difficulties in ensuring complete follow-up. All these factors will affect a clinician's ability to treat and predict a likely outcome for a condition. Prognosis is not just about mortality.

These questions are highlighted by considerations in the UK government concerning the treatment of patients with cancer. The suggestion is that oncologists need to maintain a certain level of expertise, in terms of the number of patients with a specific condition they see, before they can be considered to have sufficient expertise.

Problem 1 explores these questions. It is suggested that you think about an arbitrary number of patients required to maintain one's expertise and use the number for all parts of the section.

Prognosis of disease

When deciding how to describe the prognosis of a dis-

ease or complication, the type of disease and the reason for measuring its prognosis must be taken into account. If one hopes to intervene, measurements must be able to show whether the intervention was effective or not. There would be little point in measuring the outcome before or a long time after the intervention.

Problems

PROBLEM 1

Some clinicians become very experienced in the clinical course of certain diseases by virtue of the number of patients that they see with the disease. The exposure of a clinician to a disease will be a function of the incidence of the disease and the manner in which patients are channelled to a particular doctor. A doctor may see little of a disease because it is very rare or because he rarely sees the relevant patients.

1. Give some idea of what you would consider a reasonable number of patients that should be seen to allow a relatively accurate estimate of prognosis (clinical course). Given this number, how long will it take a general surgeon in a district general hospital to estimate the 2-year recurrence rate of urinary tract stones if a new case of urinary tract stone is referred every month?
2. How long would it take a GP to assess the response to a 1 week course of antibiotics in infants (less than 1 year old) with otitis media if two new infants with this condition are seen each week? If the same GP wishes to assess the prognosis for these patients for speech and language difficulties at the age of 5 years, how long will it now take?
3. Three partners in general practice wish to assess the clinical course of children presenting with asymptomatic systolic murmurs. They estimate that a minimum follow-up of 15 years would be required to decide if the murmur was truly 'innocent'. Together they see two cases every year. How long will it take them?

4. A hospital paediatrician wishes to assess the prognosis (over 15 years) of children with 'innocent systolic murmurs', with a referral rate of 20 such patients each year. How long will it take?
5. In the first example (urinary stones) suppose 5 of 50 patients have a recurrence of stone colic over a 2-year period of follow-up. What is the recurrence rate? Work out the 95% confidence interval for this proportion. That is within what minimum and what maximum value for this proportion (range) could recurrence rates truly occur for the population from which the patients are drawn. The confidence interval is the proportion plus and minus twice its standard error where the standard error of a proportion (p) for a sample of n patients is.

$$\sqrt{\frac{p\,(1-p)}{n}}$$

How could the standard error and, therefore, the 95% confidence interval be reduced?

PROBLEM 2

Prognosis can be expressed as a rate. In which case the time of follow-up should be specified (in practice this is not always done). If the interval of follow-up is not specified, it must be long enough for all events to occur.

Table 12.1 shows the survival time, following presentation, of 91 patients whose acute myocardial infarction was complicated by 'post-infarct' ventricular septal defect, and who were treated medically.

What follow-up period would you use in reporting a case fatality rate and what is that case fatality rate?

Table 12.1 Survival time of patients with ventricular septal defect after acute myocardial infarction (Lowe & Gall 1997)

Survival time	No. patients	(%)
Less than 1 week	49	(54)
1 week to 2 months	30	(33)
2 months to 1 year	5	(5.5)
1 to 4 years	4	(4.5)
4 to 5 years	2	(2)
$6\frac{1}{2}$ years	1	(1)
Total	91	(100)

PROBLEM 3

Table 12.2 shows the outcome of attempted prehospital resuscitation from cardiac arrest by South Glamorgan paramedics.

How would you express the prognosis for these patients?

Table 12.2 Outcome of attempted prehospital resuscitation from cardiac arrest by paramedics (Weston & Donelly 1995)

	Rhythm of arrest		
	VF	Asystole/EMD	Respiratory
Prehospital	98 (72 died)	169 (158 died)	7
Admitted to ward	26 (9 died)	11 (10 died)	7 (4 died)
Discharged	17	1	3

VF, ventricular fibrillation; EMD, electromechanical dissociation.

PROBLEM 4

Table 12.3 shows admission and discharge (transfer) figures for a fictitious coronary care unit, gathered over three 2-year periods.

1. Is the newspaper headline 'more patients are dying in coronary care' correct?
2. What is the prognosis of patients admitted to the coronary care unit (expressed as mortality rates) for each period of 2 years?
3. Why is this an unsatisfactory method of describing/monitoring the performance of the unit?

Table 12.3 Admissions and discharges for a coronary care unit gathered over two years

	1969–79	1979–80	1989–90
Admitted	300	1000	1200
Discharged	270	920	1152

PROBLEM 5

Table 12.4 shows operative mortality rates for coronary artery surgery performed in two hospitals over a 2-year period. The hospital with the fewest total cases appears to have a higher mortality rate.

Calculate total death rates and death rates for the three types of patient stratified by preoperative risk (e.g. age, sex,

Table 12.4 Operative mortality for coronary artery surgery in two hospitals over 2 years

	Hospital A		Hospital B	
Preoperative risk	No. Patients	Deaths	Patients	Deaths
High	500	30	400	24
Medium	400	16	800	32
Low	300	2	1200	8
Total	1200	48	2400	64

re-do procedure, emergency operation). Show why a comparison of total rates is misleading.

PROBLEM 6

Table 12.5 shows 10-year follow-up data for patients referred to a neurologist because of symptoms and signs suggestive of the first manifestation of multiple sclerosis (assuming complete follow-up).

- In disease of long duration and relatively low lethality, e.g. angina, rheumatoid arthritis, multiple sclerosis, how could prognosis be expressed?
- If follow-up is not complete, which types of patient are most likely to be lost to follow-up?
- How will this affect the neurologist's estimate of prognosis?

Table 12.5 Follow-up data at 10 years for patients with signs of multiple sclerosis (Sadovnick et al 1992)				
	Alive			
Course of disease	No disability	Disability	Dead	Total
Remission	79	1	0	80
Remissions and recurrences	10	45	0	55
Progressive	0	15	17	32
Total	89	61	17	167

PROBLEM 7

Figure 12.1 shows the survival and mobility of patients after the onset of multiple sclerosis, together with the expected survival of people of the same age and sex who did not have the condition. It is a community-based (population-based) study rather than a clinic-based study.

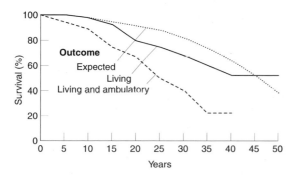

Fig. 12.1 Survival and mobility of patients after the onset of multiple sclerosis; expected refers to people of the same age and sex who do not have the condition. (Citterio et al 1989)

1. What is the approximate 10-year survival rate?
2. Why does this differ from Problem 6?

PROBLEM 8

Figure 12.2 shows the percentage survival for patients with strokes or fractured hips admitted over 8 months to a hospital in Somerset.

1. If you were expressing prognosis in terms of 4-week mortality rate, what is the prognosis for patients with stroke when first admitted, and 4 weeks after admission?
2. Why are these so different?
3. Do they reflect the true survival rates?

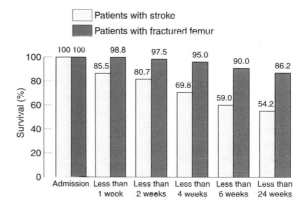

Fig. 12.2 Survival of patients with stroke and fractured femur. (Malmgren et al 1987; Ions & Stevens 1987)

PROBLEM 9

In a study of surgical treatment for morbid obesity, 123 patients were studied between 19–47 months after surgery. Only 103 patients could be located. In these the success rate (>30% loss of excess weight) was 60/103 (58%).

What is the approximate range within which the true success rate for the whole sample must lie?

PROBLEM 10

Consider a group of cancer patients who are followed up from the time of presentation and diagnosis and who are found to die at an unusually constant rate of 10% of the survivors per annum.

1. Draw a figure with percentage survival on the y axis and years along the x axis. What is the approximate 5-year survival rate?
2. Suppose these same patients had been diagnosed 1 year earlier because of screening tests. If no treatment was offered or an ineffective treatment was provided

draw in the new survival curve. What is the 5-year survival rate from the time of screening. Has screening improved the prognosis in these patients?

Answers

PROBLEM 1

Pragmatically one may consider 50 a reasonable number.

1. This emphasises that it takes time to amass the 'correct' number of patients. For instance, the 50th patient will be seen at the beginning of the 50th month (49 months after the first patient). The 2-year recurrence rate can only be estimated on the total number of patients 2 years after this time.
2. This demonstrates that for relatively common conditions and short-term outcomes an individual practitioner can make a good estimate of prognosis but that it will take longer to make an estimate of a long-term outcome. Again one can discuss the likelihood of follow-up difficulties between short-term and long-term outcomes. Can the GP develop objective outcome criteria, and does this matter? What place could blinded outcome assessment have in these situations?
3. This question demonstrates that for unusual conditions and long follow-up individual practitioners or small groups of practitioners are unlikely to amass sufficient experience throughout their working lives.
4. Compared with Question 3, the specialist will see in 1 year the same number of patients that the GPs see in 10 years. This emphasises that specialist interest may allow one to gain insight into the clinical course of any given condition. It may be sensible for the GPs to rely on the clinical experience of a hospital paediatrician in making a prognosis in conditions with a small presentation in their practice.
5. The 2-year recurrence rate is 10%. The value of p is 0.1 and n is 50 so the standard error is

$$\sqrt{\frac{0.1 \times 0.9}{50}} = \sqrt{0.0018} = 0.042$$

This is 4.2%. The 95% confidence interval is the recurrence rate (10%) $\pm (2 \times 4.2) = 1.6$–18.4%. This is approximately 1 in 50 recurrences up to 1 in 5 recurrences. This demonstrates that even full follow-up of a reasonable number of patients is associated with wide confidence intervals and that the larger the number of patients (n) the tighter will be the confidence intervals.

PROBLEM 2

Ventricular septal defect is an example of a disease with relatively high death rate over a short period of time. One could discuss the usefulness or difficulty of using case fatality rate to express prognosis in these patients. Did the patients dying between 2 months and $6\frac{1}{2}$ years die because of ventricular septal defect or of other cardiac or non-cardiac causes? Generally if one is hoping to compare interventions, a fairly early mortality rate (e.g. the 1-week case fatality) makes sense.

PROBLEM 3

There are a number of ways of expressing prognosis in patients being resuscitated by paramedics. One could use fatality rate for all patients or for each of the three groups of presenting rhythm. One could express survival in terms of admission to hospital or in terms of discharge from hospital. This also shows how stratification of a given condition can be used to compare like with like for prognosis.

PROBLEM 4

Assume that all the patients that were admitted but not discharged died in coronary care.

1. The headline was not incorrect in that 80 as opposed to 30 people died. However three times as many people were admitted so absolute numbers give a false picture.
2. The crude mortality rates for the three periods are 10%, 8% and 4% using this assessment, the conclusion of the newspaper headline was incorrect.
3. The figures in Table 12.3 tell us nothing about the patients that are admitted, admission policies or discharge policies. Discharging patients at 2 hours rather than 24 hours could reduce coronary care mortality rates but not help the patients.

PROBLEM 5

This example further introduces the idea of stratification of patients. It shows that the apparent total mortality rate is higher in hospital A compared with hospital B. However, the mortality rates for each band of pre-operative risk is the same. The completed table should be that shown in Table 12.6.

PROBLEM 6

In long-term illnesses, prognosis can be expressed as a remission or a recurrence rate. The neurologist could describe a 10-year mortality rate or 10-year survival rate for multiple sclerosis. The prognosis could also be expressed for death/disability rate or in terms of the course of the disease.

Table 12.6 Operative mortality rates completed for the data in Table 12.4

Preoperative risk	Hospital A			Hospital B		
	No. patients	Deaths	Death rate (%)	No. patients	Deaths	Death rate (%)
High	500	30	6	400	24	6
Medium	400	16	4	800	32	4
Low	300	2	0.67	1200	8	0.67
Total	1200	48	4	2400	64	2.67

Apparent prognosis could be adversely affected if patients with remission and no disability failed to attend for follow-up or are discharged from follow-up. Losses to follow-up are the commonest difficulty with accurately measuring prognosis. Those not contacted usually have a different prognosis from those who are contacted.

PROBLEM 7

1. The approximate 10-year survival rate is 98%.
2. In Problem 6 the neurologist is being referred the more severe cases.

PROBLEM 8

1. The 4-week prognosis on admission for stroke is 100 – 69.6 = 30.4% chance of dying; 4 weeks later there is 69.8 – 59 = 10.8% chance of dying. For fractured femur on admission there is a 5% chance of dying, 4 weeks later a 5% chance of dying.
2. These figures emphasise the importance of the clinical progress with different diseases. There is also a difference in the referral patterns of the diseases, which will affect prognosis. A proportion of people with stroke will be treated at home. It is likely that those with a poor prognosis are admitted. Virtually all cases of fractured femur are admitted to hospital, for rehabilitation.
3. Prognoses are difficult to estimate from teaching hospital or specialist centre experience compared with patients presenting in primary care.

PROBLEM 9

If all those lost to follow-up were successes, the overall success rate would be 65% whereas if they were all failures the success rate would be 49%.

PROBLEM 10

1. The figure should look like Figure 12.3. The survival

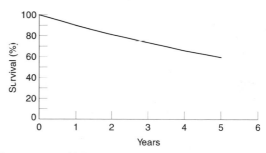

Fig. 12.3 Survival following detection of cancer at clinical diagnosis.

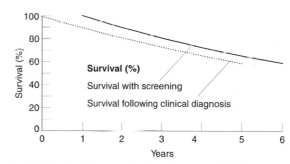

Fig. 12.4 Survival following detection of cancer at clinical diagnosis and with detection 1 year earlier at screening.

after 5 years is 59, i.e. 90, 81, 73, 66, 59% at years 1, 2, 3, 4 and 5, respectively.
2. The effect of early diagnosis (but no effective treatment) is shown in Figure 12.4. The effect of early diagnosis has been to increase the apparent survival rate over 5 years from 59% to 66%. The reason for this is that there is usually a 'volunteer effect' of people coming forward for screening (who do better prognostically than those who refuse screening). There will be a difference in the effect of early diagnosis in diseases of short and long duration. Screening will tend to detect more slowly progressive diseases than acute ones with a rapid onset. The mortality rate that produces a straight line on the graph is completely hypothetical.

12

Prognosis

➤ Prognosis is the forecast of the probable cause and termination of a disease.

➤ Intervention in a disease should be assessed by measurements of outcome that take prognosis into account.

➤ The method used to express outcome can mask the true prognosis (e.g. total deaths may be higher in a unit seeing more patients or more high-risk patients).

➤ In long-term illnesses, prognosis may be best expressed as a remission or a recurrence rate. Losses to follow-up are the most common difficulty in accurately assessing prognosis: those who are not contacted usually have a different prognosis to those available for follow-up.

The assessment of medical evidence

Theoretical aspects of the critical appraisal of medical evidence

13

In this chapter the collection of clinical evidence is described:

- assessment of medical articles
- sources of data on clinical studies
- criteria for assessing reviews
- using clinical evidence to establish clinical guidelines.

Introduction

Medical practice changes constantly. The rate of change is becoming more rapid all the time. Doctors need to keep in touch with new information and ideas and to try to keep up with the best way to work in their practice. There are a number of places where doctors, nurses and other professionals can get this information.

- original articles in journals
- summaries from the medical literature, review articles, practice guidelines
- consensus statements, editorials and summary articles in journals
- the internet
- textbooks
- consult with colleagues who are expert
- go to meetings, lectures, seminars
- advertisements in journals
- conversations with representatives from pharmaceutical and medical technology companies.

Each of these approaches is useful but each has its particular biases. Problems arise when these sources of information provide different solutions to particular problems of patient care.

Evidence-based medicine

Clinicians need a way of critically appraising the information they receive. They may choose to believe the most authoritative expert or a colleague, but they will often have difficulty coming to a conclusion. To help with this the Department of Clinical Epidemiology at McMaster University in Canada published a series of Guides in 1981, summarising appraisal methodology for busy clinicians. The series became very popular and has been reprinted in several foreign languages. Subsequently the guides have been modified by an even more intense focus on using the medical literature to solve patient problems. This approach has been called 'evidence-based medicine' and is defined as the ability to access, assess and apply information from the literature to day-to-day clinical problems.

The best care for patients in the 21st century requires an ability to use the medical literature to solve clinical problems. Health-care professionals should be able to address clinical dilemmas more often through:

- a careful definition of the problem
- an efficient literature search
- a brief and efficient screening of the articles to find the most relevant and valid information.

We should be able to use a quantitative approach in our thinking, asking:

- how big an effect can we expect from our treatment in this patient
- how much does the probability of disease increase as a result of this diagnostic test result.

It is important to differentiate clearly between clinical practices based on sound evidence from studies in human beings and those that are based on physiological principles or traditional practice. Most important is the ability to ask the right questions of a new medicine, technique or approach to care when faced with enthusiastic reports in the media or from patients.

Clinical information comes from patients and research. Information about patients comes from history, physical examination and investigations. Information from scientific research is gathered in a number of ways but is of great importance to the quality of care that patients receive. The way doctors or nurses use this information is greatly influenced by their training, which has been influenced in turn by the beliefs and research findings available at the time they were trained.

Limitations of expert opinion

Apart from scientific information obtained directly, clinicians rely on professional standards or opinion leaders to guide them. It is often assumed that the needs of clinicians for scientific information are met in this way and that community standards and the recommendations of clinical experts reflect the best available scientific information. However, variations in clinical practice, comparisons of practice with evidence-based standards and evaluations of the recommendations of clinical experts suggest that expert opinion does not always lead to rational and standard practice. Expert opinion often lags far behind the evidence and is sometimes inconsistent with evidence.

Having said this, of course, evidence in medicine is rarely cut and dried. Even careful meta-analyses require subjective judgements to be made about which trials to include and which to exclude or whether outcomes that are similar but not identical should be included together. There are, after all, greater and lesser experts at defining the clinical effectiveness of an intervention. The clinical effectiveness movement has simply tried to develop a more objective approach by codifying the methods used. The ultimate aim is to standardise the method as far as possible.

Examining medical literature

The proponents of the 'clinical effectiveness' approach suggest certain tools for evaluating and using the medical literature in day-to-day clinical practice. Three central questions are:

- what are the results?
- are the results of the study valid?
- will the results help in caring for patients?

Most clinical decisions consist of two choices, for example whether to start a treatment or not. Research articles rarely give evidence that can be used directly. Methods of measuring the validity of studies focus on identifying flaws in study design or implementation. These flaws may weaken the study so much that clinical decisions based on them are of no advantage or are even dangerous for patients. Table 13.1 shows the

Table 13.1 Guide for selecting articles that are most likely to provide valid results

Study area	Assessment factors
Original studies	
Therapy	Were the patients randomised to different treatments?
	Were all the patients in the trial accounted for?
Diagnosis	Was there an independent, blind comparison with some standard?
	Were the patients from a cross-section of those who will be receiving the diagnostic test in practice?
Harm	Were there clear comparison groups that were similar in other outcome measures (other than the one examined)?
	Were the outcomes and exposures measured in the same way in both of the groups?
Prognosis	Were the patients representative and were they chosen at a well-defined point in the course of disease?
	Was follow-up sufficiently long and complete?
Collections of studies (e.g. reviews)	
Overview	Did the review examine a clear question?
	Were the criteria used to select articles specified and reasonable?
Practice guidelines	Were the options and outcomes clearly specified?
	Did the article use an explicit process to identify, select and combine the evidence?
Decision analyses	Did the analysis follow a clinically important decision?
	Was good evidence used to develop the probabilities?
Economic analysis	Were there clearly described alternatives?
	Were the expected outcomes of each alternative based on good evidence?

things that have to be remembered before deciding whether an article is to be trusted.

Asking questions that are pertinent and answerable

Questions arise continuously while caring for patients. Most clinical questions are fairly simple. We can state them in terms of something happening to the patient. This may be a treatment, a diagnostic test or a potentially harmful agent and the effect it has on that patient. For example:

- Would treatment with streptokinase reduce the severity of a myocardial infarction? This is about the effectiveness of therapy.
- Would breast screening decrease a woman's risk of dying from breast cancer? This is about prevention through early diagnosis.
- Does a febrile seizure in a 6-month-old infant increase the likelihood of its developing epilepsy? This is about prognosis.
- Does anticoagulation increase the risk of death in a patient with an early stroke? This is about whether the therapy causes harm?

Setting up a literature search makes it easier to clarify the question when one is screening the titles and abstracts of articles. It is worthwhile identifying the type of patient and the outcomes of interest before beginning to look for an answer.

- is the patient seeking treatment for a distressing symptom or are they asymptomatic?
- if asymptomatic, are they wondering if they should take a preventative treatment, such as aspirin to prevent a stroke?
- are they concerned about the possible complications of such treatment over a long period?

It is sometimes more useful to look for published clinical practice guidelines instead of tracking down the evidence paper by paper.

A strategy for finding the evidence

Once a clear question has been devised, the best available evidence can be collected. The most accurate method of finding evidence, unless one is very expert, is the use of existing databases, such as the *Cochrane Centre* data. If a subject within the database does not exactly fit the problem, it may be necessary to search using Medline or a similar searching method. There are five ways of searching for data; these are given in order by the amount of time taken to perform each, shortest first:

- ask someone who is expert
- check the references in textbooks
- find a relevant article in a good international journal and search its references
- look up an existing published search if one exists in the subject in a suitable database
- use a bibliographic database, e.g. *Index Medicus* or its computerised system (Medline), to find meta-analyses, or failing that randomised controlled trials, or failing that any clinical trials.

The central problem is that most seniors doctors read material relevant to their work for only 30 minutes a week. Whatever approach is used, therefore, it must be efficient. Asking a colleague or consultant is highly efficient and, for doctors in training, the most common method of finding answers to problems. For more senior doctors, this also makes sense when the question concerns a problem or patient that are unlikely to be met again. It is usually clear, from previous encounters, whether a colleague is well versed in a subject. If a recent textbook is at hand, the appropriate passage may cite references that can be checked.

Reading weekly journals can often be confusing, as different ideas are tested and re-tested in these forums. It is relatively uncommon for an important change in treatment to occur rapidly without some time elapsing. An example where this did occur recently was in the debate about the prevention of sudden infant death syndrome by lying babies on their backs, rather than their stomachs. However, anyone who made more than a cursory glance at the journals or, indeed the newspapers, would have been aware of the change in approach. Memos from the Department of Health to all professionals usually accompany such rapid changes to emphasise their importance.

Some new 'subscription' textbooks address these problems by providing periodic updates and often cite the evidence used in making the changes. There are prototypes of textbooks that are based on systematic reviews of validated evidence for obstetric and neonatal problems.

A third starting point may be an article in a journal. The amount of time required to keep and cross-reference all such clinical articles is formidable. New methods for retrieving the current medical literature are rendering personal filing systems non-essential, if not obsolete. Nevertheless, everyone has his or her particular interests and a personal filing system is useful, if only to indicate where an article is stored.

Searches of the medical literature can be carried out by hand, looking at the vast tomes of *Index Medicus* year on year or by using electronic access with Medline, the computerised form. This is available in most teaching and other medical centres in a variety of on-line and CD-ROM formats. Doctors who are members of the BMA have access to their own system, which is excellent, except that viewing the final output is only possible 10 at a time. This can be time consuming if one has many papers to assess.

Professionals can easily acquire the basic skills and learn to search for citations in most medical libraries. The structured abstracts in Medline make the task of retrieving information from the medical literature even easier. Recruiting a librarian to help with the first few searches may help you to learn to avoid searches that are too broad and unfocused, or too narrow, thus missing key articles.

The final method is to look at databases that have screened articles for their validity and clinical relevance, such as the Cochrane Centre and its related group the Oxford Database of Perinatal Trials. These are increasingly available. Some of these can be reached using the Internet, though most require a subscription.

Deciding if an article is likely to provide valid results

The first question that should be applied to any article used to answer a clinical problem concerns its closeness to the truth; are the results of this article valid? Table 13.1 presents two key guides to assess the validity of studies. The busy professional who has tracked down a number of articles on a question can use the guides to choose the one or two articles most likely to provide a valid answer. We can also use these criteria to reduce the clinical literature to a manageable size when trying to keep up with new advances.

Assessing review articles?

Review articles are useful for two reasons. First, They are one way of coping with huge volumes of published reports (the number of biomedical journals worldwide is increasing exponentially, with a doubling time of about 19 years). Second, systematic reviews provide reliable answers to important questions. Impressive examples are reviews on the effects of systemic treatment on early breast cancer and of corticosteroids given to women expected to deliver prematurely.

Problems with the scientific quality of review articles

Until recently, a double standard has operated in published articles. Authors, journal editors and journal readers have expected a structured approach to reports of original research, but the same has not been true of review articles. People have not seen reviews as an extension of scientific reporting and little effort had been put into ensuring their quality, despite the fact that they are widely used to draw conclusions about research.

There is plenty of evidence of problems with review articles. This is perhaps nor surprising, given the number of review articles published. Mulrow looked at 50 review articles published in 1985–86 and assessed how they performed against eight criteria

- was the specific purpose of the review stated?
- were the sources and methods of the search for articles identified?
- were explicit guidelines provided that determined the material included in and excluded from the review?
- was a methodological validity assessment of material in the review performed?
- was the information systematically integrated with an explanation of the data limitations and inconsistencies?
- was the information integrated and weighted or simply pooled?
- was a summary of pertinent findings provided?
- were specific directives for new research initiatives proposed?

Only one review satisfied as many as six of the criteria. Other authors have looked at the recommendations of clinical experts (in review articles and textbook chapters) in the acute treatment and secondary prevention of myocardial infarction. Using the technique of cumulative meta-analysis, they used evidence from randomised controlled trials to calculate, retrospectively, the benefit associated with treatment. They identified important discrepancies between the experts' recommendations and what people might have known from systematic reviews. They concluded that clinical experts needed access to better databases and new statistical techniques. Another conclusion must be that readers would make more accurate inferences if they could assess reviews' scientific quality.

What is a review?

Journal editors have been reluctant to introduce structured abstracts for review articles, even though this would make it easier for readers to assess them. One reason is the feeling among editors that this is too pernickety. There is also confusion between the idea of a scientific review and a book review, which tends to be a generalised opinion of the subject. It is probable that we should see review articles, like book reviews, as the author's opinion of a body of knowledge, rather than a systematic weighing of the evidence. To this extent perhaps systematic reviews should be named as such and thought of as a separate entity.

The important thing is for readers to be able to distinguish a subjective opinion from a less subjective approach in a systematic review. One should never pretend to complete objectivity, of course. The methods of systematic review are open to bias and pre-judgement, though a structured approach may reduce this and help readers by providing structured abstracts and checklists. Just as important is improving the quality of reviews. This has been catalysed by the establishment of the UK Cochrane Centre in 1992. Its main purpose is to facilitate systematic, up-to-date reviews of randomised controlled trials of health care, such as those already conducted in the fields of pregnancy and childbirth. Together, the developments of high-quality reviews and of readers better able to assess their quality suggest that reviews in the future will have a major impact on knowledge, practice and policy in health services.

Getting evidence into practice

Once the evidence has been collected, weighed and a decision made of the course to follow, the next, and much more difficult stage, is to get it widely used in practice. There are a number of problems here.

Clinical guidelines: integrating the evidence into patient management

Systematic reviews, using meta-analyses to derive their data, rely on scientific papers for developing the review. Research evidence of this type is, by its nature, concerned with relatively discrete questions. There may be evidence for the best drug to use for hypertension or evidence on a broader issue such as the use of conventional or keyhole surgery for cholecystectomy. There may be good evidence for an even broader issue such as home or hospital treatment for people with serious mental illness. However broad the issues, the reviews will never cover the total management of a patient with a particular problem. For this it may be necessary to gather a number of systematic reviews and to produce **clinical guidelines** on the subject. Clinical guidelines are systematically developed statements that assist clinicians and patients in making decisions about appropriate treatment for specific conditions.

Guidelines will use systematic reviews wherever possible but there will be gaps where the evidence is not available or not yet agreed within the scientific community. In addition, guidelines produced centrally (the Royal Colleges have produced many of those that exist in the UK) or even in another country may sug-gest treatments and approaches that are not possible in the local setting. People usually produce guidelines locally, often customised from evidence produced elsewhere. Occasionally where there is no such evidence, the basic information has to be developed. Chapter 14 outlines methods of doing this.

Producing guidelines is time consuming and expensive. They should, in general, only be developed according to certain measures of priority:

- where there is excessive mortality or morbidity from a problem
- where treatment offers good potential for reducing these
- where there is a wide variation in clinical practice that appears amenable to intervention
- where the services are costly
- where many groups are involved, especially those crossing professional boundaries.

Clinical guidelines should specify the patient population concerned and the way in which their recommendations affect the management of the target population. We should, clearly distinguish recommendations supported by high-quality research evidence from those that have more limited supporting evidence. The guidelines should make clear both the costs and benefits of implementation. They should also identify areas where patient involvement in decision-making is essential and state the implications for all the disciplines involved, including GPs, Health Authorities and Trust managers. Ideally, guidelines should be able to be translated into explicit audit criteria.

The work leading to the publication in 1994 of the *Effective Health Care Bulletin* titled *Implementing Clinical Practice Guidelines: Can Guidelines be used to improve Clinical Practice?* suggested what clinical guidelines should aim to be:

- **valid:** leading to the results expected of them
- **reproducible:** given the same evidence and methods of guideline development, another group of developers will come to the same results
- **reliable:** given the same clinical circumstances different health professionals interpret and apply the guidelines in the same way
- **cost effective:** leading to improvements in health at acceptable costs
- **representative:** by involving the contribution of key groups and interests in their development
- **clinically applicable:** patient populations affected are unambiguously defined

- **flexible:** by identifying exceptions to recommendation as well as the patient preferences to be used in decision making
- **clear:** unambiguous language is used and readily understood by clinicians and patients
- **reviewable:** the date and process of review will be stated
- **amenable to clinical audit:** should be capable of translation into explicit audit criteria.

Clinical guidelines vary in many ways but have some common characteristics and attributes. Understanding these can help to design guidelines for care of patients with specific conditions. The biggest problem with guidelines is what to do about people who totally ignore them, despite knowing of their existence.

Appraisal and use of clinical evidence

➤ Evidence-based medicine is the ability to access, assess and apply information from the literature to day-to-day problems.

➤ The question to be asked should be clearly defined and then studied using colleagues, textbooks, original articles, reviews and databases.

➤ Clinical guidelines are statements that are based on medical evidence and that are intended to assist clinicians and patients to make decisions regarding treatment options.

Practical aspects of the critical appraisal of medical evidence

14

This chapter extends the information in Chapter 13 by describing available sources of material including:

● databases on CD-ROM
● source material in printed forms
● practical advice on how to access and search for material.

Introduction

There are an increasing number of sources of data available for a critical appraisal. The first thing to bear in mind is the reason for performing the appraisal. There are generally three main reasons for carrying one out:

● in order to discover the right way to treat a particular patient
● in order to increase basic knowledge of the treatment of a condition
● as a teaching exercise to learn the process of searching.

The first of these is by far the most difficult because individual patients, in our experience, rarely fit neatly into the categories where the most extensive searching has been done. This is not just Murphy's law (if something can go wrong it will) in action. Problems that have been researched and written up in detail will most likely be well known, so there will be no need to look them up. All patients are unique and have a unique set of problems. A patient with diabetes and heart disease, for instance, may well come into the ward or surgery but the literature is very sparse indeed on the treatment of heart disease in people with diabetes, for they are usually excluded from trials of therapy in heart disease.

The second reason for conducting a search is less specific and, therefore, easier. There will probably be at least one or two trials and possibly even a meta-analysis on a general subject.

The third reason is the easiest of all, for any subject can be chosen. It makes sense to choose one that has been well researched with meta-analyses and where others have picked out the trials that are of the best quality. These may, for instance, be available from the Cochrane database, when the criteria used to pick the evidence will be available and the conclusions well described.

Whatever the reason for doing a critical appraisal, the general rules are:

● make use of the large number of good sources of ready collected systematic reviews and overviews
● failing that, try to find a review from an expert in the field: if two reviews from two experts exist so much the better; they can be compared and, with luck, will largely agree
● use a computerised search, such as Medline or some of the others described in the rest of this chapter if reviews are not available; training from an expert will help to get the best out of this approach.

Sources of evidence

If you are convinced about the usefulness of using scientific evidence in practice, it makes sense to see if someone else has had the same problem and has collected together the evidence for you. There are a number of databases that can be accessed. These are listed below with their main characteristics.

High-class systematic reviews of evidence

1. **CDSR: Cochrane Database of Systematic Reviews**

● This is produced by the Cochrane Collaboration.

- It contains only systematic reviews carried out to very high standards by Cochrane Review Groups using high-quality randomised controlled trials only.
- It contains only the highest grade evidence only.
- It is fairly cheap to buy.
- It comes on a CD–ROM combined with DARE (see below).
- It is available in all postgraduate medical libraries in the UK.
- It contains a good bibliography of evidence-based methods.

2. Cochrane Collaboration for Pregnancy and Childbirth

As CDSR but includes good single randomised controlled trials in the field of pregnancy and childbirth.

3. DARE: Database of Abstracts of Review of Effectiveness

- This is produced by the NHS Centre for Reviews and Dissemination.
- It contains the INAHTA (International Network of Agencies for Health Technology Assessment) reviews and other reviews identified from the published literature.
- Most of these reviews have details of how their quality has been assessed.
- Some, though not all, meet the Cochrane criteria for classification as 'systematic'.
- Others have not been screened and need critical appraisal by the user.
- Their status is made clear in the database.
- It is fairly cheap.
- It is available in most postgraduate medical libraries.
- It contains only high-grade evidence.
- It has relatively small number of records because the systematic review methodology is fairly new.
- It is a new type of literature and database, so searching is still quite crude but improving.

Effective Health Care

- These are written bulletins describing the outcome of systematic reviews funded by the Department of Health in the UK.
- They include a wide variety of topics, such as screening for osteoporosis, treatment of glue ear, implementing clinical practice guidelines, etc.

Other sources of evidence

There are a number of other collections of data, some of which may provide systematic reviews.

Bandolier

- This is a printed news sheet reporting on published reviews; it is intended to promote evidence-based practice and methods and is, published monthly.
- It is produced by Oxford and Anglia NHS Region.
- It is a quick and easy way to get access to evidence generally, so it is a useful way of keeping up to date across the board.
- The subjects covered are printed in no particular order; as a result, it is not easy to find information on specific topics of interest.
- There is an index on the Internet, which makes it easier to find subjects relevant to your own problem.

Evidence-based Purchasing

A booklet similar to Bandolier produced by South and West R&D Directorate.

ACP Journal Club

A supplement to the *Annals of Internal Medicine*, providing commentaries and syntheses of research evidence.

Evidence-based Medicine

- A new journal similar to *ACP Journal Club*, which covers a wide variety of topics.

The do-it-yourself approach

If possible, it is better to avoid trying to decide upon the strength of evidence on a particular topic for ourselves. Groups of experts spend much of their time collecting the evidence and weighing it on virtually every medical topic under the sun. Having said this, it is sometimes necessary to weigh up a topic for oneself, either because the experts have missed it or in order to put a new single piece of work, which may look persuasive, into context.

Assessing the strength of evidence

A useful way of deciding on the strength of evidence is

to grade it in the following manner; the best sources followed by progressively less strong sources.

1. Strong evidence from at least one systematic review of multiple well-designed randomised controlled trials. Examples of good-quality reviews are those using methods outlined by the Cochrane Collaboration, the NHS Centre for Research and Development and the US Agency for Health Care Policy and Research. The quality of reviews can be appraised using checklists based on McMaster (University of Hamilton in Canada) principles.
2. Strong evidence from at least one properly designed randomised controlled trial of appropriate size. Evidence should meet criteria laid down in checklists based on McMaster principles. Evidence in this category is usually about therapy.
3. Evidence from well-designed trials without randomisation, single-group pre–post cohort, time series or matched case-controlled studies. Evidence in this category often concerns prognosis or cause of disease. McMaster checklists are available.
4. Evidence from well-designed non-experimental studies from more than one centre or research group. Evidence in this category often concerns the prevalence or cause of disease.
5. Opinions of respected authorities, based on clinical evidence, descriptive studies or reports of expert committees.

Methods of searching for scientific papers on a topic

There are a number of methods available to help to collect data on a particular subject if it is not possible to find the subject covered by the standard sources. First, there are databases that contain published data in a format which makes it possible to search for topics.

Index medicus and Medline

- This is produced by the National Library of Medicine in a CD–ROM format. It is found in print form as *Index Medicus*.
- It is an extremely large database covering journals printed from 1966 to the present, with over 12 million records.
- It gives references and abstracts to journal articles only from about 4000 health-related journals.
- It is an extensive but not exhaustive coverage of primary medical, nursing and veterinary literature.
- Medline does not guarantee the quality of the

original articles. It is not easy to pick out the different grades of evidence except by fairly complex search strategies.
- It allows very sophisticated searching by cross-referencing different headings.
- The central core is a highly structured hierarchical organisation of information based on MeSH (Medical Subject Headings) to aid searching.
- It can be a little out of date because of the complexity of the indexing procedure.
- It needs some training to make the most efficient use of the database, though it is possible to access it without prior help. Training considerably increases the number of relevant articles a searcher obtains.
- There are a variety of forms available, although the information remains the same
- Medline is available at most postgraduate libraries and can be used free by BMA members on the Internet who have a PC and modem.

Embase

- This is similar to Medline but does not completely overlap. A search on both systems will usually uncover more papers on the same subject (60–70% are common to both systems).
- It is European based (the print equivalent is *Excerpta Medica*).
- It is not as widely used as Medline but its use is necessary if exhaustive searching is being carried out.
- It is available via JANET (Joint Academic Network) and the BMA.
- It uses structured index terms but these are not the same as Medline.

ASSIA: Applied Social Science Index and Abstracts

- ASSIA covers the social sciences and is not restricted to health care.
- It covers well the sociological aspects of health care, e.g. health promotion, socioeconomic status as a health factor, community care, ageing and patients' rights.

ERIC: Education Resources Information Center

- This is a database of educational materials from 1966 to the present.
- The references are taken from educational journals and research reports.
- It is not restricted to health care. It includes

curriculum development, communication, evaluation and adult and child education.

● Hospital libraries often have access to this information service.

Other databases

Other databases can be accessed for specific disease areas and types of information. A few of the many examples are:

CINAHL: Cumulated Index to Nursing and Allied Health Literature
CANCERLIT: cancer journals, books and reports
AIDSLINE: HIV / AIDS information
PSYCHLIT: psychiatry / psychology literature
AMED: complementary medicine.

Internet

● This provides access to reports, guidelines, discussion lists, home pages, etc.
● The quality of the material is very variable (e.g. the US Agency for Health Policy and Research Guidelines are very good, others are not reviewed by experts and some are just odd).
● Access to information is haphazard, although attempts are being made to organise it (e.g. using OMNI (Organising Medical Networked Information) in the UK.
● There are discussion lists that may be of interest especially those on evidence-based-health, public health and primary health care.

Problems with the Internet

It is difficult to assess information on the internet: is the origin of work on the the Internet from a bone fide expert, rather than simply the views of an individual? This can be quite difficult if the authors are not well known.

Searching for original articles on Medline

Searching for original articles requires some expertise. Initially it is best to be taught directly by an expert. The general idea is that, when looking up a topic, one uses the indexing system of the database to improve the search where possible. It is worth looking up the list of medical (MeSH) subject headings to get an idea of the types of subject that are included. The headings have a bias towards words and phrases used in the USA. For example, a text word search for 'general practitioner', the usual UK phrase, gives 1229 'hits'. If one uses the medical subject heading for 'Physicians – family' one

gets 1693 hits. This is because the indexers have screened the articles and included general practitioner(s), GP(s), family practitioner(s) and family physician(s) under the same MeSH term since they mean the same.

It is not essential to know what all the MeSH terms are. Medline allows a subject to be entered in any words and tries to match it to the appropriate MeSH word or phrase. Apart from MeSH headings, searches can also use text words or phrases. There are problems with this type of searching: if the search is for free text words in the title or abstract, all possible spellings must be used (anemia / anaemia). It is also wise to truncate words to include singular and plurals and alternative word endings (hypervent: for hyperventilate / hyperventilating / hyperventilation).

It helps to think laterally. There are many ways in the English language to describe the same thing (pressure sore / bed sore / decubitus ulcer). If the first attempt fails try an alternative term. Sometimes asking for the opposite helps, e.g. patient non-compliance is covered by the MeSH term 'patient compliance'.

There are about 12 000 MeSH terms in Medline and the differences between them can be subtle. 'Family practice', 'physicians, family' and 'primary health care' are all different subjects in Medline. If you want them all you have to ask for all of them. Searching for liver will yield different results to a search for liver diseases. Medline gives the most precise term it can to the subject. These terms are arranged in a **tree structure** and the *most specific rule* is crucial to the correct use of the tree. One cannot retrieve an article about the brain by searching for central nervous system. If you search for NSAIDS you will not retrieve all the articles on aspirin but you will retrieve general articles on NSAIDS. Only searching for aspirin will give you specific references.

Exploding the tree

The EXPLODE option

Medline uses a branching system in its use of headings. For example, a search for NSAIDS including specific articles on individual drugs that are NSAIDS must use the option EXPLODE. Exploding within a search means that all of the subgroups are included in the search as well as the main line that you have been following. Exploding, therefore, broadens the search if there have been subgroups which you have ignored:

NSAIDS. 4554 results
aspirin: 3223 results
NSAIDS exploded: 13877 results.

Combining searches

The OR option

The OR option allows a search to be broadened by using more than one topic that could cover the subject, e.g. family practice OR physicians, family OR primary health care. All the results in any of the three sets will be found.

The AND option

If a search initially produces a great many results, the AND option will narrow the search, retrieving fewer results and being more specific, e.g. aspirin AND myocardial infarction. Only results appearing in both sets will be retrieved.

The GREAT BRITAIN option

Another option is to use the phrase GREAT BRITAIN to restrict the articles to those which have a British origin.

The LIMIT option

The LIMIT option narrows down the results further, e.g. English language only, specific age groups such as aged, human only. 'Major headings only' gives fewer results but increases the relevance of the articles to the area of interest.

Further restrictions

Use further classification of MeSH terms where available and appropriate to narrow search results (e.g. asthma – diagnosis, asthma – therapy, communication – methods, medical education continuing – evaluation). Use this facility cautiously.

A search-strategy for information retrieval

Having decided what result is needed a search pattern can be established, e.g.

1. MeSH heading etc. 1: think of possible alternative terms
2. MeSH heading etc. 2: think of possible alternatives
3. Other ideas (if appropriate): work out relationships between concepts (AND/OR/NOT)
4. Use any other existing information, e.g. references, authors' names etc. to help the search.

Figure 14.1 suggests a simple strategy overall for getting started.

> **Practical methods of accessing data**
>
> ➤ Systematic reviews provided by various organisations can be accessed and provide the most efficient method of finding up-to-date information on how to care for patients with a particular condition.
>
> ➤ Abstracting services, both in print and as CD-ROM databases, enable literature searches using headings, which may often be cross-referenced for a more sophisticated search strategy.
>
> ➤ Using medline, searches are based on database subject headings. Various options allow the search to be expanded or narrowed down depending on the type of information required.

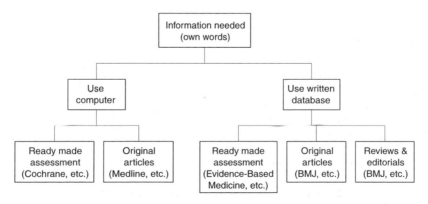

Fig. 14.1 Strategy for obtaining data.

Too many results?

Too many results can be reduced by limiting the search, e.g. to English only, by year, to reviews, AIM journals, etc.; limit the level of emphasis given to the topic (e.g. major heading); use more precise terms to define the concepts; link to other topics using the AND facility.

Too few results?

Too few results can be improved upon by widening the search using alternative sources, searching more years or using alternative terms to broaden your search using the OR option. Use fewer AND links.

What form do you require your results in?

The results can be retrieved in various forms: with or without abstracts, including author affiliation; printed out or kept on a file.

Environmental and occupational health

4

The epidemiology of environmental and occupational health

This chapter covers general aspects of environmental influences on health:

- air pollution
- water pollution
- food pollution with microbes, natural toxins and chemicals
- food additives.

Introduction

Environmental epidemiology is about identifying and measuring the influence of environmental factors on human disease in different communities. Environmental factors are usually considered as those in our general environment whereas occupational factors are those to which we are exposed because of our occupations or those of others close to us. Environmental factors may be:

- **Physical**: these may be naturally occurring, such as heavy metals, or result from human activity, such as ionising radiation or noise.
- **Chemical**: these may be related to unusual but naturally occurring toxins or synthetic toxins, often waste products, which may cause contamination.
- **Biological**: bacteria and viruses living in a reasonably symbiotic relationship with humans may be affected by environmental factors, such as overcrowding, poor general health of the population or a rapid change in life style (e.g. sexual contacts) and become pathogenic. Pathogens may also have more opportunity to spread if these environmental factors come into play.

Environmental epidemiology also aims to provide scientific evidence, based on epidemiological research, for sound environmental and health policies and practices. The main areas of concern are:

- environmental factors causing or promoting the spread of infectious disease
- environmental toxins leading directly to disease.

Poor environments as a spur to public health in the UK

Rapid industrialisation in the UK in the middle of the 19th century caused rapid changes in the environment, with crowding and poor health due to poor nutrition. This, in turn, resulted in increases in the death rate from a number of infectious diseases, especially typhus, cholera and tuberculosis.

People did not understand the mechanism of infection because microorganisms had not been discovered and public health measures relied on epidemiological observations of the relationship between sickness and bad living conditions. Only later was the effectiveness of the measures explained through the science of bacteriology. Part of the power of epidemiology is that it can detect associations between possible causes and disease and outline ways of avoiding those causes even when we do not understand the exact mechanism linking cause and disease.

A number of highly lethal infectious diseases increased in importance as a result of the poor housing and nutrition common when there was rapid increases in population following jobs made available through industrialisation. Typhus was endemic in the UK but occasionally broke out with increased virulence, as in 1846–8. These outbreaks occurred whenever a group of susceptible people came within its reach. Cholera was another highly lethal and contagious disease widespread at that time. It was usually transmitted through food or water contaminated by the excrement of cholera patients. The bacillus causing the disease, *Vibrio cholerae*, reaches the intestine and causes diarrhoea, which is often fatal through dehydration of the patient.

The greatest pandemic of cholera started in the valley of the Ganges in India in 1826. It spread until it first appeared in the UK in Sunderland in October 1831; it then spread northward to reach Glasgow in February 1832, where there were over 3000 deaths. It then spread southwards through Liverpool and Manchester to hovels of the new industrial districts of the Midlands. In south Wales, the towns of the coalfield experienced severe outbreaks of the disease in 1832 and in the epidemic years of 1849, 1854 and 1866. In the 1832 outbreak, the death toll in England and Wales was 22 000 out of a population of 14 million. In 1849, Merthyr Tydfil had a population of 50 000, having experienced a mushroom growth as an iron-smelting centre. The result resembled a large labour camp. From May to November of that year 1400 people died. In Chapter 1 we described the early efforts of John Snow to link cholera deaths to consumption of contaminated water.

Pulmonary tuberculosis was the most widespread and persistently deadly disease of the 19th century in the UK. It existed in ancient Egypt and was prevalent in the 18th century but it thrived in the 19th century because of overcrowding in factories and slums. The first analysis by the Registrar General for England and Wales in 1839 revealed that tuberculosis (consumption) accounted for nearly a fifth of all deaths. *Mycobacterium tuberculosis*, discovered by Robert Koch in 1882, is the specific cause of tuberculosis. People catch the bacterium from drinking infected milk from tubercular cows or by inhaling the bacilli from a person with the disease.

In the slums of the industrial towns of the UK in the 19th century, one in every five children did not live beyond a year. A further one in five that survived infancy died before they were 15 years old. Children suffered severely from bronchitis, pneumonia, summer diarrhoea and the common infectious diseases of childhood. The last, such as scarlet fever, measles and whooping cough, led often to fatal complications. Death from measles was often caused by secondary bronchopneumonia.

The conditions of life among the industrial poor and the part that environmental conditions played in predisposing to disease stimulated the development of the specialty of Public Health. The doctors working in the specialty advocated:

- improved water supplies
- improved refuse disposal
- sewage disposal
- better housing
- cleanliness

- ventilation
- disinfection.

Early measures to improve public health

Edwin Chadwick's *Report on the Sanitary Condition of the Labouring Population of Great Britain (1842)* forced people to face the problems of the public health. This led to political action, with the first Public Health Act in 1848. Later in the century, rejection of almost half of the army recruits for the Boer War in South Africa alerted the country to the poor health of much of the population. A number of surveys followed. One of these, in Leeds in 1902, showed that half of the children examined had marked rickets. The material progress of the 19th century for well-off people was bought at the cost of deterioration in the health of poor people. Despite this, there was overall a gain of 10 years in the expectation of life at birth during the century.

In developed countries, the improvements in infectious disease rates caused by sanitary measures in the 19th century have improved still further because of better living conditions and nutrition. Health was also improved, to a lesser extent, in the 20th century by immunisation and antibiotics. Life expectancy at birth has increased from approximately 50 years in 1900 to well over 70 years in men, nearly 80 years in women at the end of the 20th century. Infectious diseases still present some problems in developed countries but their impact upon the public health is much less than in the past.

Modern times

In the 1990s, the threat of the major infectious diseases has reduced, though not disappeared completely. Tuberculosis has shown a slight increase, though the reasons for its growth revolve around decreased resistance to infection in certain groups of people, especially those with AIDS and people on drugs that reduce their resistance to infection. Most concerns these days revolve around the effect of industries themselves and the industrialisation of the processes that produce food. There are concerns that the pace of industrial growth may be polluting the environment to an extent that it will overturn the benefits the manufactured goods bring. It is not clear whether these changes will be compensated for by technological developments like antibiotics to improve health. Some toxins may be obviously dangerous if their effect is poisoning, allergenic or teratogenic. Others may present a long-term and unclear effect if they are mutagenic or carcinogenic over a longer term.

Environmental pollutants

The external environment can affect human health through:

- air breathed
- food eaten
- water drunk
- physical means, e.g. ionising and non-ionising radiation.

As a result, it is convenient to consider environmental health risks presented by these various environmental categories.

Air pollution

Suspended particles, particularly the smaller particles with a diameter less than 10 micrometres (μm), together with gases in the atmosphere can have an adverse effect upon people's lungs. It was apparent in the middle of the 19th century that black smoke in urban areas was a problem and that gases emitted from industry killed the vegetation in the area. It seemed likely that these were also damaging to humans. The Smoke Act and the Alkali Act in the mid-19th century were aimed at reducing this. There were many deaths caused by the London smogs in the late 19th century, but people were not as conscious of pollution as a problem. Heavy smog in London in 1952 provided a turnaround in ideas and resulted in action to reduce air pollution.

The smog episode in 1952 contributed to the deaths of several thousand susceptible individuals (Figure 15.1), especially people with asthma and chronic bronchitis. It led to the passing of the Clean Air Act and of an Alkali Act in the late 1950s. The former sought to reduce the ground level concentrations of air pollution. Pollution from domestic fuel burning was to be prevented by the introduction of smokeless zones in populated areas and industrial pollution would be reduced by building higher chimneys, which would permit dispersal beyond the highly populated areas. The latter, although locally effective, led to effects upon the environment in European countries to the east, since taller chimneys led the prevailing winds to transport sulphur dioxide emissions and deposit them as acid rain. The result of this policy was that smoke concentrations at urban sites in the UK fell by half between 1960 and 1975. Some, at least, of this reduction resulted from a lucky coincidence. The general population began to change from burning house coal to gas and electricity for heating. The period coincided with a time of relative prosperity, just after the post-war austerity, so that although these were more expensive they were cleaner and more convenient to use.

More recently, the increasing use of cars has increased air pollution in cities. Approximately one tenth of exhaust gas can be carbon monoxide. It combines reversibly with haemoglobin when breathed into the lungs so the physiological effects are related to hypoxia. It is worth bearing in mind that smokers acquire much higher concentrations of these substances than non-smokers breathing city air.

Control of air pollution

In the UK, responsibility for control of air pollution is shared between central and local government. Approximately 2000 industrial sites have physico-chemical processes that are potentially highly toxic and are overseen by Her Majesty's Inspectorate of Pollution. Monitoring and control of the less toxic sites, of which there are tens of thousands, is the responsibility of the Environmental Health Departments of local authorities.

Improved monitoring of air pollution is required before we can be sure about its effects upon chest diseases. A WHO expert group in 1995 concluded that short-term pollution episodes accounted for 7–10% of all lower respiratory illnesses in children living in cities. Each year, 1% of deaths can be linked to short-term peaks of air pollution and 3–7% of new cases of obstructive airways disease can be expected to occur when pollution is high. The increasing prevalence of asthma in children is causing concern and studies have looked at the rôle of indoor pollution. A possible cause is a build up of house dust mites and fungal spores because of better insulation, more carpets and more central heating in houses. At present no one knows the cause. There has been a considerable change in the way that asthma is diagnosed in the past few years, which has also confused the issues considerably.

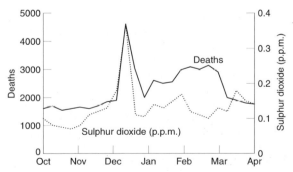

Fig. 15.1 Registered deaths and atmospheric pollution levels in London 1952–3. (Griffith & Levin 1989)

Water pollution

The preventive measures of filtration and chlorination of the public water supply has virtually eliminated water-borne disease of bacterial origin in the UK. However, while billions of *Vibrio cholerae* need to be present to cause infection, much lower doses of viruses, perhaps fewer than 100 may cause viral diarrhoea. The presence of susceptible individuals (i.e. infants, elderly and immunocompromised) in the population, therefore, places the most stringent requirements upon the safety of the public water supply.

Some organisms that are resistant to chlorination, such as *Cryptosporidium* and *Giardia* spp., can cause significant outbreaks of disease. The general improvements in the water supply system in developed countries is altering the types of disease caught from water.

The Water Act of 1973 established ten regional water authorities covering England and Wales and responsible for water resources and supply as well as sewage treatment. These have since been privatised. In the UK, 99% of homes have piped water supply and 95% are connected to the sewage system. The majority of the UK population drink water from river systems. The Thames exemplifies the potential problems of river water. The people of London drink water previously ingested and excreted by the people of the up-river towns, such as Reading. Under average weather conditions, the Thames contains about 14% of its volume as effluent from up-stream discharges (sewage, industrial and agricultural) and in a dry summer as much as 30% by volume of the river is not water.

Nitrogenous fertilisers from agricultural land are run off into rivers and the nitrate levels in many rivers have been rising. Infant methaemoglobinaemia caused by nitrates in water is rare in the UK but occurs in areas of Eastern Europe. There is also concern about possible carcinogenic risks from chemical contaminants such as pesticides, detergents and oils as well as from inorganic compounds. The greatest risks in this connection are associated with accidental spills. The chemical contamination of ground water is of even greater significance since its regeneration is extremely slow.

Bathing water contaminated with sewage can lead to infections such as hepatitis A, shigellosis and leptospirosis, but most of the morbidity from moderately contaminated water is of an unknown cause. Outbreaks of Legionnaires disease have been associated with water-cooling systems of air-conditioning plants and amoebic meningoencephalitis with swimming pools, but both can be prevented through appropriate disinfection.

Some shaky evidence has suggested that chlorinated water supplies may be associated with the higher cancer rates in populations consuming chlorinated compared with unchlorinated supplies. The suggested mechanism is an interaction between chlorine during water treatment with organic precursors, leading to the formation of chlorinated hydrocarbons, shown to be carcinogenic in the laboratory. Nevertheless, the risk of serious illness from pathogens that exists in the absence of chlorination dwarfs the risk that may be attributable to chlorination.

Food pollution

The microbiological contamination of food has increased in the 1990s in Europe. The microorganisms may multiply in the food before ingestion (e.g. salmonella) or may produce toxins in the food (e.g. botulism). Gastrointestinal infections caused by campylobacters and salmonellae predominate, although there has also been an increase in infections caused by *Escherichia coli* and *Listeria monocytogenes*.

There is a great diversity in the microorganisms and foods involved and the faecal–oral cycle (e.g. *Shigella sonnei* in children) can be broken with hygienic improvements. Outbreaks of hepatitis A in the UK in 1982 caused by eating shellfish were the spur for improving the cleansing and cooking of cockles. The withdrawal or treatment of contaminated food usually prevents the transmission of disease by food. However, an important part of the food chain can become extensively contaminated. In the late 1980s, it was discovered that bulk whole egg products and chicken flocks were extensively affected with salmonellae.

Natural toxins

There are many natural toxins (including carcinogens) in foods. There have been notable disease outbreaks associated with metabolites of fungi. Several toxic alkaloids produced by the ergot fungus can cause gangrene of the extremities if ingested. In the 1930s in the Ukraine, a fungus on grain and straw caused fatal stachybotryotoxicosis in humans and horses, and in the late 1940s in the Orenburg district of the USSR there was an outbreak of fatal haemorrhagic alimentary aleukia following consumption of bread made with contaminated grain. In the 1970s, epidemiological study showed that aflatoxin, a fungal metabolite, was associated with the high incidence of liver cancer in a district of Kenya.

In England in 1961, thousands of turkeys were affected when fattened on groundnut meal from Brazil containing aflatoxin, which is also a widespread contaminant of grain. Nitrosamines were first shown to be hepatotoxic, then carcinogenic. They are incriminated in cancer of the gastrointestinal tract and can be formed in the body by the reaction of amines and nitrites. In China's Lin Xian province, a soil deficiency of molybdenum leads to a high nitrite content of green leaf vegetables, a stable diet in this area. This environmental factor in combination with a local preference for mouldy bread (the source of the amines) is believed to be responsible for an increased incidence of oesophageal cancer.

Our knowledge of the significance of these natural toxins and also of the production of natural mutagens during cooking is at an early stage of development. Most public concern relates to food additives, and chemical contamination of food introduced by agricultural practices, food processing or packaging.

Regulation of additives

There is a huge demand for processed foods and these require the use of many chemical additives. Chemicals are used to inhibit bacterial and fungal growth as well as to limit enzymatic reactions, which affect the appearance and palatability of the food. We now have a powerful tool for screening additives in the form of rapid tests for carcinogens and mutagens. Ames devised some of the early ones in the early 1970s based on measurement of mutagenic changes in exposed salmonella bacteria.

The regulatory agencies (e.g. the Food and Drug Administration in the USA) are strict and there is little evidence of adverse health effects from permitted chemical additives. However, vigilance is constantly required, particularly for susceptible groups. In 1965 in Quebec, cobalt was added to beer to improve the head of foam. The effect of the cobalt was increased in people on a low-protein diet and having a high alcohol intake. This led to 48 people developing cardiac insufficiency. There were 20 deaths. Some groups of humans are likely to be more susceptible to any abnormal food additive or processing. This is especially the case if a substance acts upon the metabolising enzymes. For example, sulphite is added to control microbial growth in food and beverages. In most individuals the sulphite oxidase enzyme system is able to oxidise this to sulphate. However, a small proportion of the population may be less able to do this and are at risk from sulphite toxicity.

The past use of antibiotics, such as chlortetracycline to prevent spoilage of fresh fish catches and nystatin to inhibit rot on bananas or as growth promoters for farm animals is no longer permitted. It has been recognised that resistance to these drugs can be transferred to bacteria, which are pathogenic. There are concerns about genetically engineered foodstuffs, which are being developed to alter a characteristic of the foodstuff in question. This may be to reduce its liability to discolour or rot or to make its shape more uniform.

Assessment of food-borne risks

In common with many other issues in epidemiology, the risk of additives and other changes in food production has to be weighed against the benefits of increased production or better lasting qualities. More marginal benefits, such as maintenance of colour or uniformity of shape, should have fewer risks attached to them than those that improve production.

Epidemiology of environmental and occupational health

➤ Environmental factors may be physical, chemical or biological and may be naturally occurring or result from human activities.

➤ Air pollution results from gas and small particle production from industrial activities; vehicle exhaust fumes are a serious problem for cities in the 1990s.

➤ Water pollution with biological agents is reduced by chlorination in most cases. Chemical contamination with nitrogenous fertilisers and industrial waste affects ground water particularly.

➤ Food pollution from microorganisms can be reduced by hygienic measures. Natural toxins can cause serious disease in animals and humans.

➤ Modern food processing methods have resulted in the use of additives and genetic engineered products. For both, the risk-to benefit ratio must be assessed when deciding what processes to accept.

➤ Certain sections of the population may be at increased risk of certain pollutants, e.g. children are generally more susceptible, adults with particular genetic make-up may be unable to tolerate some food additives.

Environmentally linked diseases

In this chapter environmental hazards are discussed in terms of their scale of effect including:

- widespread air pollution
- contamination of the food-chain
- contamination of the public water supply.
- industrial products: local contamination and industrial accidents
- natural hazards.

Introduction

Events can affect the environment on varying scales, which can be divided into three groups:

- events that are prolonged in time and of widespread geography
- events that are limited in geography but prolonged in time
- events that are limited in time and geography.

The first type of event is the most difficult to identify and control.

Events prolonged in time and of widespread geography

Air pollution

The pollution of air from industrial sources continues to decrease in developed countries but the increase of road traffic poses a possible risk to health. Motor car exhausts are the main source of urban nitrogen dioxide, which gives rise to ozone by chemical reactions in air. Episodes of high ozone may cause respiratory symptoms in sensitive people. They occur a few days a year in European cities. Governments are introducing catalytic conversion of motor exhausts and have stopped the addition of lead to petrol to allay public concerns about lead pollution.

Diesel engine exhaust fumes are a complex mixture of chemicals, including known carcinogens. However, work investigating the association between urban air pollution and lung cancer has not shown a connection. The studies are beset with design problems such as looking for a relatively small increase in lung cancer against a large background of lung cancer incidence from smoking cigarettes. Similar limitations apply to seeking evidence of an association between fluoridation of the public water supply, to prevent dental caries, and cancer. Extensive investigation has failed to find any effect.

Food pollution

A number of significant events have occurred whereby the food chain has been affected in a diffuse manner. In these events, a large number of people were poisoned by chemicals in food, for example:

- food oil adulterated with tri-o-cresyl phosphate in Morocco in 1959
- wheat contaminated with endrin (an organochlorine insecticide) in 1967 in Saudi Arabia
- cooking oil contaminated with polychlorinated biphenyls in Kitakyushu City, Japan in 1968
- bread contaminated with mercury in Iraq in 1971.

In the Japanese episode, infants born to women poisoned while pregnant also displayed a syndrome of eye diseases and skin defects.

There was complacency about the possibility of such events occurring in highly developed countries until an episode in 1973–4 in the state of Michigan, USA. At a centre for the preparation of animal foodstuff, approximately a tonne of a commercial preparation containing polychlorinated biphenyls (PCBs) was accidentally put into a feed supplement for dairy cattle. This was distributed to the farms of Michigan, eaten by cattle and appeared in their milk and carcasses. As a result of ingesting the milk and meat the PCBs appeared in human breast milk and tissue. The population of Michigan was widely exposed but extensive follow-up has not revealed any evidence of disease resulting from the exposure. The scientific consensus is that the health effects reported subsequently by the population were either 'natural incidence' or psychologically determined. Follow-up is continuing.

A more tragic incidence occurred in Spain in 1981. European Community agricultural policy had resulted in a 'lake' of food oil. To prevent its human consumption, this oil was deliberately adulterated with aniline, a chemical dye. A group of gangsters had the even more imaginative idea of paying some chemists to remove the dye and then to sell the oil for human consumption. Unfortunately, the purification was not rigorous and when the food oil was subsequently sold in the poorer quarters of some Spanish cities it led to 20 000 cases of toxic oil syndrome and over 300 deaths. The symptoms and progression of the disease (pneumonia-like symptoms, gastrointestinal symptoms late in the first month and profound neuromuscular effects 100 days after onset) were thought to result from the triggering of a chronic autoimmune process.

Bovine spongiform encephalopathy

Bovine spongiform encephalopathy (BSE) is a slowly progressive and fatal neurological disorder of adult cattle. The Ministry of Agriculture's Central Veterinary Laboratory in the UK first diagnosed it in 1986, although studying earlier records suggested it might have occurred in April 1985. The spongiform changes in the brain are similar to those occurring in scrapie, which has been common in sheep for well over a 100 years. Experiments showed that the disease could be transmitted to mice and cattle by injection of bovine brain tissue from infected animals. The transmissible agent or **prion** is a bovine protein similar to that found in scrapie.

Researchers showed that the affected cattle had been given bone meal feed containing protein derived from sheep. Such bone meal had been fed to cows for decades. There were, however, major changes in the ways that it was produced in the late 1970s. From December 1986 to December 1988 there were just over 2000 confirmed cases on 1600 farms. Feeding ruminant protein to ruminants was banned in July 1988, but the long incubation period of 2–8 years ensured an increase in the incidence of BSE for some years after that. Suspect cattle offal was banned from human consumption in 1990.

Creutzfeldt–Jakob disease (CJD) is a rare spongiform encephalopathy that has been known in humans for many years, without a known cause. It is commonest in older people. Recently a small number of cases (23) of a variant of the disease have been identified. These cases have been found in younger people and have had a different clinical course from the previously known cases of CJD. There is, therefore, concern that the transmissible agent may have crossed the species' barrier from cow to humans. If the prion has been in bone meal, the transmitting agent could have been any other species that was fed the bone meal, including chickens or pigs. These have not shown signs of illness but these species tend to be killed young and might not exhibit symptoms before being killed. The British Government and its European partners currently disagree on the best control methods.

If mechanisms of transmission of BSE from cow to cow are like those of scrapie then infection could be passed to their calves before they showed signs of disease and without them ever developing clinical signs of disease. Selective slaughter of affected cattle would, therefore, not be an adequate control policy for dealing with BSE. Research is being carried out and active surveillance carried out for new cases of human CJD. The government has also instituted a scheme of identifying all offspring of cows for at least 10 years to form the basis of a BSE eradication scheme. Such a scheme would probably be directed at infected breeding lines rather than individual animals. The main concern is that the disease, when transmitted accidentally, is thought to have a long incubation period so that there is a small possibility of many more cases over the next few years, even if the control mechanisms prevent further transmission from cattle. This diffuse and long-term potential risk in the food chain will be better understood as evidence is collected, but unless a human epidemic occurs the link is unlikely to be proved or disproved.

Ionising radiation

The manner with which ionising radiation interacts with tissues is discussed in Chapter 21. Cosmic rays are produced in the upper atmosphere from the interaction of high-energy particles from the sun. There is no sensible way that this radiation can be avoided. Some rocks, soils and building materials contain naturally occurring radionuclides, which externally irradiate people. Natural radionuclides ingested in food and drink account for 11.5% of an individual's dose, while fallout from nuclear weapons testing or major reactor accidents accounts for only 0.2%.

The atmospheric deposition of radionuclides (fallout) increased to a maximum in the early 1960s but following the partial nuclear test ban treaty has declined since. The long-lived isotopes of strontium, caesium and carbon are the most important. The reactor accident at Chernobyl in 1986 led to caesium fallout in the UK, particularly where rain washed it out of the atmosphere in Wales and Southern Scotland. Milk accounted for about 80% of radiocaesium intake in 1986. Restricted areas, holding about 4 million sheep, were instigated in 1986 to ensure that meat containing radio caesium did not enter the food chain. By the end of 1991, there were still 600 farms and half a million sheep subject to restriction.

In the UK, about 1000 sites (e.g. hospitals, universities and research establishments) are authorised to discharge limited amounts of radioactive wastes. The largest discharges are, of course, from nuclear sites, but the total from all power stations is a small fraction of that discharged by the fuel reprocessing plant in Sellafield, Cumbria.

Exposure to radon and its products inside homes and other buildings makes the largest contribution to the dose of radiation that the population receives. High indoor concentrations are found in southwest England; outdoor radon is insignificant. Some 100 000 homes in the UK are estimated to have radioactivity concentrations in excess of the government safety level. Measurement and control programmes are underway and future homes are being designed to prevent the build-up of radon, usually by ensuring that the flooring is impervious to gas.

Exposure to diagnostic X-rays is discussed in Chapter 21.

Lead in the environment

Occupational epidemiology has shown a number of health effects associated with lead exposure. Blood lead in excess of about 90 µg/dl causes neurological symptoms. Moderately elevated blood lead concentrations may lead to impairment of blood formation and increased blood pressure. There has been some suggestion of an effect on the intelligence of children. A Government review of environmental lead stated that the difference between the average blood lead concentration of the UK population and that level at which neurological poisoning occurred was not huge but concluded that the effects of intermediate blood lead concentrations was not proved to cause harm.

Lead is naturally present in soil and in certain localities, notably parts of Wales, where past mining activity has contaminated the environment. Present industrial activity (e.g. smelting) may be a source of environmental lead. Lead salts are ingredients in paint

and are used in batteries. It may be present in the water supply and until recently was dispersed as a fine aerosol of inorganic lead particles from motor exhausts. In the UK before the advent of lead-free petrol, approximately 9000 tons of alkyl lead were added to petrol and 75% of this was emitted in exhaust fumes. Having said this, only 100 metres from the busiest motorways, lead levels in soil and grass are down to those found generally. Most public concern and environmental lobbying concerned petrol and its impact upon children's IQ. The epidemiological evidence was poor because of problems of measuring children's intelligence, the many confounding variables and the other exposure routes mentioned above.

Environmentalists publicised the finding of a marked fall in the average blood lead levels in the US population between 1976–82 and an associated decrease in the lead emitted from car exhausts. However, a very similar decrease in blood lead levels also occurred in Wales over the same period, when there was no lead-free petrol.

Investigation of lead exposure in Wales has shown that there is a raised concentration of blood lead in communities with lead water piping. The public health importance of this exposure remains unknown. The political decision to remove lead from petrol may itself carry an unevaluated risk by increasing environmental benzene in traffic fumes. This is known to cause aplastic anaemia and leukaemia if present in sufficiently high doses.

Electromagnetic fields

Electricity use for power and communications has increased since the 1940s by 25-fold and 70-fold, respectively. Cables in towns in the UK tend to be buried and supply transformers are at street level, whereas in the USA homes are supplied by a system of overhead cables. The transmission of electrical power gives rise to electromagnetic fields.

Theoretically, no biological effects would be expected from potentials from electromagnetic fields, for they are 100 to 1000 times lower than potentials which are likely to cause harm. However, scientific reports throughout the 1980s have suggested biological effects in cells and this has prompted work in this area. The New York State Power Lines Project spawned a number of epidemiological studies. A case–control study of acute non-lymphocytic leukaemia in the state of Washington showed no increase in cases when analysed by the number of and distance from home of overhead cables or by magnetic field measurements in the home. Cases of cancer in children under 15 years of age in the Denver area showed no difference from controls in relation to exposure in their homes. Similar case–control studies in the UK also showed no effects.

A cohort study of over 7000 people living within 50 metres of electrical substations or overhead power lines in East Anglia in 1971 was followed up to 1983. Standardised mortality rates did not show any increased risk for people close to electromagnetic fields.

Microwave frequencies (mobile phones)

To date radiofrequency and microwave frequency fields used for communications show no evidence of health effects. People have not found any toxic effects on pregnant women for females using radiofrequency plastic-welding machines. A cohort study of 40 000 American naval personnel exposed to radar microwave emissions during the 1950s did not differ from unexposed personnel when followed up to 1974. It is perhaps unsurprising that staff of the American Embassy in Moscow, who were apparently exposed to much lower levels of microwaves for the 20 or so years preceding 1975, as part of the USSR surveillance of them, also showed no adverse effects. It is interesting to reflect what we could do even if a very small risk were ultimately to be demonstrated, given how widespread electricity power lines and equipment using microwaves are in our environment.

Events prolonged in time but of limited geography

Metals

The element cadmium is less common than lead in the environment but is occasionally problematical. It enters the environment as a contaminant from chemical industries as well as from metallurgy or electroplating. It also occurs as a contaminant in oil refining and can get into water sources from petrochemical effluent. Chronic cadmium poisoning causes renal tubular damage, proteinuria and, sometimes, secondary hypertension.

A study of residents of Toyoma City in Japan, which had been built on top of an old mining complex, showed that water contaminated with cadmium had caused disease. In the late 1970s, villagers in Shipham, Somerset became concerned about the fact that their local environment was contaminated with waste cadmium from zinc mining carried out over the previous centuries. Their concern was increased when study of a volunteer sample of villagers suggested an increased prevalence of hypertension. Volunteers are not a representative sample and local hospital statistics and further measurements showed no increase of hypertension in the population. One might expect any long-term adverse effects to be evident in increased mortality. Comparison of mortality rates for residents of Shipham over the age of 40 during the period 1939–70 with national mortality rates showed that they had a low mortality rate. However, comparison of mortality rates with an uncontaminated control village showed a similar mortality. This may have been the result of the socioeconomic benefit of living in a lovely, rural environment. Thus, as with lead or any other environmental toxin, contamination does not necessarily lead to ill health, although it may be aesthetically or psychological unacceptable to the population concerned.

A more important risk is caused by exposure to mercury. It is known from occupational epidemiology that it is a powerful neurotoxin, with symptoms resulting from relatively small concentrations in blood. Interestingly the expression 'mad as a hatter' was first applied to hatters who used mercury to treat the felts used in hat manufacture. Mercury also enters the environment from agricultural practices, the plastics and electronic industries as well as from burning fossil fuels.

> ### Environmental events occurring over a long period or a wide geographic area
>
> ➤ Air pollution from combustion in burning of fossil fuels or motor car exhausts gives rise to high ozone levels and pollution with small particles, lead and other chemicals.
>
> ➤ Contamination of the food chain with toxins or infectious diseases can affect large populations before the risk is identified. The risk to the Public Health from 'New' diseases such as BSE are difficult to assess.
>
> ➤ Potentially dangerous substances occurring naturally in the environment may reach dangerous concentrations in certain geographical areas, e.g. radon gas in homes.
>
> ➤ Radioactive waste from nuclear processes can enter the food chain particularly after an accident of the magnitude of the Chernobyl reactor accident.
>
> ➤ Although excess lead in the body clearly has adverse effects, it is less clear what effect general environmental exposure to lead has.

A notable epidemic of mercury poisoning, subsequently termed Minamata disease, occurred during the 1950s at Minamata, Japan. This neurological disease with a high death rate was linked to fish consumption when the associated cat population also exhibited neurological poisoning. This led to the cause being identified. Waste from a chemical factory in the vicinity of Minamata Bay contained inorganic mercury and this was transformed by aquatic organisms into much more toxic methylmercury. This was absorbed into fish and subsequently eaten by humans and cats.

Industrial toxic waste

The Toxic Substances Control Act in the USA and similar legislation in the UK regulate disposal and waste treatment. However, the situation in the recent past is recognised to have been unacceptable, with a casual attitude to disposal and the proliferation of toxic waste. The greatest risk is probably ingestion of water from contaminated water reserves, but food contamination or inhalation around sites or processing plants is also possible.

The firm Rechem established a plant for high-temperature incineration of toxic waste in Pontypool in South Wales in 1974. There was little local opposition when it was set up as traditional industries in the area were in decline and the new employment was welcomed. Torfaen Borough Council under the Control of Pollution Act 1974 licensed the plant. Concern was later raised that the plant was causing congenital malformations locally. The Welsh Office investigated by making a comparison of local rates of microphthalmos with rates based on the standard notification scheme and also rates from data held by the Gwent Health Authority and the Institute of Medical Genetics at the University of Wales College of Medicine. These data are shown in Table 16.1 and reveal no excess of congenital malformation at birth around the Rechem plant.

There are particular problems with environmental epidemiological studies of congenital malformation. One is that reporting defects at birth as a way of monitoring environmental teratogens is very insensitive.

The true effect would be best shown by a rate for abnormalities divided by all conceptions. From ad hoc studies it seems that about 40% of conceptions are normally lost at an early stage of pregnancy as miscarriages; 60% of these show chromosomal abnormalities. It is likely that any environmental hazard would have an effect upon these early abortions.

A second problem is the incompleteness of routinely collected data, which may be biased if local interest and detective work selectively unearths cases compared with a lack of such effort in other areas. In Scotland, a report on the incidence of microphthalmos found that over the previous 15 years 49 cases were reported to the routine notification system. However, if they linked all possible sources of data for congenital malformations a further 50 cases were unearthed.

Such biases were also shown by a survey of birth defects and cancer near the Drake Superfund site, Pennsylvania. Male bladder cancer rates were increased over national rates but not female rates. Environmental carcinogens would be expected to present the same risk to both sexes. The observed male excess no doubt related to exposure in local chemical industries and perhaps to committed and educated industrial medical officers looking for this known risk in their workforce.

Nuclear power plants

Nuclear power plants are increasingly seen as an environmental risk. This may be because of their association with nuclear weapons. The geographical distribution of nuclear sites in the UK is shown in Figure 16.1. No general increase in cancer mortality has been observed near nuclear sites in the UK during the period 1959–80, but lymphoblastic leukaemia in populations within 5 miles of sites operating before 1955 appeared to be increased in young people less than 25 years old. There have been suggestions of an increased incidence of childhood leukaemia in the town of Seascale, which is about 2 miles from the reprocessing plant at Sellafield, Cumbria. This led to the formation of a Government Advisory Group in 1983. A subsequent follow-up of over 1000 children

Table 16.1 Cases of anophthalmos and microphthalmos in Wales and Gwent

Area	Cases		Rate per 10 000 births	
	Notifications	Specific enquiry	Notifications	Specific enquiry
Gwent	–	2	–	0.4
Wales	13	21	0.4	0.6

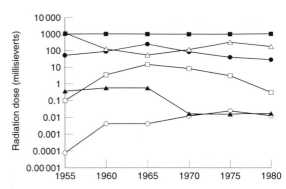

Fig. 16.2 Dose equivalents to red bone marrow of 1-year-old children near nuclear installations: ■, natural; O, fall-out; ▼, Sellafield; ◆, Downreay; ▲, Harwell; ●, Aldermaston. (Bithell et al 1994)

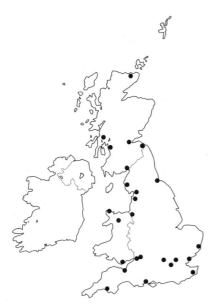

Fig. 16.1 Main nuclear sites giving rise to radioactive waste in the UK. (Bithell et al 1994)

born in the town revealed five leukaemia deaths compared with 0.53 expected on the basis of national mortality rates. There were 60 000 children aged 0–14 years living within 8 miles of the Atomic Weapons Research Establishment at Aldermaston, the Royal Ordnance factory at Burghfield or the Atomic Energy Research Establishment at Harwell during 1972–85. The normal expectation of leukaemia in these children was two cases per year whereas the recorded incidence was three cases per year.

It has been suggested that radioactive discharges may be responsible for these increased rates of childhood leukaemia. However, it has been concluded that the increase in childhood leukaemia near Dounreay could not be accounted for by radioactive discharges from the site unless doses to the stem cells have been grossly underestimated. Dose calculations have been based on measured discharges using mathematical models for radionuclide migration in the environment and absorption in tissues and contain some uncertainties. Typical radiation doses to the red bone marrow calculated at 5-year intervals for 1-year-old children living near installations are shown in Figure 16.2. The doses resulting from discharges are less than those from natural radiation except for Sellafield in the mid 1950s. No correlation with dose or dose effect is observed however, and the doses around Aldermaston and Harwell are over a 1000 times less than at Seascale. Other aetiological factors have been suggest-

ed to explain the increased incidence, such as infectious disease or, more recently, that the observed geographical excess near Sellafield can be explained by paternal employment and external radiation dose at the plant before the conception of the child, i.e. occupational exposure.

Events limited in time and geography

Events that are limited in time scale and area tend to be technological disasters, often caused by explosions or other catastrophes. They are not a new phenomenon, as evidenced by the sinking of the Titanic. However, the scale and complexity of industrial plant and the hazardous substances produced or manipulated on such sites increase all the time. If uncontrolled, these may pose risks at some localities exceeding those of more recognisable hazards such as infectious disease.

> **Environmental events occurring over a long time period in a limited area**
>
> ➤ Relatively rare heavy metals (e.g. cadmium, mercury) can accumulate in local areas and may cause poisoning, particularly at processing plants or near waste tips.
>
> ➤ Organic chemicals in toxic waste maybe teratogenic and/or carcinogenic.
>
> ➤ Ionising radiation from nuclear power plants could be a hazard.

Industrial accidents

The Seveso incident

The Icmesa chemical plant near Milan was involved in the synthesis of a compound used to make herbicides and bactericides. Industrial synthesis is simple. However, if the temperature is allowed to exceed 225°C then a contaminant, dioxin, is formed. In addition the reaction can 'run-away'. On the 10th July 1976 this happened and a chemical reactor in the plant exploded and distributed dioxin in a cloud of droplets over the surrounding area, including parts of the towns of Meda, Cesano, Maderno, Desio and Seveso.

Dioxin is toxic. A common feature seen in occupational exposure is chloracne, a persistent and disfiguring form of acne, which appears about 6 weeks after exposure. There can also be liver malfunction. The treatment of dioxin poisoning is symptomatic. The half-life in the body is long since the molecule is metabolically stable and it concentrates in the liver. Screening of all children under the age of 15 in the affected areas revealed 164 cases of chloracne. More importantly, dioxin is known to be a very potent teratogen and a number of pregnant women in the affected areas, upon learning this, sought abortions. Dioxin is firmly bound to soil and in contaminated areas it proved necessary to remove it by burying the topsoil and vegetation. The Seveso incident exposed the need for emergency planning since evacuation of the affected area was not undertaken until 14 days later.

The accident at Bhopal

Union Carbide, an American multinational company, had a plant near Bhopal, the industrial capital of the central Indian State of Madhyar Pradesh. The plant was synthesising the pesticide carbaryl (Sevin), an organic isocyanate. A tank at Bhopal held over 17 000 litres of an isocyanate, which has a low boiling point and in gaseous form is heavier than air. At the time, no occupational exposure data existed although it was known that some forms of isocyanate could induce asthma. The high reactivity of the isocyanates, which makes them so attractive to the chemical industry, also makes them toxic.

Safety measures at the plant were poor. The isocyanate in the tank polymerised and the heat released caused the tank to explode. In the early hours of December 3rd 1984, the vapour escaped and a creeping yellow and deadly vapour cloud some two to three miles wide invaded the crowded shantytowns of Chola Nagar and Jayaprakash Nagar. Over 2000 people were killed. Pulmonary oedema and corneal ulceration were the most common severe effects seen. The long-term effects have also involved the lungs and the eyes. The ignorance and unpreparedness of the local population and the health authorities highlighted the lack of information and planning between the industry and local government.

This disaster and similar lessons learnt from the Seveso incident acted as a spur to the UK government, in collaboration with the Health and Safety Executive and local authorities, to adopt schemes for information disclosure and emergency planning for protecting public health.

Contamination of the Lowermoor water reservoir

On 6th July 1988, 20 tons of concentrated aluminium sulphate solution was accidentally emptied into the Lowermoor water reservoir near Camelford, Cornwall. In the first few days following the incident, the water was discoloured and had a poor taste but the water company advised consumers that it was safe. Some people felt unwell, others had an apparent worsening of pre-existing conditions such as eczema, arthritis or digestive problems. Symptoms included vomiting, diarrhoea, fatigue, rashes and mouth ulcers. Public concern and media interest resulted in the Government setting up independent advice. The experts reported their assessment of the public health implications of the incident in July 1989. They drew several conclusions.

- For 1 to 3 days, most consumers received water of pH below 5 (guide values for pH are set at a minimum of 6.5 to minimise corrosion of plumbing systems).
- Aluminium concentrations of 10 to 50 mg/l occurred over the same period.
- Up to 1 month later, aluminium concentrations in water were above the Maximum Admissible Concentration in the European Commission's Water Directive.
- Early symptoms were mild and short-lived, as general practitioners saw no increase in consultation rates over the month from the incident.
- It is extremely unlikely that long-term effects from copper, sulphate, zinc or lead would result from the level of doses experienced.
- Toxic effects of aluminium are associated with

chronically elevated exposure, but most aluminium ingested would have been rapidly excreted.

They made several recommendations based upon the lessons learned.

- Water companies must notify the directors of Public Health and the Environmental Health Department of the local authority if any untoward event occurs.
- If significant chemical contamination occurs, arrangements should be made for an alternative public supply.
- The public and the media should have medical and scientific information and advice as soon as possible.

Environmental events

➤ Exposure causing disease can occur over a prolonged time scale and wide geographical area, e.g. motor care exhaust gases.

➤ Some events are very limited in time scale and area affected; these tend to be technological disasters caused by catastrophes such as explosions at industrial sites.

Occupationally linked diseases

17

In this chapter the concept of occupation health is discussed:

- industrially related disease notification and benefits
- identification of potential hazards
- monitoring methods to detect early signs of ill health
- monitoring methods to detect hazard levels that are becoming dangerous.

Introduction

Occupational health is concerned with:

- diseases that are unequivocally linked to work
- diseases of multifactorial aetiology in which occupational factors are involved.

Examples of diseases unequivocally linked to work are:

- coal worker's pneumoconiosis
- asbestosis and mesothelioma in workers exposed to asbestos
- angiosarcoma of the liver in workers exposed to vinyl chloride monomer.

Workers who are especially susceptible to exposures which are not a problem to the working population in general are a subgroup of those where occupational factors are only part of the cause.

Hazardous materials

The computer registry of the Chemical Abstracts Service contains references to more than four million different chemical compounds. Some 5000 new chemical compounds are produced annually, including pesticides, food additives and drugs. It is estimated that about 60 000 compounds are in common use but only

of the order of 4000 have been subjected to toxicological testing. Surveys in the USA showed that more than seven million workers are involved with products containing toxic substances that are regulated by the Occupational Health and Safety Administration and another half million with products containing regulated carcinogens.

The strategy used to try to control these hazards to health occurs in several discrete steps:

- toxicity: measured in model systems
- risk assessment: from toxicity measurements and exposure estimates
- risk evaluation: from assessment of risk and benefit and the alternatives available
- epidemiological surveillance: to guard against unsuspected risks and as verification
- evaluation: responsibility and resources for safe handling.

To get some idea of the scale of a hazard a programme of toxicity testing is set up. High risks can be identified at an early stage and prevent a toxicant being used on a large scale. For example additives to baked beans, beer or cosmetics are potentially more significant than those to yacht varnish! People use bioassays and related studies to identify occupational carcinogens. This may need 2–3 years of experiments using animals. However some clues can be gained in a few weeks or months using a battery of laboratory methods based on the detection of genetic damage (mutations in bacteria and mammalian cells).

Adverse health effects

Most adverse health effects have been discovered through epidemics of disease in exposed workers. In most of these epidemics, the connection between occupation and disease has been made only because a large number of workers were affected. If the disease in question is rare in the general population, then recognising the occupational connection is relatively easy. A very high incidence of cancer of the nasal septum in workers at a nickel refining plant in South Wales before the Second World War revealed the hazards of nickel carbonyl because the cancer was uncommon in the population.

In 1974 only three cases of liver angiosarcoma were diagnosed among workers at a single plant in the USA involved in the manufacture of vinyl chloride for polyvinyl chloride. Despite the small number of case, studies have confirmed this risk for exposure to vinyl chloride. Other examples of diseases linked to occupational exposure include:

● exposures to engineering oils can cause skin cancer
● particular dyes can cause bladder cancer
● hard wood dusts can cause nasal cancer
● asthma is commonly related to industrial exposures.

Asthma

The various dust-related diseases are declining except for occupational asthma. Asthma is common in the community, with a prevalence among adults of approximately 5%. Occupational asthma accounts for approximately 10% of adult asthma cases. Over 200 agents are suspected of causing the condition, although only 14 are recognised under the Industrial Injuries scheme. Three main categories of agents account for over 75% of cases within this scheme: isocyanates, solder flux flume and flour/grain dust. The high-risk occupations for industrial asthma are shown in Table 17.1.

Other diseases

Some of the adverse occupational health effects, such as cancer, pulmonary diseases and neurological deficits, have long latency periods as well as relatively high background incidence levels in the general population. For these, large study groups and extended follow-up periods are required. Exhaustive follow-up over decades of the male population in the mining valleys of South Wales has demonstrated that pneumoconiosis, caused by exposure to coal dust, was a very significant public health problem.

Identifying hazards

A cohort approach can often be used in occupational epidemiology. Many environmental factors produce effects only after a long period of exposure. This is the case for chemicals that accumulate in the body (i.e. cadmium) or hazards that have a cumulative effect (i.e. radiation or noise). For these hazards, the past exposure levels and the exposure duration may be more important than the current exposure. The **total exposure** (or external dose) needs to be estimated. It is often approximated as the product of exposure duration and exposure level. Examples of identifying hazards in this way include the effects of exposure to carbon disulphide, asbestos and noise.

Carbon disulphide

An example of the cohort approach is the identification of a possible hazardous effect of carbon disulphide. This is used in the manufacture of artificial silk (viscose rayon). Wood pulp is treated and dissolved in carbon disulphide and extruded as viscose. The process has been of industrial importance since early in the 20th century. Italian workers exposed to high levels of carbon disulphide in the 1940s exhibited neurological symptoms and in some cases psychosis. Until the 1980s, several thousand workers were employed producing viscose in factories in North Wales. A cohort of exposed workers was compared retrospectively with a cohort of unexposed workers and a small excess of heart disease was identified amongst those exposed.

Asbestos

Asbestos was used as a fire retardant between floors in buildings. Asbestos is a generic name for fibrous silicates of different chemical composition. Epidemiological studies have shown that exposure can cause asbestosis, a progressive lung disease that, in severe cases, can lead to death in 5 to 10 years. Crocidolite, one of the forms, has been shown to be the cause of

Table 17.1 High-risk occupations for asthma (Cartier 1998)

Occupational group	Cases	Population	Rate/million per year
Welders/solderers/ electronic assemblers	35	220 068	159
Laboratory technicians and assistants	26	127 478	204
Metal making and treating	14	56 270	249
Plastic making and processing	27	66 005	409
Bakers	29	70 839	409
Chemical processors	31	73 189	424
Coach and spray painters	35	54 737	639
Other painters	21	201 255	104

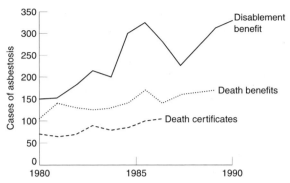

Fig. 17.1 Incidence of asbestosis by disablement benefit, death certificates or death benefits. (Ennals 1991)

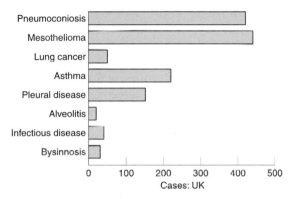

Fig. 17.2 Incidence of occupational lung disease per year. (Ennals 1991)

Table 17.2 Occupations associated with asbestos-related disease in males (Mossman & Gee 1989)			
Occupational group	Cases	Population	Rate/million per year
Electricians and power plant operators	40	354 579	113
Building and construction workers (includes laggers)	100	728 202	137
Plumbers and heating engineers	33	184 872	179
Boiler operators	14	9 862	1420
Shipyard and dock workers	77	47 792	1611

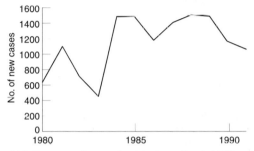

Fig. 17.3 New cases of occupational deafness. (Ennals 1991)

lung cancer and mesothelioma. Fibre size and durability seem to be the determining factors. The trend for asbestosis is shown in Figure 17.1 and the occupations associated with the highest risk of asbestos-related disease in Table 17.2. The current incidence of occupational lung disease is shown in Figure 17.2.

Noise

Another significant occupational exposure is that of noise. Noise-induced hearing loss occurs as a result of prolonged and repeated exposure to higher intensity sound at work. If the ear is exposed to high levels of noise for a short period, a test of the sensitivity of the ear (audiometry) taken immediately afterwards reveals a small hearing loss; this is known as temporary threshold shift. However, in industry the periods of exposure to high-intensity noise can be long and when these are repeated daily for a number of years a permanent hearing loss occurs. This, in conjunction with the natural progressive hearing loss owing to age can result in severe disability in later life. The trend for

---

Occupational risks

➤ Modern industries use a vast array of chemical compounds for which toxicity and risk: benefit ratios can be assessed.

➤ Exposure to asbestos is associated with asbestosis and mesothelioma.

➤ Asthma is associated with dust-generating industries. Isocyanates, solder flux flume and flour/grain dusts are major causative agents.

➤ Some diseases have long latency periods and may be identified by cohort studies.

---

occupationally induced deafness is shown in Figure 17.3.

Surveillance in occupational health

Health care in the workplace includes:

● identification of diseases known to be associated with working in particular industries

- identification of potential hazards in industry likely to cause illness
- ensuring that those who suffer industrial disease receive compensation.

Reporting of diseases

In the UK, there is a statutory responsibility to report certain prescribed diseases (Table 17.3) and there are also special benefits for people injured or absent from work because of industrial injuries.

The Health and Safety Executive provides statistics relating to occupational ill health. The official data come from three main sources:

- benefit payments made
- prescribed diseases reported
- deaths in which a prescribed disease is mentioned.

Epidemiological surveillance

The search for previously unrecognised health effects, sometimes called epidemiological surveillance, may use a number of sources. Records collected for other purposes, such as accident and illness records, insurance data, workers' compensation claims, absenteeism data, retiree death certificates, or even city, county or state vital statistics records may be analysed for illnesses related to the workplace. Routine physical and laboratory examinations and symptom questionnaires

Table 17.3 Occupational diseases for which benefit is paid through the National Insurance (Industrial Injuries) Act 1965 in the UK

Disease group	Individual diseases
Poisoning	Poisoning with Pb, Mn, As, Hg, P, CS_2, Be, Cd, Ni (CO_4), benzene and derivatives, etc.
Chest disease	Pneumoconiosis, byssinosis, occupational asthma
Infections	Viral hepatitis, anthrax, glanders, leptospira, farmer's lung, brucella
Damage caused by physical agents	Electromagnetic radiation, ionising radiation, heat cataract, decompression sickness, miner's nystagmus
Mechanical damage	Hand cramp, beat hand and knee, bursitis, inflammation of tendon
Cancer	Cornea, skin, etc. (tar and pitch), nose and lung (nickel), bladder (dyes etc.), mesothelioma (asbestos), nose (wood), angiosarcoma of the liver and osteolysis (VCM)
Other diseases	Dermatitis, ulceration of mouth, etc.

for medical screening purposes can be used to detect a cluster of unusual findings.

A workplace surveillance programme should be designed actively to search for new, previously unreported adverse effects so that aetiological relationships can be detected early and, preferably, at a reversible or treatable stage of disease. Information on spontaneous abortion, stillbirth, birth size, congenital malformation and infant mortality in relation to maternal and paternal occupation provide vital clues to the extent of reproductive hazards of work.

Health monitoring and screening

Preplacement and periodic clinical examinations play an important role in occupational health.

Preplacement medical examination
This should enable

- proper job placement to be made according to the physical and mental capabilities of the worker
- identification of people likely to be vulnerable to certain exposures.
- baseline data to be collected for use in assessing early adverse effects of exposure (e.g. lung function tests and audiometry).

Periodic health examination
This allows

- evaluation of the effectiveness of preventive measures; a group of workers may show clinical or biological evidence of excessive exposures
- identification of workers showing undue susceptibility to a particular type of exposure.

Monitoring reproductive health

There are growing concerns about possible risks to reproductive health. Certain hazards during pregnancy are already known, e.g. exposure to benzene; toluene, chlorinated hydrocarbons, compounds of lead and mercury, etc. There is a certain dichotomy in the UK legislation in this area. On the one hand, the Employment Protection Act 1975 safeguards the right of the pregnant worker to continued employment during pregnancy. On the other hand, the UK Congenital Disabilities Act 1976 states that an employer may be sued by a disabled child where the disability is believed to result from exposure of either of its parents to a toxic chemical in the workplace.

It has been suggested that exposure of males may actually present a greater risk than exposure of females since sperm production involves division of cells throughout the reproductive life of males and, therefore, the chance of chemically induced mutations may be higher. Recently, workers involved in the manufacture of dibromochloropropane, a soil pesticide, have been shown to suffer infertility problems.

Occupational screening

Screening in occupational medicine is aimed at secondary prevention through the early detection of ill health. Detection of early changes might serve as a warning of conditions in the workplace even if the individual cannot be helped. Examples of various types of occupational screening are listed in Table 17.4.

Biological monitoring

Biological monitoring techniques are designed to measure chemical agents, their metabolites or early, nonpathological indicators of exposure. The aim is to detect evidence of absorption before any adverse effect occurs. Examples include monitoring

- blood for lead levels
- adipose tissue for polychlorobiphenyls (PCBs)

Table 17.4 Occupational screening

Screening method	Function
Chest X-rays	Diagnosis of overt disease, e.g. pneumoconiosis
Physical examination	Looking for signs of disease, e.g. dermatitis, nasal perforation in chromium workers
Questionnaires	To elicit symptoms such as headache in solvent exposure
Laboratory testing	To identify pathophysiological and biochemical abnormalities, e.g. nerve conduction studies to detect early peripheral neuropathy (Csi); liver function tests to detect early hepatotoxicity in hydrocarbon exposure; blood cell examination to detect early haematotoxicity in benzene exposure; solvent concentrations in expired air; solvent metabolites in urine

- red blood cell cholinesterase in workers exposed to anticholinesterase pesticides.

Environmental monitoring

The aim of environmental monitoring is to limit exposure to levels that impose no serious threat to health during a normal lifetime of work. There are permissible levels of chemical substances known as Occupational Exposure Limits. These refer to airborne concentrations of substances and represent conditions under which it is believed that nearly all workers may be exposed day after day without adverse effect. Because of a wide variation in individual susceptibility, a small percentage of workers may experience discomfort below the exposure limits. Aggravation of another condition or development of an occupational illness may seriously affect a smaller percentage. Environmental monitoring aims to:

- detect unsafe/unhealthy conditions
- identify an emission source
- aid the design of control measures and assess their effectiveness
- record changes and relate these to consequent changes in disease occurrence
- ensure compliance with regulations
- assess serious hazards in confined spaces before people enter.

Occupational health

- ➤ Certain prescribed diseases must be reported and there are special benefits available to those with industrially related disease.

- ➤ Health care in the workplace includes identifying potential hazards and compensating those affected by industrial disease.

- ➤ Screening for industrial disease involves monitoring workers by medical examination before commencing work and regularly during work (e.g. by blood tests) and monitoring the working environment for the presence of hazards in dangerous quantities.

Infectious disease

18

The impact of infectious disease is discussed in terms of:

- surveillance of communicable diseases
- modes of disease transmission
- sources of disease
- disease in developing countries.

Introduction

The impact of communicable disease upon the health of the public has declined considerably, in developed countries, from that found at the start of the 20th century. Nevertheless, it is still responsible for significant morbidity and mortality.

Definitions

There are a number of terms that are used to describe the development and spread of infections.

Incubation period. This refers to the time elapsed between infection and the onset of symptoms. Each organism has a characteristic incubation period, although this can vary somewhat depending upon the status of the host, e.g. age and susceptibility, etc.

Host response. There is a spectrum of clinical response in an exposed population depending on factors such as host immune status, underlying disease, etc.

Communicability. The infectious agent may pass to carriers who are symptomless.

Epidemic. An increase in incidence above that which may be continuously present in a population (endemic).

Outbreak. Two or more cases of infection with a suggested relation, i.e. transmission between cases or exposure to a common source of infection. There is usually a clustering of the cases in time or space, though the extent of this will vary with the disease in question.

Attack rate. The proportion of the population at risk that fell ill during an outbreak.

Reservoir of infection. The habitat of the infectious agent, which may be in humans (e.g. measles), animals (e.g. *Cryptosporidium* sp.) or the environment (e.g. *Legionella* sp.).

Source of infection. May be the reservoir or, for example, may be contamination of food or water (termed the vehicle for infection).

Mode of transmission. The method by which the infection spreads.

The control of communicable diseases

In the health authorities in the UK the Consultant in Communicable Disease Control (CCDC) is responsible for prevention and control as well as surveillance of communicable diseases. The Public Health Laboratory Service (PHLS) provides support to these consultants at a national level. It has approximately 50 laboratories distributed throughout England and Wales and about 20 reference and special laboratories at the centre in Colindale. It has national responsibility for investigation and control through provision of advice and assistance to the health authorities as well as for surveillance and immunisation programmes. There is a legal requirement to notify the health authority of those infectious diseases shown in Table 18.1. The incidence of notifiable diseases changes with many factors, such as improved therapy and environmental control reducing incidence and lifestyle changes, which may increase it.

Anthrax, brucellosis and bovine tuberculosis

These diseases have virtually been eliminated. Anthrax has been developed, in the past, for germ warfare.

Viral hepatitis

Infection from hepatitis A virus, as measured by notifi-

Table 18.1 Infectious diseases requiring notification

Acute encephalitis
Acute poliomyelitis
Anthrax
Cholera
Diphtheria
Dysentery (amoebic or bacillary)
Food poisoning
Leprosy
Leptospirosis
Malaria
Measles
Meningitis
Meningococcal septicaemia (without meningitis)
Mumps
Ophthalmia neonatorum
Paratyphoid fever
Plague
Rabies
Relapsing fever
Rubella
Scarlet fever
Tetanus
Tuberculosis
Typhoid fever
Typhus
Viral haemorrhagic fever
Viral hepatitis
Whooping cough
Yellow fever

patients. Carriers may transmit the virus sexually, parenterally or perinatally. Infection may progress to chronic liver disease and hepatocellular carcinoma. It is estimated that there are 200–300 million carriers worldwide, primarily in the Far East, where the carrier rate may be 20%. Perinatal transmission is probably the primary mode of transmission there.

Modes of transmission of disease

An outbreak or epidemic of infectious disease requires not just a source but also transmission. There are a number of transmission methods and infections may spread by one or more of the following methods:

- airborne, e.g. tuberculosis
- foodborne, e.g. salmonellal, listerial infections
- waterborne, e.g. typhoid rotavirus
- direct contact, e.g. sexual (gonorrhoea) or wound contact
- indirect contact, faecal–oral route, e.g. shigellae infection
- insect-borne, e.g. malaria
- through the skin, e.g. schistosomiasis or leptospirosis
- contaminated blood, e.g., hepatitis B.

This transmission, in turn, involves environmental and social factors, which we have to consider for investigation and control. Some infectious agents use several modes of transmission, however, it is convenient to describe infections by their main method of transmission.

Direct spread from patients or carriers

Many serious diseases of the past that were spread by direct contact have drastically declined. Table 18.2 describes some of these and their characteristics.

cation of infections, has fallen since the mid-1980s to 4000 per annum in the UK. Small outbreaks associated with contamination of shellfish have occurred and travel to areas abroad where hepatitis A is endemic carries some risk. Hepatitis B (HBV) virus infection increased in the mid-1980s amongst intravenous drug abusers and it is about five times more frequent in health-care staff than in the general population. Immunisation of health-care staff reduces the risk to

Table 18.2 Diseases with direct transmission from patients or carriers

Disease	Comment
Smallpox	The greatest success in infectious disease control has been the worldwide eradication of smallpox, with no cases since 1978
Poliomyelitis	Salk vaccine was introduced in 1956 and then live attenuated (Sabin) vaccine in 1962. The maintenance of immunisation rates of 70–80% has stopped epidemics of poliomyelitis in the UK since the mid 1960s. However, the virus remains endemic in many parts of the world and UK experience in 1977 revealed that even in well-vaccinated communities wild virus may spread in unvaccinated groups
Diphtheria	In the UK, 84% of children complete three doses of diphtheria toxoid by the age of 2 years. The number of cases per year in the UK is less than five but the disease could still be imported, especially from the Russian Republic, where numbers are rising
Scarlet fever	This is a manifestation of acute haemolytic streptococcal infection; it has declined by a factor of 20 since the Second World War, with approximately 6000 cases occurring per annum in the late 1980s

Table 18.2 *(cont'd)*

Disease	Comment
Measles	Immunisation was introduced in 1968 and the subsequent trend in notification is shown in Figure 18.1. Notification of measles rose in 1994 (Fig. 18.2), with three-quarters of the cases being of school age
Rubella	Immunisation of schoolgirls aged 10 to 14 years was introduced in the 1970s in the UK. Uptake in 1995 was approximately 95%
Tuberculosis	Before the First World War there were over 100 000 cases per annum with 5000 deaths, but this has declined to less than 6000 cases and 600 deaths per year in the early 1990s. Incidence is increasing in susceptible groups such as immigrants from Asia and people immunocompromised by HIV infection or medicines
Chickenpox	Remains endemic, with up to a quarter of a million cases in peak years
Meningococcal infection	This has a case fatality rate of about 20% for those less than 1 year old. It is lower in young adults and rises again to 33% in old people. It appeared as group A epidemically during the periods of the First and Second World Wars, but group A has almost disappeared now in the UK. In 1986, over 1000 cases were reported with the emergence of a group B strain, type 15, which causes more infections in teenagers and young adults. The nasopharyngeal carriage rate in the population of pathogenic strains associated with outbreaks is between 10 and 25%. Recent trends in incidence and the number of deaths are shown in Figure 18.3. Viral infections of the nervous system cause considerable morbidity, with cases of meningitis and encephalitis caused by echovirus mumps and herpes simplex virus meningitis is discussed further in Chapter 19.
Respiratory virus infection	Respiratory syncytial viruses and parainfluenza virus cause pneumonia in young children, with a peak incidence in the winter. They are commonest in the very young (Fig. 18.4). The last UK epidemic of influenza A virus was in 1976. Influenza B virus outbreaks usually occur amongst children in schools
Pertussis	Immunisation started in 1957; however, following a marked decline in uptake in the late 1970s owing to public fears about the safety of the vaccine, there were epidemics in 1977–9 and 1981–3 (Fig. 18.5). The public fears were based on a combination of poor communications between senior academics in public health and the press and scare-mongering on the part of the latter. The damage done has taken years to reverse. Those who suffered were small children
Helicobacter pylori infection	Our understanding of peptic ulcers has drastically changed since the first report on *H. pylori*. It is now widely accepted that *H. pylori* is the main cause of duodenal ulcers and most gastric ulcers. The relationship to non-ulcer dyspepsia is less well understood. Eradication of *H. pylori* with antibiotics improves healing and reduces ulcer recurrence

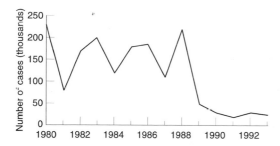

Fig. 18.1 Measles notifications in England and Wales for 10–14 year olds. (PHLS Communicable Disease Surveillance Centre 1994)

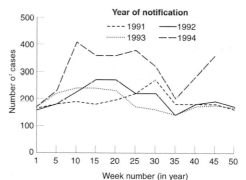

Fig. 18.2 Measles notifications in England and Wales for 10–14 year olds at varying stages of the year for a series of 4 years. (PHLS Communicable Disease Surveillance Centre 1994)

Faecal–oral transmission

Disease with faecal–oral transmission are summarised in Table 18.3.

There are many other infectious agents whose mode of transmission is by food or water. These will also spread by the faecal–oral route.

Food- and waterborne disease

Table 18.4 summarises those diseases that are food- or waterborne

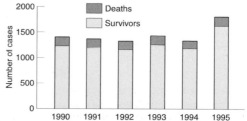

Fig. 18.3 Meningococcal disease in England and Wales. (PHLS Communicable Disease Surveillance Centre 1994)

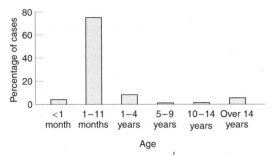

Fig. 18.4 Respiratory syncytial virus infection in children of varying age in England and Wales over the period 1990–5. (PHLS Communicable Disease Surveillance Centre 1994)

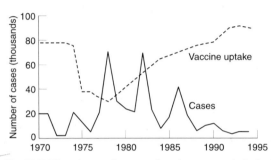

Fig. 18.5 Whooping cough cases and vaccine coverage in England and Wales over the period 1970–95. (PHLS Communicable Disease Surveillance Centre 1994)

Table 18.3 Diseases with faecal–oral transmission

Disease	Comment
Cholera	High standards of water supply and sewage disposal are responsible for the virtual disappearance of this disease in the UK; a small number of imported cases occur
Shigellae infections	*Shigella sonnei* is the most common species in infections in the UK with about 5000 cases per year; spreads mainly in family groups or children's nurseries
Rotavirus infections	There were 8000 reported cases in 1985, mainly of gastroenteritis in young children

Sexually transmitted diseases

Acquired immune deficiency syndrome (AIDS) is an example of an infectious disease transmitted by sexual contact.

However, it is just one of a number of sexually transmitted diseases that are endemic in the UK. There were approximately 100 000 cases of sexually transmitted disease per annum in the 1930s, twice this rate in the 1940s before falling back to 100 000 in the 1950s.

Table 18.4 Food- and waterborne diseases

Disease	Comment
Campylobacter infection	The most frequent cause of acute diarrhoea in the UK, with 40 000 cases reported in 1994. Contaminated poultry are suspected to be the main reservoir and vehicle but waterborne outbreaks also occur
Salmonellosis	Food poisoning notifications are increasing year by year. Salmonellosis is a common cause of food poisoning, with over 20 000 cases and 40 deaths per year. Poultry is the main reservoir and source although people have associated major outbreaks with particular foodstuffs (e.g. imported Italian chocolate and dried baby milk) or food prepared in hospital kitchens, etc. (Fig. 18.6)
Listeriosis	Foetal or neonatal death may follow infection in pregnancy. Approximately 100 cases per year occur, thought to be caused, in the main, by prolonged refrigeration of raw vegetables
Cryptosporidiosis	This zoonosis is of greatest threat to the public health through outbreaks of waterborne disease. There have been major episodes in the USA and in some areas of the UK, notably Swindon (Fig. 18.7). It is a self-limited diarrhoeal disease but presents particular problems to individuals who are immunocompromised
Giardiasis	Many waterborne outbreaks reported in the USA, and approximately 5000 cases per year of this diarrhoeal disease
Escherichia coli serotype 0157 infection	*E. coli* 0157 produces a cytotoxin. This type was responsible for an outbreak in Lanarkshire (detailed in Chapter 22) and later cases in Scotland. It causes a form of haemorrhagic colitis
Viral food poisoning	Many outbreaks are associated with shellfish contaminated by sewage

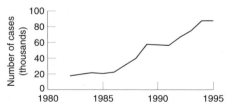

Fig. 18.6 Food poisoning notifications in England and Wales. (PHLS Communicable Disease Surveillance Centre 1994)

Following this there has been a continuous increase to over 600 000 by the late 1980s.

Syphilis (caused by *Treponema pallidum*) has declined from about 30 000 cases in the late 1940s to

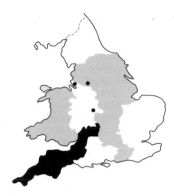

Fig. 18.7 Regional distribution of cryptosporidiosis in England and Wales; grey, more than 10 cases, black more than 20 cases per 100 000 population. (PHLS Communicable Disease Surveillance Centre 1994)

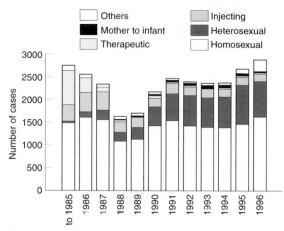

Fig. 18.8 Cases of HIV-1 by exposure category in the UK. (PHLS Communicable Disease Surveillance Centre 1994)

about 3000 cases in the late 1980s. However, **gonorrhoea** (caused by *Neisseria gonorrhoea*, the gonococcus) rates increased through the 1950s and 1960s to peak at 66 000 cases in 1973 followed by a fall in rate to just over 50 000 by the late 1980s.

Non-specific genital infection was first recorded in the early 1970s since when it has increased in males to approximately 100 000 cases per annum and in females to about half this rate. Infection with *Chlamydia trachomatis* is probably responsible for the doubling in pelvic inflammatory disease observed in the 1980s and 1990s. Clinic returns show cases of herpes simplex virus increasing since the early 1980s and 50 000 cases of human papillomavirus. The latter is associated with the development of cancer of the cervix and an increase has been observed in the death rate from cervical cancer in women less than 30 years of age.

AIDS

In 1981 outbreaks of *Pneumocystis carinii* pneumonia (PCP) and Kaposi's sarcoma were reported in homosexual men. The Centre for Disease Control (CDC) in Atlanta, USA had identified homosexual contact as the mode of transmission 2 years before the human immunodeficiency virus was isolated and identified. Transmission could also occur through contaminated blood and blood products. This caused HIV infection in haemophiliacs until controlled by donor screening and heat treatment of blood products. Spread also occurred amongst drug abusers sharing needles and by infection of babies born to mothers with the virus.

The first UK case was reported in 1981. By 1985 there were 275 cases with 140 deaths. More than 90% of these were homosexuals with the remainder falling into other known risk categories. In Africa heterosexu-

al spread is common. Fears that this might also happen in the UK have not been realised, as shown in Figure 18.8. In 1995 there was some sign of a reduction in the numbers of cases. The disease is currently incurable, though it is thought that some forms of treatment may prolong life.

Figure 18.8 shows that the overall number of cases dropped yearly until 1988 then increased gradually. The number of men with newly diagnosed HIV infection has remained at a similar number since records began. Cases in heterosexual men and women have steadily increased, especially for people exposed abroad. The number of infected people who are injecting drugs has fallen since a peak in 1991. This may be because of the development of needle exchange schemes. Mother-to-infant transmission is a small but particularly tragic cause of infection. Careful management of the labour has greatly reduced the number of cases in the late 1990s.

Hospital (nosocomial) infections

Surveys in the USA and the UK have shown that 5–10% of patients are infected by microorganisms in hospital. Many microorganisms are becoming resistant to antibiotic treatment and multiresistant organisms such as methicillin-resistant *Staphylococcus aureus* (MRSA) are very hard to treat and almost impossible to eradicate. In addition, improvements in medical treatments have led to an increasing number of vulnerable patients, including organ transplant patients and those on chemotherapy who will be immunosuppressed. These patients are susceptible to low-grade bacterial and fungal infections. There is a particular problem of infections associated with surgical

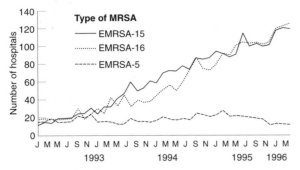

Fig. 18.9 Hospitals affected by epidemic MRSA in England and Wales. (PHLS Communicable Disease Surveillance Centre 1994)

Table 18.5 Disease spread by environmental transmission

Disease	Comments
Tetanus	Only 20–40 cases per year in the UK, but the ubiquity of the agent requires continued uptake of immunisation
Legionnaire's disease	*Legionella pneumophila* is widely present in the environment but outbreaks arise from airborne spread related to air-conditioning plants. Elderly people with underlying respiratory problems are most at risk
Amoeba	*Entamoeba histolytica* is the most important amoeba to cause disease in humans through amoebic dysentery and its complications
Amoebic meningo-encephalitis	Free-living amoebae of various species are widespread in warm fresh water and cause sporadic cases of disease similar to bacterial meningitis. It is thought to gain access to the brain by way of the olfactory epithelium

implants, which require stringent aseptic measures. *Staphylococcus aureus* is a major risk for implant patients and, more generally, MRSA may wreak havoc on a hospital ward. This is increasing in frequency (Fig. 18.9).

Intensive care units have suffered outbreaks of infection with *Klebsiella* and *Enterobacter* spp. Pneumonitis can occur when patients are immunosuppressed, for instance in cancer patients under treatment, or those with an incomplete immune system caused by HIV infection. The infecting organism is most commonly a protozoon, *Pneumocystis carinii*. These patients are also susceptible to systemic fungal infections, especially *Candida albicans*.

Group B streptococci are the most frequent causes of neonatal septicaemia and meningitis. The former occurs within a few days of birth and has a 50% case fatality rate even with early treatment. The organisms isolated from the babies are identical to those carried in their mother's vagina. Where clusters have occurred in neonatal units, no common source has been identified.

Environmental transmission

A number of infectious organisms have reservoirs in the environment:

- geonoses: residing in soil
- zoonoses residing in animals.

These can be spread by a variety of transmission modes.

Table 18.5 shows a summary of the main diseases spread by environmental transmission.

Zoonoses

Zoonoses are diseases which are spread from animals to humans. The spread of *Salmonella* sp. to from poul-

try has been described above; other important zoonoses are described in Table 18.6.

Changing human activities can alter the exposure to microorganisms, for example the increase in water sports results in more people being exposed to contaminated water. In addition, human activities may create an infectious threat where one did not previous exist. The possible transmission of the prion disease bovine spongiform encephalopathy (BSE) to humans may have occurred as a result of changes in the preparation of foodstuffs for cattle to include sheep protein. This may have allowed the prion to pass from sheep to cattle (see p. 116).

Infectious disease in developing countries

Although we have reduced the burden of infectious diseases in developed countries, they are still of great significance in developing countries. In addition to the profound social and economic effects these diseases have in the countries in question, the increase in movement between countries and speed of travel means that these infections can present in travellers from endemic areas. Table 18.7 shows the disease picture for the under 5-years-of-age group, which suffers most from infectious disease. Diarrhoeal diseases are the most significant. About 70% of young children who die could be saved if widespread low-cost oral rehydration therapy was available. The lack of adequate sanitation and clean water is also a cause of considerable disease from snail-borne schistosomiasis and river blindness as well as the worm diseases. The exotically sounding tropical diseases such as lishmaniasis, onchocerciasis and trypanosomiasis, although very important, are dwarfed by the public health impact of respiratory infections and measles.

Approximately three million children per year die of the complications of measles, tetanus and whooping cough. Malnutrition and diarrhoea have compound effect upon each other. Both render a child susceptible to the above complications but a protective course of vaccination only costs about £2.50 per child. Malaria continues to be a serious problem particularly in Africa, where it is estimated to cause over a million deaths per year. The life cycle of the malaria parasite involves passage between *Anopheles* mosquitoes and humans, and in Africa the difficulties and cost of pre-

Table 18.6 Common zoonoses in the UK

Disease	Comments
Lyme disease	Caused by the spirochete *Borrelia burgdorferi* and transmitted by ticks, primarily on deer. This multisystem disease with chronic sequelae has progressed from Lyme throughout the state of Connecticut, USA and has now established itself in parts of the UK
Toxocariasis	It is estimated that the *Toxocara canis* roundworm affects approximately 10% of dogs in the UK. It is transmitted to humans via contaminated hands. It continues to be an important infection in children. One must consider it in the investigation of a child with eosinophilia or endophthalmitis
Kawasaki disease	First recognised in Japan but now known worldwide, it mainly affects young children. The coronary arteries are involved and it may pose a risk for coronary atherosclerosis later in life. It is thought to be transmitted by a virus from cat fleas
Leptospirosis	Possibly the most widespread zoonosis in the world, being common in rodents but livestock is also affected. Animal urine can contaminate the environment, particularly rivers and canals and leptospires enter the body through mucus membranes or cuts. Farm workers have the greatest risk, but approximately a quarter of cases arises from water sports.

Infectious diseases

➤ Certain infectious diseases must be notified to the health authorities.

➤ The mode of transmission varies, some organisms spreading by more than one method:
  - direct contact, e.g. smallpox
  - faecal–oral route, e.g. shigellae infection
  - foodborne, e.g. salmonellosis
  - waterborne, e.g. typhoid
  - insect-borne, e.g. malaria
  - sexual transmission, e.g. syphilis.

➤ Hospital (nosocomial) infections are increasing because more organisms are becoming drug resistant and hospitals have increasing numbers of vulnerable patients, particularly those who are immunocompromised by disease or treatment.

➤ Zoonoses are diseases that have their reservoirs in animals from where they can spread to humans by various modes of transmission.

➤ In developing countries infectious diseases have a much greater impact particularly diseases such as measles and respiratory infections in children.

Table 18.7 Infectious diseases in children under 5 years of age in developing countries (Open University Press 1984)

Disease	No. children affected (millions)	No. children dying (millions)	No. children saved by intervention	Intervention: preventative or treatment
Diarrhoea	14	5	3.5	Oral rehydration
Malaria	9	1	Reduced	Drug treatment
Measles	8	1.9	All potentially	Vaccination
Respiratory (including pertussis)	6	2.9	0.6	Immunisation
Tetanus	3	0.8	All potentially	Immunisation
Other diseases	2	2	Avoided	Education

ventive environmental measures allied to emergent resistance to prophylaxis continue to cause concern.

It is also clear that HIV infection and AIDS is a hugely significant public health problem in developing countries. The WHO estimates that there are 15 million HIV-infected adults worldwide. Ten million of these live in sub-Saharan Africa. There are also just under two million people with the infection in each of Latin America and south-east Asia.

The solutions to these problems in the developing world will have to take roughly the same route as that taken by the developed countries. The nutrition, living conditions and wealth of the population need to improve. Education of the population must also improve so that they realise what needs to be changed. They will have to have the will to change those politico-economic circumstances both internationally and nationally that impede improvements to public health.

Viral haemorrhagic fevers (Africa, South America)

The viral haemorrhagic fevers occur in certain areas of the world. These are serious diseases often transmitted by insect vectors.

Lassa fever, Ebola and Marburg diseases
These are occasional seen outside Africa in travellers. They require nursing in isolation facilities.

Application of epidemiology to environmental problems

Investigation of disease outbreaks

In this chapter the methods used to investigate disease outbreaks are discussed with examples of their application:

- identifying a disease outbreak
- identifying affected individuals and treating them
- prevention of transmission
- investigation to draw conclusions regarding the epidemiology of the outbreak.

Introduction

The frequency with which the media report disease outbreaks associated with, for example, meningococcal meningitis, salmonellosis, cryptosporidiosis, Legionellosis gives some idea of their importance to the public. Since the media tend to report only the newsworthy, then one can conclude that the reported incidents are only a proportion of the outbreaks. Films such as 'Outbreak', about viral haemorrhagic disease, have been used to fill cinema seats with the potential horror of infectious diseases in our, supposedly safe, developed countries.

These messages suggest that modern developed societies should not suffer from such epidemics, but that they can occasionally break through. In real life, infectious diseases are constantly with us, but usually as sporadic cases. There is clearly a need to be able to identify cases and any resulting outbreaks, control them and then hopefully, by using the knowledge gained, prevent future occurrences. Epidemiological investigations are crucial for this. In particular, a close knowledge of the suspected disease and its characteristics is essential. An example of this is the incubation period of smallpox. The great majority of cases showed an incubation period of 12 days from exposure. One could, therefore, concentrate on people in contact with the index cases 12 days before.

If a number of cases of disease are reported the first steps are to:

- establish if an outbreak is occurring or has occurred
- define what constitutes a case and to decide if the provisional diagnoses fit with this definition
- act with some speed in case the outbreak is genuine
- treat and isolate suspected cases
- start contact tracing
- initiate microbiological testing, if available.

In some instances a decision will have to be made about whether to declare an outbreak before laboratory confirmation, bearing in mind the severity of the suspected disease, the unpleasantness or dangerousness of the treatment and the danger of panicking the local community. Ultimately, it is essential to confirm the diagnosis and to attempt to trace the sources and vehicles of infection.

Analytical epidemiology

The sequence of events occurring in the assessment and control of disease outbreaks can be considered to include:

1. Defining the event, identifying cases and collecting data
2. Control of disease: identification and treatment of patients
3. Management: prevention of transmission
4. Investigation: to allow conclusions regarding the epidemiology of the outbreak and prevention of future occurrences.

Obviously these steps will overlap and some actions will contribute to more than one area, for example prevention of transmission will assist control and management aspects.

1. Data collection

The first cases reported in an outbreak are only a fraction of the number of people who may be ultimately affected and the total population who are or were at risk from an infective agent is initially unknown. Detailed analysis of the initial cases is, therefore, very important in order to unearth things that they have in common. These may involve direct contact with particular people, food, drink or places. This will help to decide the size of the exposed population and, therefore, help to track down other cases. If, for example, the initial cases have been in a school or hotel, then other cases would be followed up from that setting. If the cases have all been in touch with a particular person then that person and their further contacts would need to be traced.

Once the population at risk has been identified then both the affected and unaffected individuals are given a standardised questionnaire. Information gathered may include age, sex, time of onset of illness, food eaten or drink taken, occupation. Attack rates can then be calculated using these parameters and this may give clues about the source of the disease or how it spread. This work can sometimes be delayed if the initial (index) patient is critically ill.

An example of data collection: acute asthma in Barcelona

Figure 19.1a shows the number of attacks of acute asthma in Barcelona during January 1986 reported to emergency rooms and Figure 19.1b shows that people were affected during certain hours of a particular day. Analysis of the area of the city in which presenting patients lived showed that cases were clustered around the vicinity of the docks regions of the city (Fig. 19.1c). This spurred further investigation of activities in the port during the working day. Later analyses showed an environmental allergen associated with the unloading of soybean.

2. Control

Treatment of the patients and prevention of further cases is more important than the investigation of the outbreak. Once a vehicle or source of infection is suspected then action may be taken to limit the outbreak before scientific proof is obtained or sometimes even if rigorous proof is lacking. For example, a manufacturer of infant dried milk voluntarily withdrew the product from the market when a preliminary outbreak investigation showed an association between its consumption and infant salmonellae infection. The source was ultimately shown to be contaminated factory machinery.

(a)

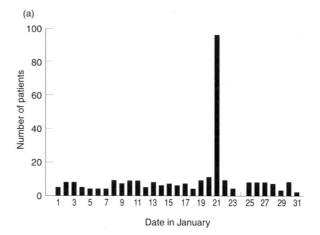

(b)

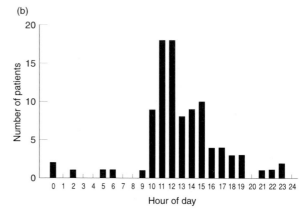

(c)

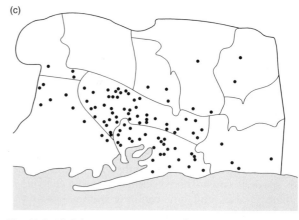

Fig. 19.1 Admissions to emergency rooms for patients with acute asthma in Barcelona, January 1986. (a) Admissions on varying days of the month; (b) admissions by hour of the day on 21 January; (c) city map showing distribution of cases. (Anto et al 1989)

3. Management of outbreaks

The Consultant in Communicable Disease Control in a health authority manages small outbreaks with assistance from local departments of microbiology and environmental health. An epidemiologist from the nationally based Public Health Laboratory Service is available for serious outbreaks. Foodborne outbreaks from zoonoses (diseases affecting humans from animal carriers) are controlled by identification of the infecting animal or species. Person-to-person outbreaks rely for their control upon isolation and treatment of cases or carriers. For example, isolation and treatment of typhoid cases and carriers or for institutional measles a vaccination programme of institutional contacts will prevent spread to susceptible individuals.

Issues of science, judgement, ethics, economics and politics are all involved in this aspect of public health practice. Sometimes these can be dealt with straightforwardly, but sometimes interests conflict. For example, in the late 1980s Edwina Currie, then Minister of Health in the UK, drew attention to the risk of salmonellosis associated with eating eggs. This was rapidly taken up by the press and had severe repercussions in the egg industry. It also ultimately resulted in her resignation, as the carrier of bad news.

The interplay between the economics of the livelihoods of those associated with different aspects of food production and particular food risks to the public's health is becoming increasingly obvious. This has led to calls in the UK for the separation of food safety from the Ministry of Agriculture Fisheries and Food to a ministry of its own to protect the public health where serious economic counterforces may operate. The UK government has now agreed this.

4. Analytical investigation

Investigations will involve extensive questionaries, laboratory tests (including blood tests, serology, microbial identification and sensitivity testing) and analysis of environmental sources.

Ideally public health actions are based on evidence of an association between exposure and disease as well as the strength of the association. This evidence is obtained by carrying out case–control or cohort studies. The usefulness of this approach has been demonstrated time and again in outbreak investigation. Salmonella outbreaks in which case–control or cohort studies were carried out in Wales between 1986 and 1990 are shown in Table 19.1. In all but one of the outbreaks a statistically significant association with a suspected cause was found.

An example of an investigation of a disease outbreak: meningococcal disease

We now describe a local outbreak of disease to point out the importance of the methodological issues we have described.

Table 19.1 Salmonella outbreaks in which case–control or cohort studies were carried out in Wales 1986–90

Place of outbreak	Cause	Case–control studies			Cohort studies			
		Cases	Control	Odds ratio	Exposed	Not exposed	Relative risk	p
Pub	Egg sandwiches				3/7	0.24	–	0.007
Home party	Scrambled egg				17/35	3/40	6.5	<0.001
Hospital staff	Scotch eggs	16/17	5/37	102				≪0.001
Home party	Cheesecake				5/6	0/5	–	0.015
Restaurant	Egg sandwiches	6/36	0/57	–				0.003
Pub	Egg mayonnaise				27/31	16/30	1.6	0.009
Home party	Sea trout with raw egg				12/12	0/2	–	0.01
College	Egg mayonnaise	16/19	0/47	–				≪0.001
Hospital	Beef rissoles with egg binding				87/190	13/82	2.9	≪0.001
Campsite	Lemon meringue				40/40	1/7	7.0	≪0.001
Hospital staff	Chicken				182/213	15/54	3.1	≪0.001
Shop	Custard slices	27/34	9/57	20.1				≪0.001
					15/25	13/48	2.2	0.01
Golf club	Eggs				23/48	5/25	2.4	0.04
Hotel	Beef and turkey				21/24	0/1	–	0.16

Investigation of disease outbreaks

➤ Disease outbreaks are declared once sufficient data are collected to indicate that more than a sporadic case is involved.

➤ Control includes treatment of patients and prevention measures to reduce the spread of disease. An outbreak team may coordinate measures.

➤ Epidemiological assessments assist in identifying causes of the outbreak and in analysing future public health measures.

Table 19.2 Cases of meningitis in Cardiff students

Patient	Admitted	Notified	Confirmed	Microbiology
1	16 Oct.	16 Oct.	5 Dec.	Blood culture negative Rising serum antibody Untyped
2	16 Nov.	17 Nov.	18 Nov.	Latex A, C, Y positive on blood culture supernate Blood culture negative Group C on PCR
3	26 Nov.	28 Nov.	28 Nov.	Latex A, C, Y positive on blood culture supernate C2a P1.5 on blood culture
4	28 Nov.	28 Nov.	30 Nov.	C2a P1.5 on blood culture Died on 28 Nov.
5	27 Nov.	29 Nov.	30 Nov.	Latex A, C, Y positive by enhanced agglutination Group C on PCR
6	29 Nov.	29 Nov.	1 Dec.	C2a P1.5 on CSF and blood culture Died on 1 Dec.
7	2 Dec.	2 Dec.	5 Dec.	CSF and blood culture negative CSF positive on PCR Untyped

1. Data collection

There was an outbreak of seven microbiologically confirmed cases of meningococcal disease among students at the University of Wales, Cardiff between mid-October and early December 1996. The initial patient became ill on 15 October while at home in Newport, a nearby town. A clinical diagnosis of meningococcal meningitis was made. Following treatment, the student recovered. Subsequent cases and their date of admission to hospital and association microbiology are shown in Table 19.2.

The public health department gave antibiotic prophylaxis to the close contacts of patients 1 and 2, both residents of the same university hall of residence. More than 4 weeks had elapsed between the two cases and in the absence of any common close contacts no further action was taken. The cases were only just over 4 weeks apart but it was assumed that the national guidelines, which say 4 weeks, erred on the side of caution.

Patient 3 lived in private rented accommodation and no close contact was identified with the hall of residence so once again action was again limited to giving antibiotic prophylaxis to close contacts. The occurrence of case 4, a patient who lived in the hall of residence, was confirmed within 12 days of case 2. This meant that the patients now officially constituted an outbreak as defined by the Public Health Laboratory Service guidelines. An outbreak team was constituted on 29 November. Patient 5 had been admitted to hospital on the 27 November with a provisional diagnosis of vasculitis secondary to viral infection, but the team prudently considered him to be a potential case which was subsequently confirmed.

2. Control measures

Initial control measures in the treatment of existing patients were already instituted by the time an outbreak was declared and a team constituted. The outbreak team set up measures to identify and alert the population at risk to ensure that further cases are quickly identified and treated.

● the immediate at-risk population was defined as all staff and residents of University Hall
● further urgent enquiries were instigated regarding the hall of residence social network and the law school as possible settings for transmission of infection
● a meeting was convened immediately at University Hall to inform students and staff of the situation, to alert them to the symptoms of meningococcal infection and to advise them how to obtain prompt medical assistance
● GPs serving University Hall residents were immediately appraised of the situation by

telephone so as to ensure vigilance in case finding and prompt admission of all potential patients

- all GPs in Bro Taf (the area) were alerted by fax
- a twice daily check was carried out by University Hall wardens personally visiting each student's room
- the University Hospital of Wales was placed on alert, an open access policy to receive ill students was instituted and arrangements were made to admit all potential cases immediately to the Infectious Diseases Unit
- the university doctor would be available for consultation on site over the weekend during daylight hours
- the public health team was available on site to monitor the response by GPs and provide advice where necessary.

3. Management: prevention measures

To prevent further spread of infection among hall residents and to provide longer-term protection the following measures were carried out:

- antibiotic prophylaxis with a single dose of ciprofloxacin 500 mg was issued immediately to all students and staff at University Hall in order to eradicate nasopharyngeal carriage of meningococcal organisms
- the University Hall bar was closed until further notice because of its potential as a focus for spread of meningococcal infection
- throat swab specimens were obtained from all students at University Hall prior to the antibiotic dose for later use in ascertaining the meningococcal carriage rate and for investigating possible risk factors and mechanisms of spread of the organism
- immunisation with meningococcal A and C vaccine (for longer-term protection) was arranged for all students and staff at University Hall before the end of term.

The Infectious Disease Unit at the hospital was set up to evaluate and treat any suspect cases. In the 10 days following the declaration of the outbreak 82 students were admitted of whom two were confirmed as cases. The seven cases in total consisted of:

- three patients from whom isolates of *Neisseria meningitidis* were isolated and characterised by the Public Health Laboratory Service as serosubtype C
- two patients confirmed as serogroup C by antigen detection

- two patients with untyped but confirmed disease.

As many of the patients had type C *N. meningitidis* and immunisation is available for this subtype, a mass immunisation programme was started on Sunday 1 December. By 2 December all but 70 students at the hall of residence had been accounted for. Over 1000 vaccine doses had been given. By Wednesday 4 December all but two students at the hall had received antibiotics and vaccine.

4. Investigation

Some investigative information had already been obtained in identifying the serotype of the infection. Patients were interviewed in detail and certains common links could be identified.

- Six of the seven patients were resident at University Hall. Patient 1 did not know either Patient 2 or Patient 3 (see below) but was acquainted with (though not a close contact of) Patient 4. Patients 4, 5 and 6 lived in the same block as Patient 7. Patient 2 was not acquainted with, and lived in a different block from, any of the other patients. Patients 4, 5 and 6 lived on the same corridor of the same block at University Hall. Although resident in a different block at the hall, Patient 7 belonged to the same close circle of friends as Patient 6.
- Patient 3 lived in private rented accommodation. None of his close contacts were resident at University Hall, and he was not acquainted with any of the other patients.
- Both Patients 3 and 4 were students at the Cardiff Law School. However, after detailed interviews with their close friends and with Patient 3, it was determined that there had not been any kind of academic, social or incidental contact between the two patients.

As a result of these links, it was agreed that all control measures should be focused on the hall of residence as the most likely setting where spread of infection had occurred.

Throat swab specimens were obtained from 454 students on 29 and 30 November and 89 of these yielded cultures of *Neisseria meningitidis*, although the PHLS Meningococcal Reference Unit confirmed only three of these as serogroup C. Therefore, although the overall carriage rate of meningococcus was high, the number of group C meningococcal carriers was low.

Disease surveillance

Epidemiological surveillance is an activity in which the distribution and incidence of disease are observed by means of a systematic collection of morbidity and mortality data and possibly environmental parameters.

Data collection

The collection of data may use routine data collected by health authorities or data from specifically designed studies about an illness. In simpler forms, the history of data collection can be traced back to at least the 17th century in England. At that time, they collected disease-specific mortality data and described diseases specifically linked to occupations. The publication of *The Sanitary Conditions of the Labouring Population of Great Britain* by Edwin Chadwick in 1842 was a landmark in the collection and interpretation of data on health and related factors. People used it to decide on preventive action and in providing health care.

The government of the UK established the Office of the Registrar General at about the same time. Its purpose was to collect data on births and deaths in England, which helped to support the reform of public health. The authors soon extended these reports to include occupational and infectious diseases. The latter had to be notified by law by 1899. In 1842, the first of a series of reports were published that dealt with patients treated in six London hospitals. This developed into a national hospital reporting system by 1929. A limitation of this early work was the imprecision of the cause of death. An international list of causes of death was first produced in 1989 and the WHO International Classification of Diseases (ICD) currently provides uniformity. However, a diagnosis may be restricted to the immediate cause of death rather than the underlying pathology. In a patient diagnosed as suffering from AIDS, for example, a doctor may for social reasons certify an immediate cause rather than the underlying cause of death.

The problem of accurate case definition can be particularly acute for surveillance of new diseases. Before surveillance for AIDS could be implemented and agreed, a vigorous definition of what combination of symptoms constituted a case had to be agreed. This had implication for health provision, benefits and insurance. The working definition used initially by the Centres for Disease Control in the USA is shown in all its complexity in Table 19.3. There are now more specific blood tests for AIDS.

Table 19.3 The CDC definition of AIDS

The occurrence of biopsy-proven Kaposi's sarcoma and/or culture-proven infection at least moderately predictive of cellular immune deficiency (as below)

Infection group	AIDS-defining illness
Protozoal and helminthic infections	Cryptosporidiosis, intestinal, causing diarrhoea for over 1 month
Pneumocystis carinii on histology or microscopy
Strongyloidosis causing pneumonia, CNS, or disseminated infection
Toxoplasmosis causing pneumonia or CNS infection
Fungal infections	Aspergillosis causing CNS or disseminated infection
Candidiasis causing oesophagitis
Cryptococcus causing pulmonary, CNS or disseminated infection
Bacterial infection	Atypical mycobacteriosis causing disseminated infection
Viral infections	Cytomegalovirus causing pulmonary, gastrointestinal or CNS infection
Herpes simplex virus causing chronic mucocutaneous infection for more than one month or more disseminated infection
Progressive multifocal leukoencephalopathy

Objectives of disease surveillance

Surveillance may have one or more of the following objectives:

● the early detection of changes in disease distribution to enable immediate investigation and subsequent control
● collection of data about new diseases so that their epidemiology can be described and aetiological hypotheses identified
● evaluation of disease control measures
● determination of the prevalent infections in a population so that clinicians can be alerted and preventive measures undertaken
● surveillance of immunisation programmes.

The early detection of changes in disease distribution

There are a number of examples where surveillance of disease statistics, enabled control measures to be identified and instigated.

Notifications of infective jaundice increased in the early 1980s and adult incidence peaks in 1981 and 1982 (Fig. 19.2) were associated with outbreaks of

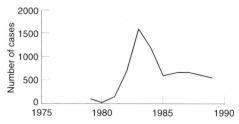

Fig. 19.2 Cases of hepatitis A in Great Britain in 1979–90. (PHLS Communicable Disease Surveillance Centre 1994)

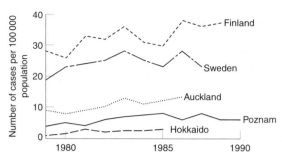

Fig. 19.3 The incidence of insulin-dependent diabetes in different parts of the world. (Alberti 1993)

hepatitis A. This was considered to be transmitted by the consumption of shellfish. This ultimately resulted in improvements in the cleansing and cooking of shellfish and subsequent surveillance revealed a decline in incidence.

However, continuing surveillance of infective jaundice demonstrated an increase in hepatitis B infections and there were outbreaks amongst intravenous drug abusers. The control measures implemented in this instance were the promotion of immunisation for hepatitis B and the direction of health education at the group at risk.

An example of this type of surveillance was the observed increase in asthma deaths in the 1960s. This declined once the use of prescribed aerosols was controlled.

Surveillance also pinpointed an increase in reports of *Salmonella napoli*, which was subsequently controlled by removing a make of imported chocolate from the food chain.

Collection of data about new diseases

Information on environmental factors and on drug use can be helpful in establishing a time cause–effect relationship for new diseases.

Toxic shock syndrome was a 'new' disease that occurred in young women in Minnesota and Wisconsin in January 1980. Between 1st January 1980 and 18 October 1981 the Centre for Disease Control was notified of over 1000 cases of toxic shock. The great majority of the reported cases were associated with menstruation. A number of case–control studies showed that the increased risk was associated with the use of new synthetic super-absorbent tampons with marked changes in chemical composition, which had been marketed over the previous 3 years.

The decline in reported cases in late 1980 and early 1981 (Fig. 3.6, p. 28) followed great publicity surrounding toxic shock syndrome and is thought to have been caused by withdrawal of one make of tampon and changes in tampon use by women. It is possible that

changes in the prevalence of toxin-producing *Staphylococcus aureus* might also be involved. Since toxic shock syndrome still continues to be reported, it is desirable that research is undertaken to work out if tampons are responsible.

The thalidomide tragedy described in Chapter 5 spawned the development of another aspect of this type of surveillance. This is sometimes referred to as pharmaco-vigilance since it is concerned with identifying new problems of drug safety. This is underpinned in the UK by the Committee on Safety of Medicines Reporting Scheme for Adverse Drug Reactions. Doctors use a confidential 'yellow card' to inform the committee with details of suspected reactions to new drugs and serious reactions to established ones. We know that no more than 10% of serious reactions is reported and only about 2% of non-serious reactions. Hospital doctors appear to be the worst offenders. Nevertheless, reporting has improved with time and the scheme has provided some useful early warnings of drug hazards.

Chronic disease may also be amenable to this approach. The incidence of insulin-dependent diabetes in children alters in parallel in many countries for which data has been collected (Fig. 19.3). Such alterations in incidence are not consistent with the long incubation required by current immunological views. It has, therefore, been suggested that this disease should be incorporated into national surveillance systems so that epidemics can be identified. Once identified, direct intensive analysis could be directed at finding possible international environmental factors.

Evaluation of disease control measures

In 1983 the Public Health Service in the USA recommended that members of groups at high risk of AIDS should not donate blood. In 1985, they first set up screening of the blood supply for HIV. They assessed the effectiveness of these control measures at the Centre for Disease Control. Surveillance for AIDS is based on

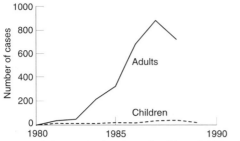

Fig. 19.4 Transfusion-associated AIDS cases in adults and children. (PHLS Communicable Disease Surveillance Centre 1994)

doctors reporting cases to state or local health departments using a standard case report form to ensure uniform data collection. Cases of AIDS were classified as transfusion associated if there was a history of having received a transfusion of blood or blood components after 1977 without other reported risk factors for AIDS.

The trend of adult and paediatric transfusion-associated AIDS cases is shown in Figure 19.4 for the period 1981 to 1989. This surveillance showed that the largest number of infected children was transfused in 1983 and of adults in 1984 and that the control measures outlined above resulted in a decline thereafter. However we will continue to diagnose cases among children transfused between 1978 and 1985 because of the long incubation period.

Determination of the prevalent infections in a population

Infection surveillance in hospital infection control is a well-known example of surveillance to identify prevalent infections. The national prevalence survey of 1980 reported that 19.1% of patients in hospital suffered infections and that half of these were hospital acquired (nosocomial). Some hospitals and infection control teams use selective surveillance to save time and money. In this approach they examine selected patient groups or hospital units. A survey of surveillance methods in UK hospitals revealed that less than a fifth were producing infection rates and less than half performed analyses of the data collected. Large studies in the USA have demonstrated that active surveillance and control programmes reduce nosocomial infection rates by half and that dissemination of results to doctors and nurses is critical.

Surveillance of immunisation programmes

Surveillance of immunisation programmes encompasses all the objectives so far described. However, because this activity is so widespread and important, it is worthy of separate categorisation. One of its most

important uses is in monitoring mutation of microorganisms to resistant forms. Influenza virus changes with time; as a result, it is necessary for the WHO to collect and study antigenic types from all over the world. They use these data to estimate which strains of vaccine should be produced. Such antigenic change was responsible for the decreased efficacy of pertussis vaccine in the UK in the 1960s. Surveillance of the prevalent serotypes helps us to modify vaccines and keep the incidence of the infection low. Serological surveillance can also show when immunity in certain groups of the population is getting low. We can then target immunisation campaigns at these groups.

Passive surveillance of adverse vaccine reactions uses the 'yellow card' system mentioned above.

We can use active surveillance in certain circumstance, for example looking for all cases of paralytic disease associated with polio vaccination. The uptake of immunisation programmes is passively surveyed using data from district health authorities to the Department of Health.

Non-communicable disease surveillance

Although surveillance is most widely practised for communicable diseases, it is increasingly being applied to other fields, such as primary care, cancer, perinatal morbidity, occupational health, injuries and poisonings. A large number of different organisations now monitor non-communicable disease. The best-known and most widely organised of these are the regional cancer registers, which collect data on identified cases of cancer, mainly from hospital diagnostic units and from death certification. Others, for example the National UK Perinatal Epidemiology Unit, founded in 1978, monitor trends over time and identify outcomes requiring research or control.

Disease surveillance

➤ Surveillance data can be used to detect changes in disease distribution and new diseases and to evaluate control measures.

➤ Surveillance is most often used for infectious diseases, but it is increasingly used for other areas such as cancer registers and perinatal morbidity.

➤ Surveillance may involve the collection of data regarding possible environmental parameters linked to a disease.

Environmental health surveys

20

Two approaches to a potential health risk from local exposure are discussed:

- epidemiological approach, monitoring ill-health
- environmental survey, monitoring the presence and level of pollutants.

Introduction

Chronic health risks associated with environmental exposures that are limited in geography but prolonged in time were discussed in Chapter 16. The most common example of such risk is that presented by industrial plant. Public concerns and demands for assessment of the risks these places pose as well as for ways of reducing their risks are a feature of modern life. This often requires an environmental survey. The survey methods used in practice are discussed using as an example, the risk posed to health by living close to a coking works.

Epidemiological approach

In Chapter 15, the success of the smokeless fuel policy in decreasing urban levels of atmospheric pollution was described. To produce smokeless fuel it is first necessary to drive off volatile substances. This in itself presents an environmental problem. In 1942, the Disticoke Company of Paris designed a plant for the middle of the Cynon Valley in South Wales, as shown in Figures 20.1 and 20.2. This processed small fine coal, which was wasted in tips nearby, and converted it into a solid smokeless fuel. The process essentially consists of mixing liquid pitch with the waste coal to form briquettes and then carbonising these at 900°C for several hours to drive off the volatile substances.

It was well known that coke workers exposed to such volatile substances get more lung cancer if their exposure exceeds set limits. Aromatic polycyclic hydrocarbons are the prime suspects. It is much more difficult, however, to decide on the risk to respiratory health from long-term exposure to low levels of pollution. The plant was producing 15% of the UK demand for smokeless fuel in the late 1980s. As time has passed, there has been a general increase in awareness of environmental pollution and worries about adverse effects from the local population.

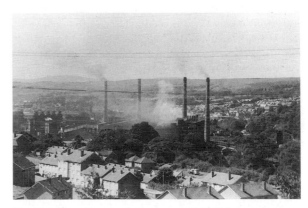

Fig. 20.1 The coking plant in the cynon valley in Wales.

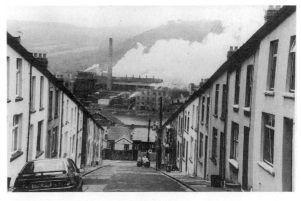

Fig. 20.2 Housing around the coking plant.

Researchers set up a series of epidemiological surveys to answer to the questions:

- Is there more ill health in the people near coking works than might be expected?
- A more difficult question: whether exposure to emissions from the plant had caused the ill health discovered.

Such surveys can never be conclusive about a cause and an effect, but they might suggest an association so strong that the cause seems very likely. These data might then be used to agitate for better environmental control.

Survey of health status

Researchers from the Medical Research Council did an investigation around the plant. They carried out two studies in the villages of Aberdare and Mountain Ash at the upper and lower parts of the Cynon Valley.

In one study they examined 12 boys and 12 girls in a secondary school in Aberdare and the same number of boys and girls in a secondary school in Mountain Ash. They took respiratory peak flow measurements from these. The researchers made the measurements each morning. There was much variation in individual subject measurement and, because of high absenteeism, there was not a single day when all 48 children were available. They made measurements for 2 months but observed no statistically significant change for individual subjects or for the group as a whole. A north-west wind would bring pollution from the plant towards Mountain Ash School and a south-east wind towards Aberdare School. Because of this, wind patterns over the period were investigated and compared with the peak flow measurements. There was no evidence that peak flows were reduced on the days when the wind direction may have posed a risk. The peak flow measurements and respiratory symptoms compared favourably with those of other children of the same age surveyed at the same time in Kent.

In another study, people with established bronchitis were requested to complete a daily diary and record whether their daily symptoms had changed. Completed diaries were returned by 138 subjects from Mountain Ash and 78 from Aberdare. The mean condition of each group each day showed large variation, but there was no consistent relationship with pollution measurements (smoke and sulphur dioxide) made at each location.

Researchers, in response to a similar problem near a coking works in Monkton in Tyneside, had analysed patterns of consultation with GPs. This showed that consultation rates for respiratory disorders were higher on days when air pollution, as indicated by sulphur dioxide levels, was higher. These rates did not diminish, however, when production stopped in Monkton in 1984–6 or after the plants final closure in 1990. The GP records showed a higher prevalence of respiratory disease among children in the area close to the plant than in the control area but no similar excess was observed among adults. However, the gradient in prevalence was outer > inner > control and not, as hypothesised, inner > outer > control and the numbers involved were small.

An analysis was also carried out of routine statistics of mortality, cancer and stillbirths in South Tyneside. Mortality rates and cancer registration rates were highest in the outer areas. The inner area had rates close to the average for South Tyneside and there was no evidence of a greater proportion of stillbirths in the population near the Monkton Coking Works. The investigators concluded that the Monkton Works was associated with a marked excess of reported symptoms and a small excess of diagnosed respiratory disease but no association with cancer or other mortality.

Factors limiting the epidemiological approach

Despite good planning and epidemiological expertise, the surveys undertaken in Wales and Tyneside were not able rigorously to test the hypothesis that living near to a coking plant adversely affected people's health. The reason does not concern design and execution of the surveys but basic factors of the disease prevalence, the magnitude of the expected clinical effect of exposure and the size of the populations for study.

Air-borne emissions from such processes could cause additional ill-health in the neighbouring community. This is likely to take the form of an excess in respiratory morbidity (i.e. illnesses from chest diseases) or mortality (i.e. deaths from chest diseases). Even if the process increased the respiratory mortality of the population by as much as 20% then the 'excess' deaths, compared with communities without the process, would remain far too small to allow us to find a statistical association.

The problem is further confounded by the fact that year-to-year variations from the diseases in question will almost certainly be much larger than rates between two communities. To make matters worse the people in the communities around industrial sites are usually poor, tend to be heavy smokers and work in industries likely to cause high morbidity. In the unlikely event of a statistical association being demonstrated between respiratory morbidity and the closeness to the process, it would be virtually impossible to conclude, with confidence, that the difference resulted from the process and not the circumstances of the population. Environmental problems of a local nature do not lend themselves to an epidemiological approach unless the risk is very high. However, there is a different approach, which can offer a constructive way to assess such problems.

Environmental health survey

It is important to separate the aesthetic concerns of the public, although legitimate, from the health risks. In the vicinity of the coking plant in South Wales, the most frequent and vociferous complaints made by residents were along the lines of 'I had to re-wash all the clothes I put out to dry', 'The paint is ruined on my car' or 'We were all made to feel sick by the atrocious smell'. The complaints of the community are perfectly valid on quality-of-life grounds, whether there is a measurable objective effect upon health or not. The community and their elected representatives are right to make such complaints but they do not need an environmental health survey. The aim of an environmental health survey is to determine the doses of relevant pollutant to a population and relate these to what is known about health effects, usually at higher doses, or to statutory standards for ambient pollution.

Pollutant assessment

In order to assess health effects it is first necessary to assess the types of pollutant associated with the process. If the process is complex then the technical personnel employed by the plant and scientists from Her Majesty's Inspectorate of Pollution in the UK may be able to supply such information. The various pollutants that could be identified with the coking plants were:

● dust
● polycyclic aromatic hydrocarbons (particulate and gaseous)
● various gases and vapours such as carbon monoxide, sulphur dioxide, hydrogen sulphide, hydrogen cyanide and oxides of nitrogen, benzene, toluene and xylene.

The local community was concerned with the dust that they could see on their washing and cars but this presents little risk to health. However, dust with an aerodynamic diameter of less than 5 μm can be respired deep into the lungs and does present a risk to health. Similarly the community were understandably ignorant of the potential risk presented by polycyclic aromatic hydrocarbons (PAHs). It is known from occupational epidemiology that these are carcinogenic above certain dose levels.

In order to determine the dosage of pollutants received by the local community it is necessary to set up good monitoring. This must take into account the centres of population density as well as local topography and meteorology. The coking works in South Wales was situated on the floor of the Cynon valley at a point that is about 500 metres wide. The valley is separated from neighbouring valleys to the west and east by mountain ridges 300–400 metres high. As shown in Figure 20.3, the valley runs from north-west to south-east and contains the towns of Aberdare (population 22 000) 3.5 km north-west of the works, Aberaman (6500) 1.5 km north-west of the works and Mountain Ash (16 000) 2 km south-east of the works. In the vicinity of the works, a number of populous terraces descend into the main valley from either side less than 1 km from the works.

The topography of the Cynon Valley favours the formation and persistence of inversions. Inversion is the name given to atmospheric conditions where a parcel of rising air enters a layer of air at a higher temperature so its upward progress is retarded. Figure 20.4 shows a temperature inversion of the whole Cynon Valley in which the warm gases from the coking oven chimneys are unable to break through. Pollutants build up to higher concentrations in the valley during such a period, which in winter may persist for several days.

Effects of weather conditions

Rainfall is very effective in purifying polluted air. Suspended solids are washed out and sulphur dioxide

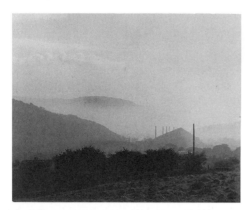

Fig. 20.3 Temperature inversion over the Cynon Valley.

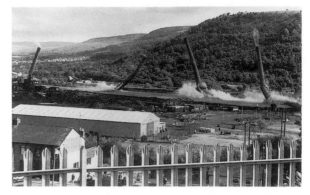

Fig. 20.5 Eventually the local populace had their way—the thermosite plant was closed.

and hydrogen sulphide are dissolved. The importance of wind speed and direction are obvious. The topography of the valley is such that the wind direction in the valley may differ markedly from that in open country. The tendency is for the wind to be channelled up and down the valley, as is shown in Figure 20.4, where the ground winds in the open measured 15 miles away are modified in the valley.

An environmental survey for such an area should include permanent monitoring sites installed around the works, each equipped with a meteorological station to produce pollution roses based upon wind speed and direction. These aim to measure dust concentrations over successive periods of a week at each of the sites for different months of the year. The sampling method draws atmospheric air through a membrane filter to measure the concentrations in air. This is determined from the weight of particulate matter deposited, the flow rate and the sampling time. This relatively long-term sampling should be supplemented with short-term sampling. Petri dishes can be deployed for 24 hours and the dust deposited in each used to build up a profile of pollution. Particulate mat-

ter can be sampled in similar fashion and identification of the pollutants carried out.

Instruments can monitor sulphur dioxide, hydrogen sulphide, nitrous oxide and nitrogen dioxide at a site downwind of the factory. This approach can give the doses of the pollutants over 12 months. Independent researchers should be able to obtain details of plant operation on a day to day basis in order to correlate levels of activity with environmental pollution.

Use of the survey

Environmental monitoring can be used to measure the nature and concentration of the toxins in the atmosphere. These results can be used to identify potential problem substances and their levels. These can be compared both with doses known to cause respiratory ill-health and with environmental air-quality standards. Surveillance can then concentrate on reducing the risk and on identifying specific health problems rather than looking at general mortality and morbidity.

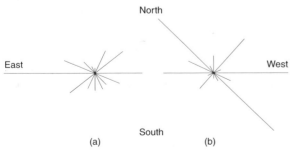

Fig. 20.4 Frequency of wind direction at the regional weather station (a) and at the coking works (b).

> **Environmental health survey**
>
> ➤ An environmental health survey determines the doses of a relevant pollutant to which a population is exposed.
>
> ➤ These doses are related to known health effects or statutory standards.
>
> ➤ Measures can then be instituted to reduce pollutant levels if necessary and for continued surveillance of pollutant levels.
>
> ➤ Local health-care personnel can be alerted to potential health problems, perhaps by improving early monitoring to detect disease.

Ionising radiation

21

Ionising radiation is discussed in terms of:

- its biological effects
- its use as a diagnostic tool
- the implication of nuclear accidents.

Introduction

The potential risk of exposure to ionising radiation was the first hazard to occupy wide public concern. This came about, in large measures because of the traumatic effect on the public psyche both at the time and since of the nuclear destruction of Hiroshima and Nagasaki at the end of the Second World War. People fear the potential risk in nuclear power generation as well as in the uptake of diagnostic X-ray procedures. It is worth considering the evidence on which risk estimates are based, the magnitude of these estimates and their consequences for the public health.

Radiation interacts with matter at the atomic level by colliding with atoms and losing energy by ionising the atoms (i.e. knocking electrons out of atoms). These secondary changes can, in turn, produce further ionisations. Radiation can exert a direct effect where the radiation interacts directly with a biological molecule (e.g. causing a chromosome break) or it can act indirectly.

The indirect actions of radiation occur through the formation of aqueous free radicals, which damage biological molecules. The very high water content of living tissue underlines the importance of the radiation chemistry of water. Free radicals are electrically neutral atoms or molecules having an unpaired electron in their outer orbit so they are very reactive. The increased effectiveness of radiation in the presence of oxygen, made use of by radiotherapists, is caused by the greater yield of damaging free radicals.

The relative biological effectiveness of the different types of radiation to cause damage depends upon their **linear energy transfer** (LET) capabilities. Neutrons and particles cause much more localised deposition of energy than do X-rays or gamma rays. (The word 'rem' is an acronym for roentgen equivalent man/mammal. The rem is now being superseded by the sievert, which is equal to 100 rem.)

Biological effects of radiation

Genetic effects

By the 1920s it was known that radiation exposure produced genetic changes in insects. No genetic defects than can unequivocally be ascribed to the effects of ionising radiation have ever been found in the children of irradiated humans. The most extensive studies are those carried out on the children of the survivors of the Hiroshima and Nagasaki bombs. No significant differences, either in mortality or in the incidence of chromosome anomalies, have been found between the children of exposed parents and suitable control groups. Almost all the evidence comes from studies on mice and a great many assumptions have to be made in extrapolating from mouse to humans. On the basis of evidence from animal experimentation, the risk of serious hereditary ill-health in subsequent generations following the irradiation of either parent is estimated to be 100–200 per million people per rem.

Radiation carcinogenesis

Eight years after Röentgen demonstrated that X-rays would expose photographic film, a report was published in 1903 in the *New England Journal of Medicine* that revealed that mice exposed to large doses of X-rays died soon afterwards. It was also observed that human skin chronically exposed to X-rays, as on the hands of dentists, would ulcerate and eventually develop cancerous growths. When Madame Curie and a number of other early radiation workers developed leukaemia, it became clear that bone marrow as well as skin was sensitive to malignant changes following excessive radiation exposure.

Cancer can be induced in practically all tissues by radiation but certain types of cancer predominate in radiation carcinogenesis:

- leukaemia
- thyroid cancer
- breast cancer
- bone cancer

In general, tissues with proliferating cells can be induced to cancerous change whereas non-dividing cells are not as easily transformed. The latency period in radiation-induced cancer varies from 10 to 40 years, except in the case of leukaemia where the latency period can be as short as 5 years.

Radiation protection agencies were set up in the 1920s to provide guidance for occupational exposure but by the close of World War Two many fundamental aspects of radiation effects were still unknown:

- how much radiation is required to produce adverse effects?
- are there differences among the various kinds of radiation?
- are diseases other than cancer increased by radiation exposure?
- are children more or less sensitive than adults?

Following World War Two, with the likelihood of the introduction of nuclear energy into the peacetime economy, an enormous scientific effort was undertaken to answer these questions. Billions of dollars were expended and extensive studies carried out with laboratory animals and exposed human populations. There was a recognised need to assess risk and to provide guidelines for permissible exposure to the public.

Evidence on adverse effects

Epidemiological evidence

There is overwhelming evidence that persons exposed to large doses of radiation (>100 rem) suffer an increased risk of death from leukaemia and from other cancers. The risk can now be estimated approximately from several sources of epidemiological evidence, both for exposure of the whole body and for that of a number of organs or tissues. The first evidence came from groups of people who had received gross exposures. Uranium miners breath in radon gas, a product

of the radioactive decay of uranium. Unfortunately, radon emits alpha particles, which are particularly damaging. Many years ago, before the hazard was recognised, the lungs of uranium miners were irradiated internally and the incidence of lung cancer in this group was very high.

Another unfortunate group of workers was employed to paint luminescent radium onto the faces of watches and clocks. They were in the habit of getting a fine point on their paintbrushes by placing them between their lips. Ingestion of radium led eventually to a high incidence of cancer of the bone in these people. The follow-up of the Japanese survivors of Hiroshima and Nagasaki under the auspices of the Atomic Bomb Casualty Commission also revealed excess cancer incidence.

In 1955 the Medical Research Council established a unit to research the clinical effects of ionising radiation. The units' researchers, Professor Court Brown and Richard Doll sought to test:

- if repeated small doses of radiation received in the course of occupational exposure could result in a loss of life from such a wide variety of causes that they might be regarded as resulting in a non-specific increase in the rate of ageing
- if the same sort of dose could cause an increase in mortality from cancer other than cancer of the skin.

Doll published the results in 1981 on the mortality of men who joined the British Radiological Society (i.e. radiologists) between 1897 and 1954 compared with:

- all men in England and Wales
- men in social class I
- male medical practitioners.

Radiologists who entered the profession before 1921 suffered a death rate from cancer 75% higher than that of medical practitioners. There was a statistically significant excess of deaths from cancers of the pancreas, lung and skin and leukaemia. No excess was found for those joining after 1920. For all non-cancer causes of death combined, the death rate among radiologists is lower than that among all men in England and Wales, men in social class I and male medical practitioners. There was, therefore, no support for a non-specific effect of radiation on mortality.

In 1982 Doll also reported on the mortality of over 14 000 patients with ankylosing spondylitis given a course of X-ray treatment in the mid-1930s. A nearly fivefold excess of deaths from leukaemia and a two-thirds excess of deaths from cancers of sites that would have been in the radiation field were discovered. The excess death rate from leukaemia was greatest 3 to 5 years after treatment and was close to zero after 18 years. In contrast, the excess of cancers at heavily irradiated sites did not become apparent until 9 or more years after irradiation and continued for a further 11 years. The number of cancers at sites not considered to be in the radiation beams was a fifth greater than expected.

Dosage levels

As a result of a number of studies, a consensus was reached on radiation risks. A cut-off line of 10 rem was indicated. For doses above this level, a clear cancer risk was identified and this was estimated to be 300–400 per million per rem. For doses below 10 rem, there was more debate. Scientific studies indicated that ionising radiation has an effect on the human body that remains directly proportional to the dose *even* at very low levels. There is, therefore, assumed to be no threshold below which such radiation can be ignored and policy-makers decided that this should be accepted when considering doses below 10 rem for both occupational exposure and that of the general public.

Epidemiological evidence supporting effects of low-dose radiation

There are a number of observations that indicate induction of malignancies in humans at doses of less than 10 rem.

Bomb survivors. For bomb survivors the death rate from leukaemia for the period 1950–72 exceeds that expected; this is also the case for the group of people estimated to have been exposed to doses of less than 10 rem.

Medical irradiation. During the first 12 years of mass immigration to Israel (1949–60), nearly 17 000 children were irradiated for tinea capitis, a fungal scalp infection. A retrospective follow-up of these subjects was carried out in 1973 and the development of a significantly greater number of cancers of the head and neck were reported in the irradiated children than in two matched control groups. The rate of thyroid tumour induction per rem is consistent with that reported by a follow-up study on children irradiated for thymic enlargement, who were estimated to have received a thyroid dose at about 350 rem, which tends to support the hypothesis.

Irradiation in utero. The Oxford Childhood Cancer Survey was set up in the 1950s to seek an explanation for the progressive increase in the death rate from leukaemia in young children. This had taken place in England and Wales between the two World Wars and led to a series of reports. It was found that a dose to the fetus of the order of 1 rad, from X-rays, would cause a malignant tumour to develop in approximately 1 in every 2000 children. Radiologists and radiographers are now well aware of this problem and X-rays are avoided in pregnant women.

Controversial studies

There have been a number of studies that gave controversial results. The most notable of these undertook a study in 1964 of mortality among employees within Atomic Energy Commission laboratories in the USA. The publication 13 years later reported an increase in cancer frequency among employees of the Hanford, Washington facility. The study has been criticised by the National Academy of Sciences and others. Leukaemia, the disease most sensitive to radiation, was not increased and the excess was caused by other cancers not usually found to be increased by radiation (carcinoma of the pancreas).

Work published in the *Lancet* in the late 1970s suggested that leukaemia was increased seven- to eightfold among former employees of the Portsmouth Naval shipyard in New Hampshire. However, investigators found only six cases and two, it turned out, had not been radiation workers. Lyon analysed childhood leukaemia and cancer among children living in southern Utah during the period when fall-out occurred from weapons testing. In comparing with those living in Northern Utah, a significant increase in leukaemia was found. There are some reservations: mortality from leukaemia was low before and after exposure; there was an inverse relationship between exposure and other cancers; and there were poor estimates of dose.

Effects of ionising radiation

➤ Carcinogenesis: risk is about 300–400 per million per rem. Leukaemia and thyroid, breast and bone cancers are particularly linked to radiation exposure.

➤ Genetic effects: not proven in humans although clearly occurring in insects and mice.

➤ There is no lower dosage level at which biological effects do not occur but doses over 10 rem are considered to be clearly detrimental.

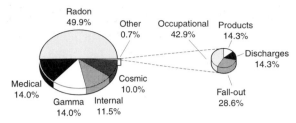

Fig. 21.1 Sources of ionising radiation in the UK. (Editorial 1989)

Diagnostic radiology

Medical irradiation is the major synthetic contributor to exposure to ionising radiation in the UK population (Fig. 21.1). Since 1957, diagnostic X-ray examinations have been increasing at a rate of approximately 2% per annum. A survey of diagnostic radiology found that 23.8 million examinations were carried out in 1977, amounting to 440 examinations per 1000 of the population.

The dose received by a patient should be as low as is possible bearing in mind the benefit the patient will receive as a consequence of their clinical management being altered by the diagnostic information obtained. There is both an associated cancer risk and a possible risk of hereditary effects on future generations.

There is a wide range of gonad dose associated with certain individual examinations. This range is still present and for some examinations extends over 3 to 4 orders of magnitude when practices throughout the UK are compared. Despite this the current situation in the UK is broadly satisfactory. Despite an increase in frequency of examinations of about 2% per annum, there has been a reduction in the gonad dose associated with a number of examinations, particularly of children, and a reduction in the frequency of certain types of examination, especially on pregnant women.

An estimate of the excess cancers attributable to diagnostic radiology in the UK can be taken from the frequency with which different practices are carried out, the average organ dose associated with a particular examination and the relevant risk coefficients. Risk estimates for individual organs are very uncertain at low doses of radiation. Approximately 300 excess cancers can be attributed to the 11 investigations listed in Figure 21.2.

It is also possible to estimate the risk for any one individual following a particular investigation. The greatest risk following an X-ray examination is that associated with examination of the dorsal spine in females. This risk is 13 in 266 800, or about 1 in 20 000.

The risk associated with any medical intervention needs to be carefully weighed against the benefits to the individual as a result of that intervention. For example, the risk of brain damage apparently attributable to the diphtheria, tetanus, pertussis immunisation is somewhere between 1 in 25 000 and 1 in 105 000. It is believed that this level of risk is acceptable in an immunisation programme. There is a prima facie case that a link may exist between immunisation and serious neurological illness and that this link spurs the search for safer vaccines. Applying the same reasoning to the risk of radiation-induced cancer in diagnostic radiology leads us to the conclusion that the level of

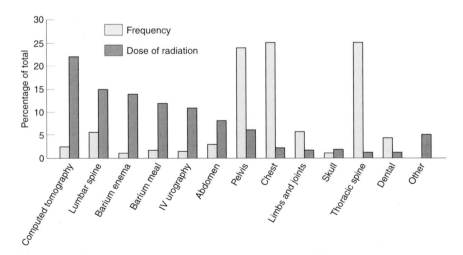

Fig. 21.2 Frequency and dose of X-ray examinations in the UK. (Editorial 1989)

risk involved is not a contraindication for clinical radiology. From the point of view of the public health, it is important that patients' exposure and the excess cancers consequently induced are minimised.

Why guidelines are needed

Studies of radiographic practice have revealed a wide variation in patients' exposure for the same examination. For example, measurements made in Swedish hospitals and the Nationwide Evaluation of X-ray Trends study in the USA in the 1970s found that patient exposures varied by more than a factor of 10 between centres for some investigations. A survey of 20 hospitals in Wales showed a similar range of variation owing to the choice of radiographic projection. If the range of this variation in patients' exposure between hospitals for the same examination were to be reduced, then a proportion of the cancers attributable to radiological practice would consequently be prevented.

A radiological investigation is only useful if the result will alter patient management or the diagnosis. The Royal College of Radiologists has drawn up guidelines on when to use different investigations for common conditions. They have pointed out that there are a great number of situations where radiology is not helpful:

- investigations where a positive finding is irrelevant because one would not treat the condition anyway, e.g. degenerative spinal disease without symptoms, which is very commonly found from late middle age onwards
- where the disease will improve or deteriorate before results can be obtained
- repeated investigations when no change could have been possible
- wrong investigation

The guideline for X-ray examination of the lumbar spine is shown in Table 21.1

> ### Diagnostic radiology
>
> ➤ Medical irradiation is the major contributor to non-natural radiation in the UK.
>
> ➤ Guidelines attempt to restrict use to situations where results will be helpful and to avoid variations associated with examination in different centres.
>
> ➤ Emphasis is placed on reducing gonad dosage levels.

Nuclear incidents

Windscale (Sellafield) 1957

In October 1957, a fire at the No. 1 Pile at Windscale Nuclear Plant, Cumbria, UK subsequently renamed Sellafield, caused a release of radionuclides into the atmosphere. Initially, the major radionuclide identified in environmental measurements was iodine-131. The most important threat was thyroid cancer, because the body concentrates iodine in the thyroid gland. Many years after the event, other radionuclides, undergoing irradiation in the pile at the time of the fire, were identified as having also been released into the atmosphere. The most significant of these was polonium-210, which is distributed fairly uniformly throughout the body.

Public concern about such incidents was less then than it is now. Nevertheless, the Government arranged for milk in the area to be disposed of and a limited programme of monitoring for radioactive iodine within the thyroids of the local population was undertaken. The lack of descriptive epidemiological data for incidence of thyroid cancer during this era did not allow estimates to be made of the significance of the exposure. Most public concern focused on possible reproductive effects and much was made of a cluster of Down's syndrome cases born to former pupils of a girls, school in Dundalk, to the West across the Irish

Table 21.1 Guideline for radiological investigation of the lumbar spine			
Clinical problem	Investigation	Radiographic Projection recommended	Comment
Chronic back pain	Lumbar spine	Single AP view	Changes common and non-specific. May be valuable in young patients with spondylolisthesis or ankylosing spondylitis or older patients with possible collapse

Sea. It has since been demonstrated that there was no difference between the prevalence at birth of Down's syndrome in the areas bordering Windscale compared with the UK as a whole.

Three Mile Island power plant accident

In March 1979 there was a potentially more serious episode when radioactivity was dispersed into the atmosphere around the plant at Three Mile Island in the USA. Two million people lived within about 10 miles of the site. Great concern was engendered concerning reproductive risks and so a detailed study of pregnancies was undertaken. Since no control population of non-exposed pregnancies were available locally, the rate of spontaneous abortion was compared with previous studies. These are shown in Table 21.2. No increase was noted. Subsequent and exhaustive measurement of environmental contamination and human exposure demonstrated that since short-lived isotopes were mainly involved, the risk to public health was small and no more than two excess cancers would be expected to occur in the whole population as a result of the event.

Chernobyl incident

Any sense of relief over the incident at Three Mile Island was exploded 7 years later by another meltdown of nuclear fuel, but this time producing the most significant nuclear event since the bombings of Hiroshima and Nagasaki. The accident primarily occurred because there were no physical controls to prevent staff from operating the reactor in an unstable regime and the shutdown system was too slow. The accident began at 1.23 a.m. on 26 April with a steam explosion that killed two people. Soviet sources did not comment in detail on the subsequent events. In particular, they did not give details of a second, larger

explosion of hydrogen gas, generated by superheated zirconium. This caused a major release of radioactivity. A fire developed in the graphite core following the explosion, producing extremely high temperatures and a burning plume 1500 feet (450 metres) high, which lifted radioactivity rapidly to high altitudes. This accounted for early fall-out in areas as much as a thousand miles away and initially less radioactivity in the area immediately around the plant.

A team from Moscow, specially designated to respond to nuclear accidents, arrived at the Chernobyl site on the morning after the accident, at a time when the fire was still being fought. In the ensuing hours, between 1000 and 2000 people were examined at the site in an attempt to:

- provide immediate medical care
- identify and remove those in need of immediate hospitalisation
- estimate the radiation doses received
- begin triage, a process of dividing injured people into three groups, those who do not need immediate help, those who need immediate help and those beyond help who may need palliative care.

In this case the process was designed to identify:

- those who had good prospects for spontaneous bone marrow regeneration
- those who would require a bone marrow transplant
- those whose radiation exposure was so high or so complicated by thermal burns, inhalation of toxic chemicals from burning plastic, or other trauma that recovery was unlikely.

Biological dosimetry was done on the basis of the following factors:

- clinical histories involving patients' location in the plant, movements about the plant, duration of exposure and recollection of inhaling dust or gases
- history and time of onset of gastrointestinal symptoms, especially early vomiting
- extent and intensity of skin burns, suggesting beta radiation exposure in addition to gamma irradiation
- the rate of decrease in the white blood cell counts.

On the basis of these examinations, 129 patients were evacuated to Moscow in three planeloads on the first day of the accident; a few others had previously been sent to hospitals in Kiev, 80 miles away. On the second day, 170 additional patients believed to be less seriously injured or irradiated were flown to Moscow. Of the

Table 21.2 Observed and expected abortions and stillbirths near Three Mile Island at the time of the accident (Tokuhata 1981)

Gestation (weeks)	Observed abortions or still births	Expected number based on population studies
5–12	11	15.6
13–20	15	7.4
21–28	0	2.8
29–36	0	2.2
37–44	1	2.4
Total	27	30.4

total of 299 persons hospitalised in Moscow, all but two were workers or fire fighters at the Chernobyl plant. Two were residents of the nearby town of Pripyat who were walking or bicycling in rapidly contaminated areas. Another two were physicians at the plant who had been contaminated while caring for patients and assisting in their removal from the reactor site in the hours after the accident.

It is now estimated that approximately 50 people were irradiated with doses greater than 500 rem and approximately 100 received doses of over 300 rem. These estimates are based on clinical dosimetry, complex calculations of radiation levels within the facility and subsequent clinical courses. Those with estimated exposures of 500 rads or more were the first candidates for bone marrow transplantation. Some patients were excluded because of the certainty of death from non-bone marrow causes. Altogether, 186 patients were hospitalised and 26 died, including the two individuals killed in the explosion. The major radioactive releases were of isotopes of iodine and caesium, with small amounts of other isotopes. The Soviet medical authorities stated they were certain that no plutonium or other radionuclides were released.

The evacuation of populations

About 36 hours after the initial explosion, a caravan of 1100 buses was sent to the Chernobyl area. The population within an 18-mile radius of the plant, approximately 100 000 persons, including 25 000 to 30 000 children, was evacuated over a period of 3 hours. All 100 000 people were examined medically and checked for evidence of radiation injury. Some 18 000 were referred to clinics and hospitals in the areas to which they were evacuated for more intensive checks, including chromosomal studies on a group of children. Thousands of studies to detect chromosomal abnormalities in lymphocytes were performed within the first week after the accident.

The delay in evacuation of the area around Chernobyl was the result of local authorities underestimating the level of radioactivity. It is thought that initial radiation readings on the surface in the affected area around Chernobyl were low because of the fire plume height. Following this, local authorities underestimated the release of radioactivity to the environment until more expert resources arrived from Moscow. The local preoccupation was with the task of containing the graphite core fire. It is believed that a substantial number of the 100 000 evacuees received doses of more than 50 rad mostly from direct exposure to fall-out and from inhalation of radionuclides.

A second, smaller and less formal evacuation subsequently took place in Kiev, a city of 2.4 million persons located 80 miles to the south-east of Chernobyl. The initially westward blowing winds apparently protected Kiev until the end of the first week in May, when for 2 days there was a short-term increase in the gamma radiation level and the evacuation of infants, children and pregnant women was recommended. The dose over 2 days was approximately 50 mrem per person.

The magnitude of medical response

More than 300 medical staff members from Moscow were involved in the care of the Chernobyl patients, in addition to those sent to the site in the initial response. Some 230 medical teams, totalling 5000 physicians and nurses, were sent to the Chernobyl region or mobilised in the areas to which residents were evacuated, to conduct the medical examinations of the 100 000 evacuees. All five of the blood centres in Moscow were used to provide platelet and the whole blood transfusion. The Soviet physicians pointed out that this effort strained the medical capabilities of the entire nation.

In addition to the direct medical effort, 188 permanent stations and 38 mobile stations were set up to monitor radioactivity in the evacuated area. Approximately 800 laboratories measured soil and water samples taken every hour in the Pipyat and Dnieper rivers, the reservoir serving Kiev, and elsewhere in the region. Milk and food samples in the Ukraine were monitored continuously. In the weeks after the accident, the Soviet press reported that large dikes had been built along the banks of the Pripyat River and 11 drainage outlets sealed. To prevent further spread of contaminated dust, vehicles inside the evacuation zone were scrubbed down at stations 6 miles from the reactor and again at turnaround points at the border of the zone.

Plans for long-term epidemiological follow-up

The 100 000 evacuated persons are now resettled elsewhere in the Ukraine and in areas of the former Soviet Union as far away as St Petersburg. They will not return to their homes for many years. Long-term follow-up and monitoring of this population and probably other populations in the Ukraine must go on for 40 years or more. The known risks include an increased incidence of leukaemia, cancers of the thyroid, lung, bone, liver, breast and stomach, colon and urinary tract, genetic abnormalities and damage to fetuses.

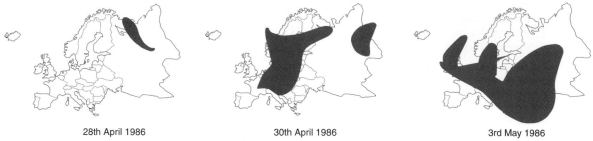

28th April 1986   30th April 1986   3rd May 1986

Fig. 21.3 Areas covered by the cloud after release from Chernobyl. (Anspaugh, Catlin & Goldman 1988)

Data on individuals will be incomplete, particularly regarding internally deposited radionuclides and specific organ doses. In addition, latency periods range from a few years to decades and vary with the age of the person at the time of exposure. To compare population-based rates of cancer incidence, non-irradiated and control populations of roughly equal size and socioeconomic and occupational characteristics must be monitored with equal intensity for equal lengths of time. The effort will be the largest since the Atomic Bomb Casualty Commission studies at Hiroshima and Nagasaki.

The governments and populations of Europe watched the weather reports with concern over the ensuing days to see where the radioactive effluent was being transported (Fig. 21.3). There was, for instance, some contamination in North Wales. Subsequent evaluation of the public health significance of the incident to the population of the European communities estimates that a total of 2000 cancers (35 in the UK) may ultimately occur and be attributable to this event. The significance to the Russian population is obviously more, but insufficient data are currently available to permit estimates.

Nuclear incidents

➤ Accidents at nuclear facilities have occurred. The scale of the radiation effects will depend on the release and spread of radioactive particles. This in turn will depend upon the size of an explosion and the weather conditions.

➤ Casualties can be reduced by a rapid response to reduce releases, to evacuate populations at risk and to provide specialised medical help.
  Radionuclides released in the Chernobyl incident in the Ukraine were deposited over western Britain 7 days later.

Application of epidemiology to health care

6

The need for health care

22

In this chapter the need for health care is discussed in terms of:

- values in public health
- need and demand for health care
- data collection to assess health provision.

Introduction

We cannot judge the need for health care objectively. At first sight this may seem a ridiculous statement. A patient in extremis with, for instance, an allergic reaction to a bee sting or a patient in great pain with a fractured upper arm needs health care. We know that, given treatment, they have an excellent chance of full recovery. Ideally those who need medical care:

- have a problem which needs expert help
- can be assisted by medical intervention
- will have a recovery that is very likely and long lasting
- require treatment that is reasonably priced for the benefit they receive.

Not all cases are so. There is a difference between demand and need. Some patients demand help when their doctor may think that they can manage without expert intervention. The most obvious example is the common cold. Some people go to their GP after a couple of days of discomfort and ask for antibiotics. These people have a demand but, in the doctor's view, no need for care.

In other cases medical intervention may not be relevant to the particular problem:

- GPs are often asked to help sort out marital difficulties where medical intervention is not effective
- some doctors would expect a daughter living at home with a disabled mother to give a considerable amount of care and would not consider that health service intervention was appropriate
- patients who have little hope of recovery, for instance with end-stage cancer, for whom treatment is no longer effective, on humanitarian grounds, would not receive treatment that might be given to an otherwise completely healthy person
- a cardiac bypass operation in a patient with end-stage cancer may be thought to be too costly for its benefit. This would have an impact upon the amount of money available for other people, for there is a fixed amount of money available for health care.

All four of these examples need one to make a judgement about the place of medicine. They also make one decide how much each patient should receive in relation to others; what is their fair share. It is estimated that it costs (in the mid-1990s) about £50 000 to save a life or avert a major disabling disease. If any one person has more spent on them, others will suffer as a consequence. Individual doctors and nurses have to make these decisions in their daily work, though they may not always be aware that they are doing so. The people who run health authorities and trusts have to do this more formally by deciding where money should be spent within the service. These decisions are not easy to make and depend upon the values held by the people making the decisions.

Values in medical care

The Oxford Shorter English Dictionary defines values as 'Ethics: worthy of esteem for its own sake; that which has intrinsic worth'.

In the UK health service, the NHS, we are dealing with values all the time. Programmes relating to effectiveness of treatment, quality improvement, equal opportunities, the Patient's Charter and rationing health care all rely on sets of values. Despite this, there is no statement of the values underlying the structure, policy and work of the NHS nationally or locally. A single code for all the professions within the health service may be asking too much. However, the board of directors of health authorities through consulting the populations they serve and the professionals they use should develop a set of values. This would provide an important backbone for the development of strategic and operational changes.

The need for values

Organisations work according to certain sets of values whether stated or unstated, agreed or not. The advantage of identifying and agreeing them is that, when crises come, the organisation has a better chance of reacting consistently and agreeing to a plan of action. If health authorities wish to pass on the utilitarian principle of 'the greatest good for the greatest number', they must, for instance, have a view of what this means for screening patients. These people have no disease, yet the money for screening is taken from the budget for treating acutely ill patients.

Priorities

Health authorities setting up contracts with hospitals will need to decide between different services and which should have priority. The UK Department of Health in its *Health of the Nation* document has suggested certain principles for the development of services. These relate to the effectiveness and efficiency of services and makes general comments about 'improving health'. It seems a bit too obvious and not very helpful to say that health authorities should aim to improve health. It would be like a shoe factory saying that it should make shoes that fit on feet. A shoe factory, when it decided upon what values it should have, would need to decide whether to make the highest possible quality shoes or the cheapest ones, or a good compromise between these two options. The company would choose to 'value' high quality or cheapness or the cleverness of its compromise.

What is health care?

One difficulty for the health service is that it is not clear about what it is meant to be doing, like a shoe factory that occasionally branches out into making hats or coats. It tends not to be very good at these other things because it does not have the skill to do so. Examples are when the health service tries to give

largely social care or tries to educate the public. They are not very good at it.

Most health authorities pretend that they are giving the highest possible quality at a very low price. However each health authority will tend towards one of the following types.

Health for all

Health in this instance is defined as in the WHO definition as a 'sense of complete mental, physical and social well-being'. This covers the whole population, with interventions in many fields beyond the traditional health areas with many groups working with the poor and ethnic minorities. It tends to clash with government policies in budgeting, always overspending.

Health promotion

Ways of maintaining health is regarded as something taught to people. The approach follows closely the research evidence for the avoidance of disease. It relies on population data and is geared to the whole population. There is some politics involved. Health educationists have clashed heavily with the government in the UK on the promotion of information about sex, drugs and tobacco. They spend a great deal of time promoting exercise for young fit people.

Health services for providing reassurance

There is an emphasis on screening for many diseases, including some that are quite rare. This gives reassurance to large numbers that they are 'normal'. It may not leave much money for patients who need acute hospital care.

Health services for 'cradle to the grave' care

Advocates of this approach suggest that 'all effective services should be free'. This diverts attention towards deciding what is meant by effective. It is difficult to prove that many of the health services we provide are effective, so the health authority tends to clash with its consultants, as the authority wants proof before it will spend money.

Health services for 'health gain'

Those in need of health care are defined as those who will gain appreciably in terms of mortality and morbidity by receiving health services. The approach tends to be a bit woolly on what to do for people who are not going to get better and on new developments that are promising but provide no health gain yet.

Acute health interventions only

There is a need to define what services provide acute

medical care. The health interventions are often described as a 'core' service. Other services are described as 'social care' and taken out of the remit of the health service. This shifts the argument to one about where the boundaries between health, social and educational care should lie. An example of the difficulty of following this approach was when some health authorities said that long-term care for elderly people was not part of the health service. The government disagreed and rapped them across the knuckles.

What values?

One expert (Andrew Wall) has suggested four values for the development of management in the health service:

- justice
- value for the community
- value for the individual
- sense of duty.

Another expert (David Seedhouse, in a book on ethics) has suggested a similar four:

- respect persons equally
- create autonomy
- respect autonomy
- serve needs before wants.

One reason for the need for values is when we have to make priorities for scarce resources. The Oregon State government, for example, had a particular problem, for many of its citizens were uninsured for health-care costs. The government decided that they would like to provide a basic package of care for all of their uninsured population but could not afford all available services for everyone. They decided to set priorities for different types of medical care, based on a set of values. The following shows the list of ethical values or areas of concern drawn up from public response at community meetings and individual phoned interviews:

- prevention
- quality of life
- cost effectiveness
- ability to function
- equity
- effectiveness of treatment
- benefits large numbers
- mental health and chemical dependency
- personal choice
- community compassion
- impact on society (e.g. infectious diseases)
- length of life
- personal responsibility (lifestyle).

The researchers grouped these into three sets:

- essential to basic health care
- of value to society
- of value to the individual

Prevention and quality of life appeared in all three. Three others described as being essential were:

- benefits to many
- an impact on society
- cost effectiveness.

Many of these are not values but characteristics of a functioning service. There will always be trade-offs between one type of service and another. Values help one to decide which of these should have priority when the trade-offs occur.

Values are needed to:

- decide if a service falls into the realm of health care or should be carried out by another agency, e.g. the family, social services, the education service
- decide priorities for two options if both cannot be taken on because of financial or other constraints
- set the style of the service, e.g. an excellent service for the severely ill or a wide spread of services for all groups.

Values in practice

One researcher highlighted the values that exist in hospitals in a piece of research. In 24 hospitals there were a large number of innovations introduced during a 6-month period. The importance given to these innovations suggested the values held by managers. The researchers classified them into four groups along two axes. The first axis had, at one end, an emphasis on flexibility versus, at the other end, control. The second related to internal versus external changes (Fig. 22.1).

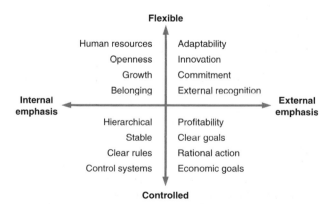

Fig. 22.1 Types of organisations and their values produced during a survey of 24 hospitals instituting innovations.

The most notable finding was that the 'flexible, internally orientated' group was good at the development of training for their staff, but this group contained by far the smallest number of innovations. Half of the hospitals questioned did not have any innovations of this type. Only three hospitals failed to introduce innovations in the 'external orientation, control' group. This suggests that hospital managers were not concerned with developing their staff. Managers were keeping close control over the way that their people worked and, while aiming to care for their patients, care did not extend to the staff working for the organisation. People have often suggested in the past that caring organisations are likely to fail to care for those who work in them.

Problems with values

There are a number of general approaches to choosing what we should do first.

Equity given pre-eminence. Expensive treatments are limited in favour of the cheaper.

Greatest potential for improving health. Purchasing is based on the greatest number of lives saved and disabilities avoided. Smoking prevention by the GP tends to be most effective here.

Accessibility. This tends to favour primary care. Acutely ill people have less priority.

Best possible service for everyone. These services are likely to run out of money because of spending on services of marginal value.

Need and demand in health care

People in most countries recognise the idea of sickness. Some researchers have suggested that the

---

The need for health care

➤ Balancing demands and needs requires a set of values upon which health service provisions can be based.

➤ Sets of values are needed to decide if a service falls into the realm of health care, to decide priorities if only some of several options are possible and to set the style (ethos) of the service.

➤ In practice, sets of values may affect the type and range of care available and there will always be deficits in care resulting from the imposition of value sets.

---

essence of sickness is an 'unwanted condition of self'. This may include any part of the person, the body, the mind, the experience or relationships. Such conditions come in degrees of severity and different people have different thresholds for how serious a condition must be to qualify as sickness. The culture a person lives in defines what constitutes an unwanted condition so that there will be differences between different societies on what is counted as sickness or health.

In developed countries, most people look for health care as a way of obtaining a better level of health. People usually see the advantages of more health in terms of function, the things they can do, rather than an abstract goal.

The four main elements of health

Health can be considered as having four aspects.

Human biology: includes genetic inheritance, the process of ageing and the robustness of our 'body systems'

Environment: includes those factors related to health external to the person and over which the individual has little or no control, e.g. adequacy of sanitation, water supply, atmospheric pollution, radiation

Lifestyle: the aggregation of decisions by individuals that affect their health and over which they have ostensibly some control, e.g. smoking, diet

Health care: includes quantity, quality and access to health care.

Demand for health care is those wants which people express by seeking the assistance of a medical practitioner or other health-care professional.

Need for health care is more difficult to define but invokes the notion that a professional judgement is involved in converting a demand into a need.

The idea of demand requires that people are aware of the alternatives available to them and that they make choices according to certain criteria. Need is paternalistic: a health-care professional 'knows best'. The individual's need for care is what the doctor thinks he ought to have. However, need is not absolute. Views about what is needed depend on a whole variety of factors to do with the relationship between the patient and the doctor and the values of the society in which they live. This leads to the 'iceberg' phenomenon of patients experiencing wants but not expressing them as demands. We would say these people had a need if they had approached the health service for help and a doctor agreed that they needed help. Sometimes such people are identified in screening processes or in surveys of the population. We can also define a need for health care by our ability to offer an effective intervention. The term effective means that the intervention does more good than harm.

Estimating the need for health care in a health authority

Traditionally, the need for health care in a health authority is estimated using various indicators and projected changes over time as proxies for more direct measures of need. Sources of information for measuring need include:

- routine data
- special local health status and behavioural surveys
- treatment and service effectiveness reviews.

Evaluation of health care is discussed in Chapter 23 and assessment of treatment and service effectiveness in Chapter 25. Here, we will concentrate on sources of routine data.

The problem with using routine data for working out the health needs of a population is that most of these data are collected after an event has happened. This may not be a good guide to what is going to happen in the future. In addition, the data tend to emphasise the importance of hospital and other institutional care, for the great majority of the information is collected in hospital.

Routine data are those data that are collected (usually by the health services) without a special request. A number of different public agencies collect and publish them in a variety of ways. There are three main groups of routine data that are useful for health purposes.

General data

- Census
- OPCS registers information; births marriages and deaths.

Health services data

- Hospital returns
- Community returns
- Notification of disease.

General practice returns

- individual records
- drug use including flagging adverse effects
- hospital referrals.

Non-health service data

- Local authority
- Health and safety, etc.

Patients' charter data.

Health services data

Health services data in the 1990s in the UK are in a state of change related to the development of the internal market and the rapid developments in technology. Before the 1990 act, the Department of Health at regional level collected and distributed most of the data. The data were standardised throughout the country with each hospital providing similar returns and there were careful checks on accuracy. The problem was that the data gave a superficial view of what was going on in the health service. Nevertheless we could, with a little imagination, make use of the basic bed use and diagnostic data. The data are still obtainable, but they are becoming steadily more difficult to obtain.

Doctors and nurses spend a third of their time directly collecting or using data. The relationship between purchasers and providers, with its requirement for detailed monitoring data from health trusts and the liberty that the trusts have to develop their own data collection systems has caused some confusion. Some attempts to bring order do exist. The National Clearinghouse project collects data from trust data systems nightly and puts together comparative statistics. These are useful bench marks against which to judge, for example, a teaching hospital with others.

Hospital data have the advantage that patients come into hospital, have something done, then go home or die. In other words, their care occurs in discrete episodes that can be easily counted. In the community, the patients are more likely to be seen intermittently over many years. Different facets of the service leading to double counting may also occur. Until recently, when patients are increasingly being given their notes to look after, it was difficult to know how many health service personnel had been to a patient at home and what they had done. People regarded recording this centrally as a low priority.

Hospital episode statistics

Hospital episode statistics are a way of collecting, for each patient admitted to hospital as an in-patient, details of age, sex, area of residence and condition treated. They also mention operations done, the time the patient spent on the waiting list and how long was

165

spent in hospital. They include data about the area of residence of patients, including their postcode. We can use this to define the catchment population of the hospital, district or region. The catchment area is the area from which people travel to be treated. It will obviously vary from specialty to specialty. This is important if one wishes to look at treatment rates on a population basis. Patients going into geriatric ward care are likely to be local. In regional centres, usually gathered around a medical school, patients are likely to travel considerable distances. This tends to be for services that are expensive or very specialist. Cardiac surgery, for instance, may have patients travelling for hundreds of miles.

SH3 or QS1

These forms traditionally contained bed-use statistics for hospitals in the UK. The data are now collected on computer as one database. The SH3 has been an administrative form containing information about numbers of allocated and used in-patient beds, out-patients and day patients. The information has been extended in the last few years by the Körner data set (see below) to include data on out-patient care and specialty-based information. This in turn is being modified by the new data-collecting systems.

Mental Health Inquiry

The Mental Health Inquiry in the UK relates to mental illness and developed separately, probably because of the separate development of the mental hospitals. It is a slightly better system in that diagnostic data is combined with administrative data. Despite this there are considerable problems with the diagnostic data. This is often because of genuine disagreement between psychiatrists on what is wrong with patients with mental illnesses. The Mental Health Inquiry includes a point prevalence of patients both for age, sex and diagnosis and for length of stay to that point. This is a census of the patients in hospital taken one evening in the year. This approach is useful where there are a lot of long-stay patients in hospital.

Körner

The Körner data set includes information on the different treatment specialties. There are more subspecialty groups and more information on in-patients and out-patients who did not attend than in the pre-existing data sets. Recently, there has been a lot more information on waiting lists, especially whether the waiting list patients were classified as urgent or not and the time patients were kept on the list. There is also information on the actions of professionals working alongside doctors, such as physiotherapists, the pathology services and suchlike.

Diagnostic-related groups

In the USA, diagnosis-related groups (DRGs) have been a popular method of categorising patients on admission for some years. They were set up to fit in with the price schedules for paying hospitals used by US organisations. Medicare, the federal safety net for poor people, and Medicaid for elderly people use them to decide on how much to pay hospitals and others. DRGs classify patients into one of around 500 categories, based on the diagnosis with added information on, for example, the age of the patient or whether there were major complications. These are set up in such a way that the costs of treating patients in any one category should be approximately the same wherever they are treated. Different DRGs relate to different levels of cost. In the UK, the costs are different but for common diseases the ratios between the different costs appear to be reasonably accurate.

In the USA, where the system is used for paying hospitals there is a temptation to overcategorise patients, in other words to assign patients on the margin between two categories to a more expensive DRG. Similar things happen in the UK with some of the contracting in the NHS at present. An example is the pricing, by hospital trusts, of specialist care compared with the price of general medical or surgical care. The superspecialty is always priced higher than the general specialty. This appears at first sight to be sensible, but when one thinks further the difference between specialist and generalist wards may be very little, except that the patients on the specialist wards have similar problems to each other. There is little proof that they cost more.

The existence of specialist wards in district general hospitals is often an accident of history or to do with the area in which the hospital is placed. Hospitals in south Wales and the Potteries in the UK, for instance, often have chest wards because the local industries were toxic to lungs. There is an argument that a general ward, expected to deal with a wide range of problems, could be more expensive than a specialist ward. Table 22.1 shows an example comparing specialties of general medicine, medical gastroenterology and geriatrics.

There is no nationally agreed distinction between the definition of one specialty against another except historical precedent, a general view on the length of

Table 22.1 Classification of patients and costs

Specialty	Code	Currency	Contract level	Trust price (£)	Marginal price (£)	Contract value (£)
General medicine	300	Cons.epis.	4657	918	246	4 275 126
Gastroenterology	300	Cons.epis	356	1092	273	388 752
Geriatrics	430	Cons.epis	2075	2335	625	4 845 125

The currency column consists of completed consultant episodes (Cons.epis.). The contract level is the number of those episodes over the year in question. The trust price is the price per episode and the marginal price the amount charged by the trust for extra cases if the trust provides more than its contracted number of cases.

stay of patients in each type of bed and the training of the specialist in charge. It is obvious that re-designation of beds or a slight alteration in the admission criteria for one type of bed against another can alter the total cost of the service considerably.

The UK government aims to develop all purchasing according to DRG categories in the future. The reason for this is that they and the purchasers will be able to compare more closely the costs of one hospital with another for a specific intervention. The theory is that, by using DRGs, like can be compared with like, in other words the approach will allow us to take account of different severities of patients in different areas. This is known as taking account of the 'case mix' in the different hospitals.

In theory it should be possible to compare, for example, death rates according to the commoner DRG categories. There is a growing tendency for people to publish this information so that patients can make comparisons between hospitals. However, we must remember that the origin of DRGs was as a way of banding patients according to their cost. Their originators did not intend them as a way of categorising the severity of one group of patients compared with another. If outcome data, deaths or morbidity are published according to DRG to make different hospitals comparable, some careful work will be needed to validate this approach. We are not aware that any has been done so far. We certainly know that the relationship between outcome and diagnosis is complex.

Community health services

The person providing the service usually collects community health service information. It tends to be rather inaccurate. The people in the service see little point in filling out forms and the feedback of the information collected is not good. Midwives and health visitors use the data to identify new mothers from their maternity records. It later identifies children of certain ages, who receive checks on their physical and mental development.

Clinics

Antenatal clinics make records of the number of their sessions and who runs them. Similar data are available for postnatal clinics. The number of women who attend relaxation classes and the number of attendances during the year are recorded. Out-patient clinics generally are part of the hospital episode statistics.

Child health services

Child health clinics record the numbers of children seen, the number of sessions held and who supervised them. The school health service also gives information on medical examinations performed, ophthalmic data, ear diseases, postural defects and skin diseases. Many health authorities are trying quietly to dismantle the school health service because of criticism that their commonest findings by far were head lice, virtually all the other information gathered being already known to the GPs. Teachers are very keen to keep the service.

Immunisation details

Records are kept of the number of persons vaccinated including BCG, tuberculosis and other immunisations. GPs have been specifically given the task of ensuring that vaccination and immunisation levels are improved year on year. This has been very successful, backed as it was with the carrot of more money for those who reached specified targets.

Communicable Disease Surveillance Centre

The centres for communicable disease surveillance in the UK and the USA have been mentioned in some detail in Chapter 18.

Staff data

Approximately three-quarters of NHS expenditure is on wages, about two-fifths on nurses' wages. Despite this, data on staffing are often hard to get hold of and are often inaccurate.

Cancer registration

Other information that is collected includes cancer registration. Cancers are registered at diagnosis whether at postmortem or when diagnosed in hospital. Some registries in the UK have fallen badly behind with collecting their data.

League tables

One result of trends in the UK to create an internal market in the health service has been the desire to provide data that compares hospitals or other health-care providers The government has published league tables on hospital performance. Until now, the greatest variation in the measures between hospitals was with cancelled operations not readmitted within a month of the second cancellation. Some regions of the UK had no patients in this category, in others over half of the patients had such cancelled operations. The UK government has also published some data from primary care including the proportion of medical records transferred urgently or routinely, the allocation to a GP and the percentage of practices who had charters. The idea of these charters is to allow people to make choices, but so far little information about clinical quality has been included in the charters.

The government has been resistant to publishing clinical information, especially about death rates. The reason is that there are differences between patients admitted by different hospitals. In some places the age, sex and severity of the disease will be different for patients with the same condition. Some of the data are not complete. For example, deaths from an episode of illness may occur after discharge from hospital, especially if people are discharged earlier in some areas than others. It may be that for some diseases death is not a reasonable way of measuring the quality of the service received in hospital. It may, for instance, just be the culmination of a series of different treatments with people admitted to hospital for the last part of their illness.

General practice data

GPs have to produce an annual report by law in the UK. The practitioners provide this for the health authority. We have had basic information on prescriptions for some time but this has recently become more detailed. Prescribing data can be very valuable for looking at trends in treating patients, especially the development of new drugs. The annual report also contains data about patients referred to hospital, though this is often not very accurate. It does allow a cross-check to the referral data held by the hospitals.

General practice records are now usually held on computer. They contain the names of the people in each practice, their address, date of birth and their NHS number. The GP's record is sometimes the only way of telling how many people of, for instance, a particular age group are present in the practice. The other benefit of the record is that it contains the NHS number. This is a unique number for every one in the UK. It can be used if necessary to trace people who may, for example, have been in a research project. These data are held at the National Health Service Central Register in Southport. Patients of interest can be flagged in the central register, so that when they die or move that information can be returned to the person who asked for the flagging. This is also a useful device for doctors or nurses wishing to follow up their patients over a long period.

Nationally representative information on consulting in general practice has been collected in the National Morbidity Studies intermittently since the mid-1970s. These studied a large number of practices and gave information on the diagnosis, and the number of consultations and referrals in those practices.

Non-health service information

Non-health service information that is relevant to health in the UK includes the local authority registration of handicapped people and notification of industrial diseases to the Health and Safety Executive. Certificates of incapacity to work are collected by the Department of Social Security. The General Household Survey gives data on a wide variety of items, including visits made to hospital services and lifestyle factors such as cigarette smoking.

Figure 22.2 shows data for the number of people certified incapable of working since 1970. The problem with the data is that people who are unemployed and have a marginal incapacity may be more likely to be signed on by their doctor in times of high unemployment. It is not clear how accurate these data are, but the figure does show the great rise in numbers during recent years. The government of the day decided that the rapid changes, without other sings of increasing illness, must be an artefact and checked all incapacity claimants and their doctors.

Demographic and social data provide background information on poverty in different areas. This has

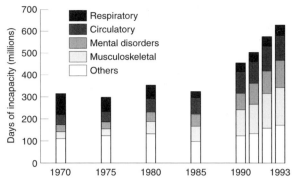

Fig. 22.2 Days of certified incapacity by selected causes. (Rates of incapacity for work. Cause OPCS, HMSO 1970–93)

implications for the need for health care, but the data do not provide information about absolute levels or even about the nature of specific services. Health-status surveys are usually about the need for health. They are not often about the need for health care unless they are designed to measure, for example, cataract opacity or hip movement and pain, for which an effective remedy is available. Rates for people visiting GPs or waiting lists are usually related to the amount of the service supplied not to the need of the patients.

The Patients' Charter

The Patients' Charter is a government provision in the UK that lays down what consumers should expect from health service providers. The Charter is produced annually by the Government which gives guaranteed standards for the NHS. These standards are reported annually by each of the local Health Authorities to Central Government and are published for the general public. Quite a lot of information

---

Need and demand

➤ Demand is considered to require an aware population who can make choices regarding their needs.

➤ Need is considered to involve a professional judgement that considers many issues.

➤ DRGs (diagnosis-related groups) are a popular means of categorising patients on admission.

➤ Information to enable needs to be assessed can be obtained from routine data reflecting past use, special status and reviews of treatment and service effectiveness.

---

is published in the UK in relation to the Patients' Charter, much of it available on the Internet as http://www.open.gov.uk/. The Patients' Charter does not lay down rights to service. It sets up standards of national performance. This encourages local hospitals, community services, ambulance trusts, health authorities and GP fundholders to improve on these with their own higher standards for the delivery of care. The Charter has so far concentrated on the time patients spend waiting for treatment in hospital for out-patients or in the accident departments or in the GP's surgery.

General rights

● Patients have a right to know if they are going to be placed in mixed sex wards.
● National standards address security and cleanliness as well as single sex washing and toilet facilities for patients in hospital.
● If a patient complains, they should receive a written acknowledgement within 2 working days and a full reply within 4 weeks.

More specific standards: in-patients

● A 3–4 hour standard for emergency admission to hospital through accident and emergency departments to be strengthened to 2 hours.
● Children should normally be admitted to children's wards under the care of a paediatric consultant rather than to adult wards.
● An 18 month maximum to be guaranteed for waiting time for all in-patient treatment.
● A standard should address hospital catering services.
● Patients when admitted should receive written information about hospital facilities.
● A coronary bypass or similar treatment for blocked coronary arteries should occur within a year of being diagnosed as needed, including the waiting time for the first appointment.

More specific standards: out-patients

● A 26 week standard for first out-patient appointments to be set, including a target of 90% for all trust out-patients to be a seen within 13 weeks.

More specific standards: other services

● Standards for home visits by community nurses in 2-hour time bands to be set and other standards addressing when their visits should be made.

- A series of standards set for ambulance arrival.
- Waiting should not be more than 4 hours in an accident and emergency department.
- Patients with serious mental illness will work with a carer of their choice and agree and keep a copy of their care plan.

Expectations of health-care provision

The data gathered in the various forms described above provide the basis for decisions on future health-care provisions. The implementation of policies in documents such as the Patients' Charter will also affect the future provision of health care.

Other things that will alter the quantity of services needed when planning health services include:

- disease incidence and prevalence, including 'new' diseases such as AIDS; incidence and prevalence measures do not automatically provide a measure of 'need' for health care
- medical technology (all kinds of care and interventions) that creates a new need and new clientele: magnetic resonance imaging scanners, coronary artery laser surgery, hospice care.

All these factors often must be balanced against what is being provided. It is difficult, for instance, to close down a large hospital, even if it does not appear to be needed. Other pressures come from public opinion, politicians, community health councils, the press and voluntary groups. These people usually have their reasons for trying to alter what is provided, not necessarily in line with what the general public wishes. Other influences include policy laid down by government departments, in the UK the Department of Health, Welsh and Scottish Offices and health authorities (again influenced to a varying extent by public opinion).

Most of the activity that takes place is forced by external factors. It is virtually never possible to reconcile the difference between these different pressures in planning.

Future expectations for health care

➤ The Patients' Charter lays down standards of national performance in the health service.

➤ New diseases and new technology may also produce new needs for health care.

➤ Data on which future planning is based is dominated by the hospital sector, where most money is spent but where a minority of patients are treated.

Evaluation of health care

23

In chapters 23 and 24 the evaluation of health care is discussed in the three areas of input, process and output. In this chapter general aspects of evaluation are examined including

- routine evaluation methods
- clinical and medical audit
- evaluation of clinical effectiveness.

In chapter 24 evaluation of output is described.

Introduction

Evaluation is the systematic and scientific process of determining the extent to which an action or set of actions were successful in the achievement of predetermined objectives. This definition implies using a rigorous scientific method and emphasises that the objectives should be predetermined. Evaluation in health care involves the measurement of the adequacy, effectiveness and the efficiency of the health service.

Areas open to evaluation

There are three main areas of interest in health services, which can be evaluated. They are shown in Figure 23.1.

Inputs

Inputs to the health service include the money and buildings. The major input from which all the others are derived is money. It is often said that the UK health service requires more money. Yet the same thing is said in the USA where they spend the same proportion of the money they have available on public health care with, in addition, one and a half times as much on pri-

Inputs ——▶ Process ——▶ Outputs

Fig. 23.1 Classification of evaluation areas in health services.

vate health care. This suggests that there is not a 'right' amount. The second problem is what to buy with the money, the inputs. There is a tendency in the health service to develop long shopping lists of things, which would possibly improve the service. But how should we decide when to stop? New technologies and equipment often have high costs but expand the areas open to treatment.

Processes

Processes are what happens within the health service. The processes of care are important to the staff, for this is what they are directly involved in. Hospital wards and community nursing departments always give an air of extreme activity. People are rushing about at all hours so that it is difficult to believe that such active processes are not doing good. Sadly this often appears to be not the case. A number of reports have suggested that out patient departments, for instance, are often extremely busy seeing patients returning to hospital for 'check ups' that are not clinically justified.

Outputs

The inputs to the service and the processes undertaken by the service are only justified by the *effect* that they have. We call these the outputs from the service. The outputs are measures of the effect the health service has on the community and on patients. For convenience we have divided the outputs into two types, the outputs themselves and a subgroup, the outcomes.

Output measures

- the effect on the staff, e.g. employment
- the effect on the country, e.g. fitter people helping the economy
- indirect effects, e.g. information about health
- research spin offs into other disciplines.

Outcome measures

● the effects on the patients: lifespan
● the effects on the patients: quality of life and fitness.

In this chapter, general methods of evaluation are discussed and assessment of clinical processes. Output is discussed in Chapter 24.

Historical precedents

Over a century ago William Farr, John Simon and Florence Nightingale were suggesting careful comparisons of historically based practices to determine the relative value of different methods of treatment. These ideas did not catch on, possibly because improving basic nutrition and hygiene were very obviously successful in combating the main scourges of the day without careful analysis. Their objectives were to reduce the death rate over a short period, which was reasonably easy to measure.

Unfortunately many of the specific treatments of disease which were developing as nutrition and hygiene improved fooled many doctors into thinking that their therapies were the thins that were having the effect. The need for evaluation is much greater these days when the dreaded diseases have long-term causes and are rarely cured. It is an old trick of epidemiologists to ask students to mention one effective hospital treatment – one form of therapy given by hospitals which unequivocally helps patients. There is usually an incredulous silence; first, that anyone should doubt that any therapies are definitely effective, then trying to think of one that is. Someone in the class will say appendicectomy if you are lucky because you have the next figure waiting (Fig. 23.2). This shows the mortality figures for appendicitis with time based on figures from the USA. We can see that the death rate from appendicitis actually increased after the operation became popular. Better anaesthetics and antibiotics

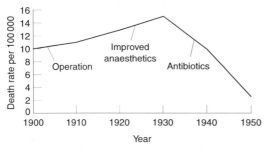

Fig. 23.2 Death rate from appendicitis. (Smith 1986)

appear to have reduced the rate over the years. Data from this period may, of course, be inaccurate. Appendicectomy became fashionable after the coronation of Edward VII in 1902 had to be postponed to allow the King to have his appendix removed. It may be that the diagnosis became popular and that more severe illnesses were incorrectly labelled, leading to the higher death rate. Whatever the reason, the existence of data showing a rising death rate did not put off the US surgeons.

Maxwell's criteria for evaluation of a service

Maxwell suggested a series of principles that should underlie any service.

Access to services. Access can mean personal access, such as the availability of the service to wheelchair users or its proximity or its times of opening in relation to the people who need to use it.

Relevance to the needs of the whole community. This brings in the need for a judgement about whether the service has been given an appropriate degree of priority compared with other services. One hopes that services that are given in greatest quantity are most needed in the community that is served. A service set up for infants might be thought to be less relevant to an area dominated by retirement homes.

Effectiveness for individual patients.

Equity. Equity is a difficult concept. One needs to clarify whether each person should have equal access to the available resources; a situation that few people would tolerate for very ill people might run out of their 'share' very quickly. Equity refers to equal access to services for people with similar degrees of illness. This is equity according to health need. Judgements are required regarding how much more resource severely ill people should receive compared with people with minor degrees of illness. There is no accepted measure of severity of illness, though attempts have been made to introduce a measure of disability in the UK, known as the SF-36 in the health service. Equity may simply mean that people, no matter what their characteristics (i.e. their age, sex, social status or race) should have equal access to the services they need, according to their state of health. Such equity does not occur at present. There are example throughout the medical literature which show that elderly people, women, poor people and racial minorities usually have less access to services than young people, men, those who are rich and those who form the racial majority.

Social acceptability. This may refer to the acceptability of a treatment. It may be embarrassing, painful or difficult to apply. It may have embarrassing side effects, such as causing loss of hair or colouring the skin.

Efficiency and economy. These aspects become of increasing importance with the rising costs of health care.

Maxwell's approach is broader than simply measuring the effectiveness and efficiency of the service. Methods of measuring such things as access, relevance to the whole community, equity and social acceptability are not at all well developed. As a result, relatively little research has covered these areas.

Evaluation methods

There are a number of methods of evaluation, some specifically assess the process – the clinical activities occurring within the health service – while others also provide outcomes, with measures of effects on patients and provision of data.

Problems with evaluating health care

It is difficult to decide if an intervention made by a doctor or nurse is effective on the results of a small number of patients. At a physiological level, patients are all different. Older patients may require a different dose of the medication from younger, other diseases or an allergy to the first choice of medication may require a different approach. At a psychological level, the relationship between the doctor and patient has a direct effect on how sucessful the treatments is likely to be. One of the most powerful ways of deciding whether the quality of health services is reasonable is to ask the patients their views on how it affected them. Some authors have shown that patient satisfaction is important because satisfied patients are more likely to co-operate with the people giving their health care. They are more likely to fulfil their part of the implied bargain that patients and doctors strike when they meet, for instance by taking whatever medication or advice the doctor gave them.

Routine evaluation in the health service

There are groups that regularly evaluate the quality of care in the health service in the UK. At the top, the Department of Health issues norms or guidelines to the NHS about the inputs or processes of care. Norms are suggestions about, for instance, how many beds that hospital specialty should have per 100 000 population. The number is usually based on a 'best guess'

somewhere between the average for the country as a whole and the maximum in some areas. The government also passes laws about some patients in the health service. For example, some patients may be detained in mental institutions for their own or others' safety and the government through parliament controls this.

Other parliamentary institutions such as the Health Services Select Committee make reports on problems in the health service. The Select Committee, for instance, suggested, some years back, that the health service was badly underfunded. The Public Accounts Committee and Comptroller suggest where there is waste and inefficiency in relation to buying, for example buying medicines from different sources for health service use.

Regional outposts of the Department of Health evaluate the performance of health authorities in England. The Welsh and Scottish Offices also take this function. The health authorities, in turn, evaluate the performance of the hospital, community and ambulance trusts, mostly by setting up contracts with them that contain set standards.

For doctors, the General Medical Council, as well as being empowered to keep a register of all medical practitioners, can use disciplinary powers against doctors and remove their names from the register. The Royal Colleges set standards for postgraduate medicine by setting up examinations for allowing specialists to practice within their own specialty. The profession make judgements about good standards of practice and may in certain circumstances evaluate the behaviour of individual members. Clinicians make judgements about the quality of the work of their colleagues in peer review and, more commonly in the UK, clinical audit. Senior nurse managers practice job performance reviews of their staff.

The following list gives types of routine evaluation in the health service:

- Norms, e.g. for the number of beds in a service: usually set up by the Royal Colleges and usually biased towards expansion of the service
- Parliamentary Select Committees
- regional outposts of the Department of Health evaluate health authorities
- General Medical Council, General Nursing Council maintain standards for doctors and nurses
- Royal Colleges maintain standards for specialist doctors
- peer reviews, e.g. the Confidential Enquiries into Maternal Deaths, Perinatal Deaths and Perioperative Deaths

- Community Health Councils monitor health authorities
- NHS Commissioner (Ombudsman) monitors NHS
- Audit Commission monitors performance in the NHS, especially efficiency
- Health Advisory Service monitors long-term care facilities
- medical and clinical audit: all doctors are required to audit their own work with their colleagues
- guidelines: becoming increasingly common for the treatment of common conditions; are often produced nationally and followed, with local variations, locally
- Patient's Charter standards: published nationally, mainly concern waiting times
- outcomes (in Scotland): measure patient mortality and morbidity.

Peer reviews

The Confidential Enquiries into Maternal Deaths, Perinatal Deaths and Perioperative Deaths are national forms of peer review. Leaders in each of the fields examine data from colleagues in the field and make recommendations about how services should be adapted to prevent further deaths.

Other bodies in the UK

Community Health Councils are composed of lay people chosen by the Secretary of State to make judgements about all aspects of care within their district. Sometimes politicians within their constituencies are called in and may raise a question about some problem in the House of Commons.

There is National Health Service Commissioner (Ombudsman) for England and Wales. The commissioner may not examine matters that involve the exercise of clinical judgement and can only look at cases that have already been investigated by the health authority; but the Ombudsman can look at administrative failures of the health authority.

The Health Advisory Service is an independent body charged by the government with examining and giving advice on the standards of long-term health facilities for the mentally ill, those with learning disabilities and the elderly long-stay patient. It looks at processes of care in two main areas. These are mainly input orientated:

- physical: are the wards suitable for purpose, do they have privacy and are they clean?
- numerical: is there sufficient staff for the purpose?

They are less concerned with whether the processes of diagnosis and treatment are being accurately carried out.

Medical and clinical audit

Since 1990, medical and clinical audit has become part of everyday life for most health care professionals in the UK. Audits weigh the use of resources against the efficiency of their use. Although they are basically concerned with the 'process' of health provision, they do provide output measures too. Medical audit is, in general, confined to the work that doctors do, clinical includes the whole team working in a specialty. Different approaches are adopted in hospital and community trusts and in primary care. The difficult part is to discover which aspects of the clinical audit movement have been successful.

Clinical audit should be central to the care of patients, bringing together professionals from all sectors of health care to:

- consider clinical evidence
- promote education
- suggest new lines of research
- develop and implement clinical guidelines
- improve information management skills
- contribute to better management of resources.

These all have the aim of improving the quality of care of patients. In primary care, clinical audit has not been compulsory, but from 1991 each health authority has set up a medical audit advisory group to support general practices making audits. The most successful medical audit advisory groups have been professionally led. They have taken a helping and educational rôle, and this approach has secured the commitment of most GPs and their teams. Audit support staff have been vital in helping busy practice teams to improve their clinical care. Doctors initially suspected managerial interference, and practices have found it increasingly difficult to find time for what remains a voluntary (and unpaid) activity in already crowded days. However, there has been an increase in the quantity and quality of clinical audit in general practice as a direct result of the activity of medical audit advisory groups. This was accompanied by improvements in care and an acceptance of audit as part of general practice.

Selection of audit topics

Current guidance states that 40% of audit projects should be chosen by the health authorities, 40% from within audit departments and the remaining 20% split between national audits and audit across the primary or secondary care interface.

Audit requires a number of things:

- the development of information systems that handle patient management and audit data at the same time, with safeguards regarding the confidentiality of patients
- health authorities to negotiate audit topics that are relevant to patient care and which are amenable to change
- mechanisms to involve patients in identifying topics for audit should be explored
- health authorities should promote audit topics that encourage health-care professions to work as multiprofessional teams
- the audit programmes should be based on a 3 yearly cycle. This helps establish audit as part of the overall contracting process.

The use guidelines

A major expectation of audit is that it will help to provide guidelines that will contribute to a more effective service.

Evidence-based guidelines, properly implemented, can contribute to good medicine. Staff are more likely to adopt guidelines produced from local discussion than guidelines imposed without modification. Work is, therefore, needed between local clinicians, purchasers and audit staff to adapt guidelines for local use. At the same time they need to define the key audit questions they need to monitor the application of these guidelines. Many existing guidelines are based on medical research. The development and adoption of multiprofessional guidelines may influence the success of clinical audit. Audit is a means by which we can judge guidelines, using the guideline as a basis for writing standards and developing criteria. Ideally, the audit package should be an integral part of the guideline, developed and tested at the same time as the guideline to make sure that it is valid and reliable.

The legal implications of using guidelines revolve around negligence. The law recognises the need for doctors to use discretion in individual cases, and a well-designed guideline will allow for individual judgement. Should doctors not comply with a guideline, it is unlikely that people would find this negligent, unless the action taken was one that no doctor acting with reasonable skill and care would take. Doctors are only guilty of negligence if a responsible body of medically qualified people do not accept that their actions were reasonable.

Standards

Work on the local adaptation of guidelines will lead to discussion of the standards against which personnel can measure their performance during the audit.

- Ideally, standards should be evidence based. Standards must not be so different from current practice that they cannot be achieved and they should reflect current best practice.
- There should be discussions between the health authority and clinicians before local standards are set. This allows them to compare their results with those of their colleagues.
- The National Centre for Clinical Audit has developed criteria for audit, which will help to set up audit protocols. This will help health-care workers to compare their work with that of their colleagues elsewhere.
- Purchaers should encourage the use of standards and audit tools, especially for developing services. They can apply these to specialties across a range of health-care activities, including management. Example of such generic audit packages include the speed of communication between hospitals and GPs and the setting by clinicians of target discharge dates for individual patients.
- Standards selected purely by consensus, unsupported by research evidence, are likely to perpetuate ineffective treatment.

Outcomes

Clinical audit aims to improve health outcomes for patients by focusing on the clinical outcomes of care. Outcome measurements are a positive way of focusing on improvements. Clinical trials identify those treatments that improve clinical outcome.

Audit can be used to measure how well people have translated research into practice. It can measure short-term outcomes. In certain chronic conditions (e.g. hypertension and diabetes), the quality of the control of the disease can act as an alternative measure of the likely long-term outcome.

Patient satisfaction can be used as an outcome measure. The most constructive data are acquired if the focus is kept on quite narrow but important aspects of treatment. An example may be a patients' satisfaction with a drug they are taking. Alternatively, we can measure the level of communication they have had with the clinicians by their knowledge of the side effect of a common drug they are taking. We know that auditing *general* levels of satisfaction does not provide such useful responses.

At present, we cannot predict population-based outcomes for many conditions with certainty. For this reason there must be some allowance made for individual clinical judgement in some cases.

Summary

Clinical audit is the process of checking whether processes known to work have been carried out in practice. It should be seen from this that it is different from research. Research is a process of trying to find the best way of doing something, whether treating a disease or managing an out-patients department. In research, there is uncertainty about which of two or more procedures is best. In audit, there is only one acceptable approach. The measurement process, which is part of audit, is aimed at discovering whether people have consistently used that approach.

Evaluations of process in the health service

The great majority of evaluations of services are carried out on process data. One feature of such data is the enormous variations in the number of processes used on the same problem in one place compared with another. Some American figures have shown that in the treatment of children there are 18-fold differences in the rate of admission to hospital for gastroenteritis and 15-fold differences for respiratory disease. Some researchers have shown sixfold differences for bronchitis and fivefold differences for pneumonia. A study comparing only teaching hospitals still showed fivefold differences for respiratory tract infection.

The risks of being admitted to hospital for surgical conditions are also markedly different. It may be argued that these differences are simply owing to some areas of the country having more sickness than others. To check this, researches looked closely at three diagnoses, bacterial meningitis, fracture of the femur and appendicitis. These are severe disease in which the diagnosis is usually verified. In these diseases the rates of admission to hospital were very similar, suggesting that where there are more objective definitions of a disease the admission policy varies less.

It also suggests that for less precise, less severe conditions, admission policies vary greatly in their approach, some of which must be extremely wasteful of resources and possibly dangerous to patients. We have known about these differences in medical practice for many years. Glover in the 1930s showed a great variation in tonsillectomy rate for schoolchildren in different areas. The doctors responsible for these variations are likely to be acting in good faith for the benefit of individual patients. Medical practice for some problems, usually the less severe ones or those where no one treatment is obviously better than others, does not have a consensus for the best treatment. This may represent a lack of agreement within medicine about the correct treatment for some diseases. It is, therefore, usually impossible to say what the 'right' rate is. People have suggested that only 10% of all admissions to hospital are related to unambiguous medical need.

There are three main causes for medical practice variations

Clinicians uncertainty. The research in the field may not be good enough. This may be because the disease is uncommon so that it is difficult to collect enough cases for a good trial, or because the treatment requires a total community approach so that randomisation is difficult. Using community mental health teams for mentally ill people is an example of the latter problem. The use of hormone-replacement therapy for the prevention of fractures in elderly women is another example where the research is not yet clear.

Clinical ignorance. The research may be good but is not known or forgotten. This is usually an individual doctor's ignorance of the subject. A further subset of this group is the inability of doctors to gather all the relevant evidence, as in the use of lignocaine for cardiac arrhythmias long after the evidence, if properly analysed, would have made it obvious that the drug was useless.

Informed preferences. There may be advocates for two or more approaches with evidence supporting each but no consensus. This often happens where new forms of therapy are vying with each other to become the preferred approach. The use of coronary artery bypass grafting or less invasive opening up of coronary arteries using lasers in an example of this uncertainty. The former has longer lasting effects but is more dangerous an operation than the latter.

Planners and economists tend to see these variations as a way of saving money. They suggest that if they can force those people who are, for instance, referring more patients to hospital, much money may be saved by reducing their pattern to the average. They assume two things by this: first, that all variation results from ignorance on the part of the clinician and, second, that the 'right' level of referral is at the average. We strongly suspect that neither of these assumptions is correct in most instances.

Where there is uncertainty in a health service, the assumption must be that the cheapest option is best until more data are available and a more accurate decision can be made.

Where there is ignorance it must be identified and rectified with the necessary teaching. Where there is an informed choice of two preferences, we need to carry out research to decide upon which is better. In this situation, there is a moral duty on everyone giving treatment to include their patients in controlled trials to help to resolve the difficulty.

Clinical effectiveness

The term clinical effectiveness is an old one but more recently has been refined to mean: 'to alter the natural course of a disease for the better'. Evaluation of clinical effectiveness tries to marry together:

- scientific evidence
- knowledge of an individual patient and their reaction to different approaches and situations
- legal and moral requirements of the society in which one works.

Scientific knowledge is important, but the other two pressures always temper it. Care must, of course, be taken to ensure that the last two pressures are not used as an excuse because of ignorance of the scientific method.

The individual patient is an essential component of clinical decisions at a number of levels. At its most extreme, someone dying of cancer would not be offered major cardiac surgery, no matter how effective. More subtly we might well offer a violinist with a traumatic injury to the hand a different treatment from someone whole job required strength in the hand

rather than rapid movements. Much of this approach is common sense, but it is easily forgotten in the move to standardisation of treatment.

The context of the treatment is also important, though more controversial. It may be that a particular therapy or investigation is not available in the area. More controversial still is the pressure to use less than optimal treatment where the general finances of the health authority do not suffice for such treatment. In this instance, it may be necessary to forgo the best possible treatment for one person to be able to give a less effective treatment to a large number.

Evaluation of health services

➤ Health services may be evaluated in terms of their input, processes and outputs.

➤ Medical audit assesses the effective use of resources in the work doctors themselves do while clinical audit includes the whole team working in a speciality (i.e. including nurses and paramedical staff).

➤ There are enormous differences in the 'process' used on the same problem in different places. Variation results from clinical ignorance, clinical uncertainty and the exercise of informed preferences between equally acceptable treatments.

➤ Clinical effectiveness is the ability to alter the natural course of a disease for the better. The individual patient and the legal and moral requirements of the society will be components in a decision on clinical treatment.

Measuring health care outcomes

24

This chapter continues the discussion of evaluation of health care from Chapter 23 to discuss outputs:

- the relationship between input and output
- patient outcomes
- quantitative assessments of outcomes.

Introduction

In order to decide if health care is effective it is necessary to classify what it produces and compare this with what is put in: are the outputs worthwhile. The aim is also to put the approach to effectiveness-based medicine into context, for we measure effectiveness, ultimately, according to the outcomes of the health service.

Archie Cochrane, in his book *Effectiveness and Efficiency*, asked a crematorium worker why he appeared so satisfied. The worker replied that he was fascinated by the way in which so much went in and so little came out of the crematorium. Archie said that this was similar to his own fascination with the health service, where huge amounts of money and people put time and effort in and so little comes out.

In this chapter different aspects of output are examined.

Evaluation of a service by its outputs

There are a number of outputs for the health service listed in Chapter 23. We can divide these into the general outputs of the service, the impact on society of the improved health of the community, the employment that the health service gives to large numbers of people and the usefulness of the data collected by the service. The services are not usually judged on these measures.

In general the **patient outcomes** (see below), the prolongation of life (mortality) and prolongation of

good quality life (morbidity), are considered to be important for evaluating services. They are not often used. The reason for this is that except in very controlled circumstances, most notably a randomised controlled trial, it is difficult to link the standard of the health care given directly with the outcome for groups of patients. This is simply because usually some groups of patients will be more severely ill than others. It is obviously impossible randomly to allocate patients to different hospitals or clinics at different ends of the country. This makes it difficult to evaluate one service compared with another by outcome.

Some attempts have been made to measure and control for the severity of the disease in question, but there are very few generally accepted measures of severity. An exception is in the staging of some forms of cancer, where severity has been codified. This makes it possible to compare results for different stages of disease between different places. Such comparisons to are normally restricted to research rather than used in the daily routine evaluation of services in different places.

A recent exception to this has been in Scotland, where a determined effort has been made to compare mortality and, to a lesser extent, morbidity between different hospitals. The aim is to help people working in those hospitals to know which are the best in terms of their outcomes. The problem of whether patients are comparable between hospitals remains, but the Scottish data have been standardised by measuring the severity of the relevant disease as far as possible. This does not guarantee comparability but it does suggest to hospitals at the bottom of the league tables that they should look at what is going on.

Outcome indicators are presented for health authorities, hospitals and psychiatric hospitals. They are:

Health board indicators

- teeange conception

- therapeutic abortion
- cervical cancer morality
- suicide
- diabetic ketoacidosis
- in-patient stays for children with asthma

acute hospital indicators

- survival after fractured neck of femur
- discharge home after fractured neck of femur
- survival after myocardial infarction
- re-operation after transurethral prostatectomy
- emergency re-admission soon after discharge
- survival after admission with stroke
- discharge home after admission with stroke

psychiatric hospital indicators

- deaths within a year of discharge
- deaths under 65 years within a year of discharge
- suicides within 1 year of discharge.

Variations in output

Figure 24.1 shows one of the sets of data, emergency in-patient admissions from diabetic ketoacidosis, a highly life-threatening complication. Differences between the health boards need to be examined because these differences may be because of a failure of support and advice to diabetic patients, learning to manage their disease. Because of the problems already mentioned about the interpretation of the data, they are merely a trigger for further work if there appears to be a problem. The researchers have standardised the figures by age, sex and deprivation, for we know that such problems are more common in poor people. It would, therefore, be a mistake to judge health boards dealing with a deprived population by the same criteria as those dealing with an affluent population. The lack of overlap between the 95% confidence intervals shows that there are statistically significant differences between health boards.

Another example, from the acute hospital section shows the data for survival for 30 days after admission for a fractured neck of femur. In this case the data are standardised for age, sex, deprivation and pre-existing morbidity (Fig. 24.2). The reason for the standardisation is that patients with problems before their fracture will have a more difficult rehabilitation, not affected by the quality of the hospital care. Again the figure shows that there are statistically significant differences between the hospitals that need to be looked at.

We can see that these data, looking at outcomes, have potentially much more serious consequences than looking at process measures. The data suggest that patients are suffering directly as a result of the actions of doctors and nurses in different hospitals, or at the least that the performance of the hospital calls into question the way that such cases are managed. Because of these serious consequences the data have to be very carefully prepared. The researchers used data over a number of years and standardised the results to try to account for differences in the severity of the cases seen in different areas.

One of the most remarkable things about health services is the difference in the numbers of procedures performed in different places, for what appear to be the same problems. Figure 24.3 shows that there is a marked difference between different places in the number of hysterectomies performed. In particular, it shows the difference between three UK regions and the USA and Canada. We can see that the rates in the English regions vary greatly, but that these rates are much lower than are those in the North American

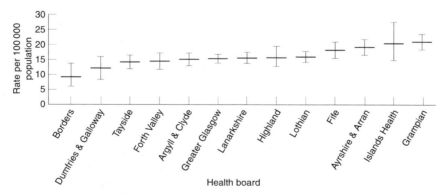

Fig. 24.1 Emergency admissions for diabetic ketoacidosis in 1992–4. The admission rate (means ± 95% CIs) was standardised for age, sex and deprivation. (SIGN 1997)

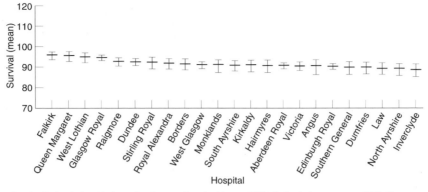

Fig. 24.2 Survival at 30 days after fractured neck of femur 1991–4. Survival as means ± 95% CIs standardised for age, sex, deprivation and pre-existing morbidity. (SIGN 1997)

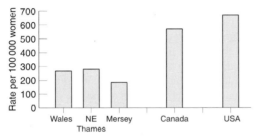

Fig. 24.3 Variation in the hysterectomy rates in three UK areas, Wales, North-east Thames and Mersey, and Canada and the USA. (McPherson et al 1982)

countries. There is no suggestion that the difference in rates is caused by differences in disease of the uterus in the countries or between the regions.

The researchers attempted to try to uncover any factors in the UK regions that may have lead to the differences in rates. Figure 24.4 shows the correlation coefficients between the hysterectomy rates in the regions and other factors. The measures which are most related to an increasing number of hysterectomies, shown as the highest positive correlation coefficients, are the number of GPs in an area and the

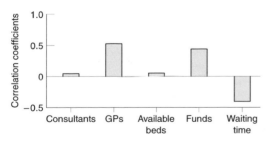

Fig. 24.4 Factors influencing hysterectomy rates in three UK areas, Wales, North-east Thames and Mersey. (McPherson et al 1982)

funds available. Higher waiting time for hysterectomies reduces the number done. These figures do not show us the correct number of hysterectomies for the best overall outcome.

Patient outcomes

The ultimate output of the service is the benefit the patients obtain from the care they receive. There are two major subsets of this final output, sometimes known as outcome. There are many ways of describing outputs that give direct benefit to patients; the simplest is as:

● mortality or more strictly, as everyone dies at some time, prolongation of life
● morbidity, or prolongation of high quality of life
● quality of life years (QUALYs): an attempt to combine prolongation of life with quality of life.

Preventable deaths

Charlton has suggested a simpler way of comparing the outcomes between different services using only death rates. This is the idea of preventable deaths. For example, all those deaths that should not occur in a well-run health service can be added together and standardised to allow comparisons between health services in different areas. Unfortunately, because such events are rare it is difficult to compare services at anything less than a health authority level. In management terms, it is not possible to decide whether one particular technique or surgeon is useless using this method. In addition, preventable deaths, like standardised mortality rates, are closely related to socioeconomic group. Figure 24.5 shows these data where there is a linear

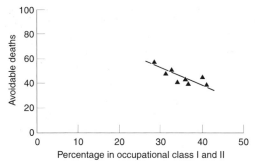

Fig. 24.5 Standardised preventable deaths by occupational class I and II in the Welsh counties.

relationship between available deaths and the proportion of people in socio-economic groups.

Another problem is that for some services mortality is not an important measure. By definition, most chronic diseases do not lead to early death, so another measure is required related to the quality of that person's life.

Morbidity

Measures of disability

The classification of impairments, disabilities and handicaps was discussed in Chapter 2. These measures are described as:

- impairment: organ based, e.g. renal, cardiac failure
- disability: person based, e.g. unable to walk, wash oneself
- handicap: socially based, e.g. unable to fulfil the functions of a student, parent.

Impairments are obviously closely related to diagnostic categories. Diagnoses themselves are not suitable for this purpose for they have grown up over time as a wide variety of descriptions using a wide variety of ways of categorising diseases. Some are based on the underlying cause of the pathological process, for example coronary thrombosis. They may describe the pathology itself, for example myocardial infarction. Some diagnostic categories make a judgement about a continuous measure, for example hypertension. In this case, one has to know the height of the blood pressure in the patient and the level considered by the doctor to be abnormal. Some categories are confusing if taken at face value, such as a stroke or even a cerebrovascular accident. In what way was it accidental? A number of diagnoses refer to organ failure: heart failure, renal failure, hepatic failure, respiratory failure. These measures depend upon symptoms initially but may rely upon investigations to show the degree of failure and whether it is improving.

Dimensions of disability

There is a further complication with the measures of disability, sometimes called quality-of-life measures, for they come in a number of different dimensions. We mention four important ones below, but there are others that do not easily fit, such as continence and the use of the special senses, such as sight and hearing.

Physical dimension

- Measures of function. Is the patient able to wash and dress? Able to go shopping or tie his or her shoe laces. Information may be collected by asking the patient. Patients may not accurately reflect what they do in practice.
- Activities of daily living. These measures usually involve watching the patient do a number of things, such as climb stairs or make a cup of tea. Therapists use these measures quite often. Patients often perform better with someone watching than when they are left on their own.
- Dependency. The extent to which patients need help to do their daily chores.

Mental dimension

- Anxiety measures
- Depression measures
- Memory measures, intended to detect early dementia
- Personality and other disorders.

Social dimension

- Seeking work
- Loneliness
- Isolation
- Poverty

Environmental dimension

- Access to buildings, shops and doctor
- Housing problems
- Violence
- Litter.

Carers

A further aspect of disability is the affects on carers:

- Strain of caring

- Loss of earnings
- Problems with family, e.g. children.

Interactions

Some interventions may improve one dimension of the quality of life to the detriment of others. For example, smoking may be harmful to physical but good for mental health. They may even cause different effects upon the same general dimension. Jogging may make the heart fit but ruin the knees and hip joints. In order to produce benefits, doctors or nurses must usually see the patients and treat them. The contacts between doctors and patients could, therefore, be seen as a sort of output, but they are best thought of as intermediate outputs for they are the means towards the end of improving the well-being of the patient.

Quality of life

The measurement of quality of life for the health service is quite complex. It is, however, what really matters to patients and, therefore, the measure by which we must ultimately judge the success of the health ser-

> ### Outcomes
>
> ➤ Patient outcomes (mortality and morbidity) are difficult to compare between health areas because other confounding variables such as severity of disease and poverty will occur.
>
> ➤ Preventable deaths is one potential comparison index but this is only an effect for large units such as health areas and does not reflect chronic illnesses where mortality is not a common outcome.
>
> ➤ Patient outcomes can be described in terms of mortality (prolongation of life), morbidity (prolongation of high-quality life) or quality-of-life years (QUALYs), a combined factor.

vice. Figure 24.6 shows Horatio Nelson, a man who was impaired (later than this picture) by the loss of an arm and later an eye. Despite this he was not handicapped. He could fulfil his rôle as an Admiral of the Fleet until his death in action at Trafalgar.

Other outputs

Employment

The health service has an effect on population health, it produces a fitter population, which can contribute more to the economy than people who are ill. It is also the biggest single employer in the UK with 10 million people on its payroll. Its effect on giving employment is, therefore, extremely important and is one output of the service. The NHS in the UK has a turnover of about 250 billion pounds per annum (1997). It is, therefore, important simply as an employer of labour and its policies for the recruitment and payment of staff will have great importance. The clashes that the government has had with workers in the health service, especially with nurses, show how importantly the government views the employment of the people in the health service. The government has seen setting wages for the people in the health service as one of the ways of controlling the rest of the public sector in this country. The attempt by the government to set wages for nurses locally has been an attempt to stop the voters from blaming them when nurses are given less money than they want.

Employment is very important for the wealth of an area so that one of the less commonly thought of outputs of the health service may be to improve health

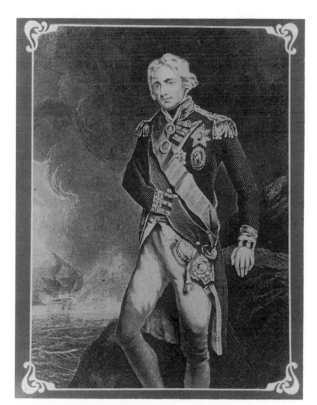

Fig. 24.6 Horatio Nelson.

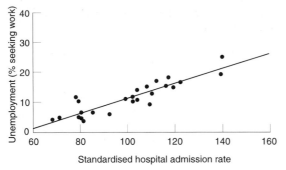

Fig. 24.7 Unemployment and admissions to hospital by electoral ward in Cardiff 1993 (Cardiff = 100).

simply by giving employment. We can see this in Figure 24.7, which shows that there is a relationship between the unemployment rates for the electoral wards of Cardiff and the admission rate of the people in those wards to hospital.

Information about health

The workings of the health service also produce a number of indirect effects, such as the collection of data about populations and making this available by publishing it. There are research findings which have an effect upon the wider population and into other related areas, such as social services, the education service and veterinary medicine.

Effect on the country

In addition because the NHS in general provides care on the basis of *need* rather than the ability to pay, it may have an effect on alleviating the effects of poverty in relation to health. This may narrow the gap between the health experiences of different social classes. This is not to say that there are not still wide differences between social classes in the use they make of the services available but at least the service is available to all.

Research

Research is an output of the health-care services. It is stimulated by clinical problems and needs and enables new treatments and existing ones to be evaluated. Basic research tends to examine the science underlying a disease process. This information is helpful in predicting and developing new treatments. Researchers evaluate new, unproved methods of working. The

function of research is, therefore, to ensure that new approaches to diagnosis, treatment or investigation are considerably better than existing ones. The term 'considerably better' is a loose one, which must include a number of elements:

● the research must show a statistically and clinically significant difference; this is a basic scientific requirement
● it must show that other factors, such as Maxwell's principles (Chapter 23), do not affect the result to the degree that the advantage is invalidated: pragmatic controlled trials may give answers to some of the Maxwell criteria
● assessment of its results must take into account the cost of 're-tooling' the new method and abandoning the old method. This may be important for a new, more accurate scanning procedure, such as magnetic resonance imaging (MRI). The costs of the machinery and running costs are such that the method should show considerable advantages over the older methods before it replaces them.

A factor that should not play a part in development of new research into a service, but often does, is fashion. Some new methods appear to appeal to some unknown sense so that we accept them on little evidence, whereas others take years to be accepted. MRI scanning has become almost universal in the UK in a short time despite a lack of evidence that it is, universally better than existing methods. A number of factors, including skilful marketing and the aesthetically pleasing images produced by the machine, appear to have been of great importance.

Although there are many jaundiced comments regarding research – it's always about something else when it's finished: there are not (quite) enough cases; the results will be largely ignored – some research does get done and does produce useful results. At the beginning we need to ask a series of very important questions.

● What is the research question?
● Is it the right question? Will the answers be useful or relevant. Will it make any difference what is shown?
● Can we answer the question at all? Are there methods available to answer it?
● Should we answer the question? Are there ethical problems with the research or potentially with the results?

Relationship between input and outcomes

One hopes that if more money is put into the health service this increases the outputs. This is not necessarily so. If all the money was spent on leeches, for example, that would certainly increase the input to the service but would unlikely have any effect on output. Figure 24.8 shows one input to the health service, the number of doctors, compared with an important outcome measure, the infant mortality rate. The data are taken from developed countries, which are part of the Office of Economic Cooperation and Development. This is similar to some research work by Professor Archie Cochrane some years ago. He suggested that countries with a high proportion of doctors had a higher infant mortality rate than those with a relatively low proportion of doctors. This suggests that simply having more doctors available in a country does not affect the infant mortality rate. Having more doctors is not necessarily the answer to increasing the outputs from a health service.

Figure 24.9 shows a similar set of data for nurses and infant mortality rate. In this instance, there does seem to be a relationship between more nurses and a lower infant mortality rate. Infant mortality falls off rapidly with an increase in the numbers of nurses per head of population.

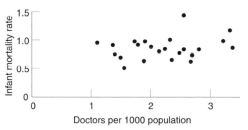

Fig. 24.8 Relationship between the number of doctors and infant mortality rates. (World Bank 1993)

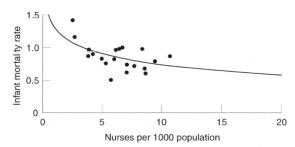

Fig. 24.9 Relationship between the number of nurses and infant mortality rates. (World Bank 1993)

Measures of health: health status instruments

Some researchers have suggested that people evaluating health care should concentrate on measures of *health* rather than measures of disease. One approach to this is the health status measure. People divide health status instruments into four main groups according to two characteristics.

First, an instrument can be 'specific' for a particular disease or condition. For example, the Arthritis Impact Measurement Scale and the Kidney Disease Questionnaire have been designed for specific use. They would be inappropriate for most other patients or for the general population.

Second, an instrument can assess wider issues. There are fewer instruments designed for use in a wide range of patient groups and health-care intervention (e.g. The Sickness Impact Profile). This type of instrument is necessarily less specific about particular symptoms or functional abilities, but it involves more general questioning on several dimensions such as physical functioning, social roles and psychological state. The focus is more on the impact of symptoms on a person's life rather than on the symptoms themselves. The advantage of such instruments is that we can use them in a variety of clinical settings and allow comparison between different patients with different diseases.

Health status instruments can also be divided according to the type of data they produce. Many of the most commonly used instruments yield a 'profile' with scales for several different dimensions. These are presented separately. For instance, people score the Nottingham Health Profile in six dimensions (sleep, energy, emotional reactions, social isolation, physical mobility and pain). One cannot normally aggregate the score. Other measures of health status produce aggregated scores.

Quality of life years (QUALYs)

There are instruments for measuring a wide range of aspects of physical health. We can readily measure height, weight or lung function. It is possible to calculate a surrogate for a person's quality of life. One approach gives each patient a score of 1 if they have 'full-quality health', and a score of 0 for 'death'. Life quality that is less than full scores less than 1. Figure 24.10 shows such profiles for two hypothetical patients. The first survives for 5 years with a quality index of 0.7 (i.e. 70% of 'full-quality health'). The second patient survives for longer (10 years) with a poorer quality of life (an index value of 0.5).

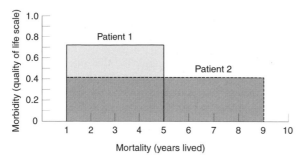

Fig. 24.10 Quantity and quality of life for two patients.

Quality-adjusted life years (QUALYs) are the units of measurement resulting from measuring the area of the rectangle in Figure 24.10, so that one QUALY results from 1 year of full-quality life. The QUALY score is derived from:

Mortality score (years) × Morbidity score (quality of life scale)

The first patient has 5 × 0.7 = 3.5 QUALYs and the second patient 9 × 0.5 = 4.5 QUALYs. Although the second patient survives twice as long as the first, the difference in their quality-adjusted life years is much less.

There are several important points about the measurement of QUALYs. The first is that the measurement is only useful for diseases that have a significant mortality and morbidity. Transient diseases and those that are rapidly fatal do not require this complexity. The second point is that we use the method for comparing treatments in a large number of patients, such as a randomised controlled trial. The scores will then be averages for one treatment over another and always, of course, after the patients have died. The measure helps when one is assessing the contribution of a treatment to patient well-being when, for one reason or another, it is useful to have a single summary measure. It is not a means of valuing the future life of individuals.

Studies have confined the measurement of quality of life using this approach to purely physical measures, such as the presence of pain and disability. There are obviously more dimensions to quality of life, including mental, social and environmental. The personality of patients may be the most important factor when they are responding to therapy and is virtually never measured in this context. Measures of mental illness, especially refractory schizophrenia, depression or obsessive disorders can be as handicapping as any physical problem.

QUALYs are most often used for weighting the costs of different services against one another. There is a problem with QUALYs when comparing treatment

for people of different ages, especially groups of elderly people with younger. The life expectancy of older people will usually, except for very lethal diseases, be more limited by their natural life expectancy rather than the relative effects of two treatments.

It has been suggested that in the economic evaluation of health-care interventions it may be necessary to describe the difference in benefit from different treatments. One might expect a patient in poor health with a quality of life of say 0.4 to live without treatment for 5 years. If they were to receive treatment then their life expectancy might rise to say 10 years and their quality of life index to 0.75. We could measure the gain from treatment in this case as follows:

Treatment option	10 years × 0.75	= 7.5 QUALYs
No treatment option	5 years × 0.4	= 2 QUALYs
Effect of treatment		= 5.5 QUALYs

For individuals a simpler and more realistic approach would be to set out a list of the likely outcomes, as in Table 24.1. This approach is much more useful and realistic when giving options to individual patients, for each patient will put different values on different aspects of their life. For example, some people will value their ability to play a musical instrument much higher than their ability to work. Women with breast cancer will vary in their reaction to, for instance, a mutilating mastectomy against the removal of a breast lump if there is a difference in the likelihood of recurrence of the cancer. The QUALY is attempting to simplify to a single number the complexity of the human condition, a very tall order.

Table 24.1 Outcome of hypothetical treatment options for a patient with cancer

Measure	No treatment	Treatment
Longevity	5 years	8 years with a 1 in 10 chance of death because of the treatment
Side effects of treatment	None	20% chance of loss of hair and libido after year 3
Quality of life		
Physical	Good for 3 years, likely to very poor for 2 years	Good for 5 years, poor for 3 years.
Mental with a robust personality	Good for 4.5 years	Good for 7 years
Social	Good while husband survives	Good while husband survives
Environmental	1 year in a nursing home	2 years in a nursing home

The measurement of QUALYs requires good survival data and an appropriate measure of health-related quality of life. We can use life tables for the general population and survival curves estimated from the results of clinical research for the disease in question.

The main use of QUALYs is in health economics. They are used to describe the relative benefits from different forms of treatment. The economists' main requirement is, therefore, for an instrument that is applicable to a range of conditions and patient groups and which produces a numerical score for overall health status. They suggest that this is the only way that we can compare such diverse treatments as cataract surgery and control of blood pressure regarding the amount of benefit patients get. This benefit is weighed against the cost of the treatment. The use of QUALYs requires an instrument that is both generic and yields a single index. These requirements severely limit the number of instruments that are available for generating QUALY data. Some assessors feel that this approach is asking too much, even when averages for large groups of patients are being taken.

The most commonly used measure of life quality is the **Rosser Classification of Illness States**, developed in the UK in the 1970s. It has two dimensions (disability and distress) and describes 29 states of health, each of which has a value representing severity. In the original works, the researchers asked only 70 respondents to estimate the severity of the 29 states. The researchers compared them and estimated how each state compared with the previous one in terms of severity. Rosser used this information to compute scores or weightings for each of the states defined in the classification.

Researchers have used these weights to generate QUALYs in studies of:

- joint replacement
- scoliosis (spinal curvature) surgery
- chronic renal failure
- psychiatry
- chiropody
- physiotherapy
- hip fracture.

The calculation of QUALYs

As an example, assume that 200 patients aged 45 with a hypothetical medical complaint complete a health status questionnaire at the start of a randomised control study. Their average score for health status is 0.75 (on a scale from 0 to 1.0 where 0 represents death and 1.0 represents full-quality health). Assume, too, that these people have an average life expectancy of 30 years. Two alternative treatments are being studied, drug therapy and surgery.

We assign 100 patients to received medical treatment – drug therapy – and they complete the same health status questionnaire 6 and 12 months later, reporting an average health status of 0.85. Among 100 patients undergoing surgery, 95 survivors also completed a health status questionnaire at the same follow-up intervals reporting an average health status of 1.00. Five patients died following surgery.

Medical treatment

$$\text{QUALY change} = [30 \text{ years} \times 0.85] - [30 \text{ years} \times 0.75]$$
$$= 25.5 - 22.5$$
$$= 3.0 \text{ QUALYs per patient}$$

Overall, 300 QUALYs gained by 100 patients on drug therapy.

Surgical treatment

$$\text{QUALY change} = [30 \text{ years} \times 1.00] - [30 \text{ years} \times 0.75]$$
$$= 30.0 - 22.5$$
$$= 7.5 \text{ QUALYs per survivor}$$

Overall, 712.5 QUALYs gained in total by 95 surgical survivors.

Surgical non-survivors

$$\text{QUALYs} = -[30 \text{ years} \times 0.75]$$
$$= -22.5 \text{ QUALYs per non-survivor}$$

This gives 112.5 QUALYs lost in total by five surgical patients who died (i.e. these patients lose 30 years of future life expectancy in the health status before surgery).

Overall gain from surgery

$$= 712.5 - 112.5$$
$$= 600 \text{ QUALYs}$$

This is 6 QUALYs per patient undergoing surgery. (600 QUALYs for 100 entering surgery).

Comparison of surgical and medical treatment

The net QUALY gain for the surgical compared with medical treatment of this conditions is:

$$= \text{QUALYs (surgery)} - \text{QUALYs (medical)}$$
$$= 600 - 300$$
$$= 300 \text{ QUALYs.}$$

This estimate represents the benefit to patients undergoing surgery compared with receiving drug therapy. We could have performed a similar calculation to compare two or more medical therapies or different surgical techniques. At this stage it is not necessary to have cost detail on the treatment options to determine their relative benefits.

QUALYs and costs

Judged independently of cost, QUALY information may be less powerful than when combined to form a new measure. In theory we can demonstrate the differential in benefit of one treatment over another (or health-care programmes) for gain in QUALYs. We can also calculate the costs of the two treatments to establish the difference in costs between them (Table 24.2).

The use of cholesterol testing and diet therapy appears to have a very low cost per QUALY compared to other interventions, for example neurosurgery for malignant brain tumour. Although we must treat this cost per QUALY with a certain amount of caution, it does reveal major differences in the cost-effectiveness of different forms of interventions. The relative perfor-

Table 24.2 Quality-adjusted life year (QUALY) of competing therapies: some tentative estimates (Morrow & Bryant 1995)

Therapy	Cost/QUALY[a] (£)
Cholesterol testing and diet therapy only (all adults, aged 40–69 years)	220
Neurosurgical intervention for head injury	240
GP advice to stop smoking	270
Neurosurgical intervention for subarachnoid haemorrhage	490
Antihypertensive therapy to prevent stroke (ages 45–64 years)	940
Pacemaker insertion	1 100
Hip replacement	1 180
Valve replacement for aortic stenosis (narrowing)	1 410
Cholesterol testing and treatment	1 480
CABG[b] (left main vessel disease, severe angina)	2 090
Kidney transplant	4 710
Breast cancer screening	5 780
Heart transplantation	7 840
Cholesterol testing & treatment (incrementally) of all adults 25–39 years	14 150
Home haemodialysis	17 260
CABG[b] (single vessel disease, moderate angina)	18 830
Continuous ambulatory peritoneal dialysis	19 870
Hospital haemodialysis	21 970
Erythropoietin treatment for anaemia in dialysis patients (assuming a 10% reduction in mortality)	54 380
Neurosurgical intervention for malignant brain tumours	107 780
Erythropoietin treatment for anaemia in dialysis patients (assuming no increase in survival)	126 290

[a]Costs at August 1990.
[b]CABG: coronary artery bypass graft.

mance of any new treatment can be judged in the context of such a league table. For example, a new cholesterol-testing programme that yielded a marginal cost per QUALY gained of several thousand pounds rather than several hundred would clearly be unattractive from the point of view of a rational health service manager. We might regard a new neurosurgical procedure that only yielded a reduction of hundreds of pounds in cost per QUALY similarly.

Cost per QUALY data can play a part, too, in helping to inform decisions about the potential gains to be derived from alternative patterns of resource allocation. A decision to invest new growth money of say £100 000 in antihypertensive therapy to prevent stroke would produce $100\,000/940 = 106$ QUALYs. The QUALY yield from investing in erythropoietin treatment for anaemia in dialysis patients (assuming a 10% reduction in mortality) would be $100\,000/54\,380 = 1.8$ QUALYs. The differences in health gain expressed as QUALYs are clearly large in this example and indicate a substantial advantage for the antihypertensive therapy. It may be less easy to identify a clear advantage where costs per QUALY values are within a few hundred pounds, as with, for example, pacemaker insertion, hip replacement and valve replacement for aortic stenosis.

Estimates of both the costs and the quality-of-life weights used in the estimation of cost per QUALY values may be widely dispersed. Therefore, we should give confidence limits for cost per QUALY values. Furthermore, since health-state valuations obtained from different reference groups may also differ, it is necessary to test the extent to which different sets of valuations produce different cost per QUALY estimates and, consequently, different rankings within league tables. Little empirical evidence is currently available with which to explore these issues.

The use of cost per QUALY is not without its critics, who have questioned its appropriateness for comparing interventions that save life with those that improve life. Others challenge the apparent emphasis on efficiency at the expense of equity. These questions are not unique to the application of QUALYs. They remain fundamental issues that face decision-makers within the health service.

The use of QUALYs in health care services

Perhaps the most well-publicised use of QUALYs to date is the Oregon experiment to prioritise the health services reimbursed under Medicaid. In its initial stage, researchers used the Quality of Well-being measure to examine the patient benefit from over 700 condition and treatment pairs. However, they considered the resulting condition and treatment pair ranking unrealistic and politically untenable (e.g. cosmetic breast surgery was ranked higher than treatment for an open thigh fracture). The main problem was that sufficient data were not available for a detailed cost-effectiveness analysis. Despite this, similar legislation in 10 or more other US states has been proposed and recently endorsed by the Clinton administration.

Measures of health

➤ Health status instruments are measures of health. They can be specific for a particular disease or condition or focus more on the impact of symptoms on a person's life.

➤ Quality-adjusted life years (QUALYs) are used to measure the composite of mortality and morbidity or quality of life (years of life multiplied by morbidity score on a quality-of-life scale with 0 for death and 1 for full quality health).

➤ QUALYs are mainly used in health economics to describe the relative benefits of diverse treatments.

➤ Cost per QUALY values can be calculated using estimates for both factors and can be used to evaluate cost-effectiveness of different interventions and new treatments. They can also be used to access gains from differing patterns of resource allocation.

Evaluation of new technologies

In this chapter new technologies are described in

- biotechnology
- genetics
- surgical and medical techniques
- information.

Introduction

The range and variety of technologies that are currently used, and those that will be used in the future, are so large that they will have a huge impact on health care. The fields of biotechnology and genetics have already made some inroads into the use of health services and this is accelerating. Many advances are outputs from health care: evaluation of care procedures indicating areas where questions need answers or new treatments are needed. The occurrence of new diseases will also stimulate research to find new methods of treatment. Some technologies are outputs from other areas of endeavour and their medical implications and use are secondary, for example carbon nanotubes to deliver drugs within the cell.

Biotechnology

Monoclonal antibody technology has already proved its worth and future possibilities seem almost endless. Antibodies are normally produced by the immune system to bind foreign materials (antigens). Monoclonal antibodies are highly specific antibodies, which are produced in the laboratory, or industrially, using hybrid cells in culture (the hybrid is formed by fusing an antibody-producing cell with another type of cell). Already a wide variety of diagnostic tests are available using commercial kits based on monoclonal antibody technology:

- pregnancy testing

- measurement of blood enzymes following myocardial infarction
- sexually transmitted disease
- susceptibility to thrombosis
- HIV virus (AIDS)
- test for ovulation
- screening for prostrate and cervical cancer
- test for viral or bacterial infection.

As well as their high specificity, ease of use, speed of result and cheapness, such kits have the major benefit of being possible to use in general practice or even in the home.

Monoclonal antibodies can also be used in therapy, and early experimental trials are underway using them against specific tumour cells. The antibodies can be tagged with radioactive or cytotoxic molecules, which then deliver damage selectively to the cancer cells. In future, doctors could use fibrin-specific antibodies to deliver thrombolytic drugs to specific sites in the cardiovascular system to un-block coronary occlusions, or to specific sites in the cerebrovascular system for people with strokes. These new techniques of biotechnology are used in the production of blood products. Plasma proteins such as factor VIII and albumin are already produced.

Genetic manipulation

Many other new ideas are being tested. Chemical synthesis or fermentation methods for the production of drugs in the pharmaceutical industry are being replaced by recombinant DNA technology. This approach is used to produce large quantities of human insulin. This helps diabetics by avoiding the problems that could arise with the animal insulin previously used. Researchers can also produce compounds that are new. Interferon, which is produced following viral infections, can now be produced in reasonable quantities using recombinant techniques. Interferon belongs to a class of substances that modify the immune response and, therefore, may be useful for treating diseases when the immune system is damaged.

As molecular biology research clarifies the way that cell receptors and biologically active molecules interact, the new technologies will produce tailored molecules. These will be both more effective and have fewer side effects.

Gene therapy

Gene therapy is still in a very early and experimental stage. A non-infectious virus is used to insert particular genes into defective cells. In the immediate future its use will probably be mainly for the treatment of immune deficiency diseases and blood disorders. Genetic engineering of vaccines will prevent many of the safety problems that occur with the use of killed or attenuated microorganisms. They may be engineered to permit them to be stored without refrigeration. The haemoglobin module has been cloned and this may revolutionise the blood transfusion service if we can also produce platelets in a similar manner.

A huge amount of money and effort is currently being expended on the *Human Genome Project*, the goal of which is to map all human genes. As genetic diagnosis and screening rapidly expands, there will be uncertainties about its moral and social implications, especially concerns about altering genetic material to make humans with desirable characteristics.

Genetic screening

Genetic screening finds most application in obstetrics. Intrauterine diagnosis of Down's syndrome, thalassaemia and Tay–Sachs disease is already undertaken. Researchers working on Tay-Sachs disease have already taken fertilised embryos from parents who were carriers and have examined them genetically, replacing only those which were not carrying the abnormal gene. This combines screening with the techniques developed for in vitro fertilisation. It ensures a normal baby for the mother and that the disease is not carried to the next generation in a carrier state.

Genes are continually being identified that may be implicated in the aetiology of a number of diseases, for example breast cancer, diabetes, Alzheimer's disease and, possibly, cardiovascular disease and even depression. Theoretically, such common diseases should not have an important, or at least a simple, genetic component. If they did they would have been selected out over the generations by evolutionary forces. The interplay between genetic and environmental factors in

---

> ### New biological technologies
>
> ➤ Monoclonal antibodies are used in a wide range of diagnostic tests.
>
> ➤ Recombinant DNA technology enables fermentation techniques using microorganisms to produce large quantities of biologically important proteins, e.g. insulin.
>
> ➤ Gene therapy where a new gene is put in to replace a defective gene is still at the development stage. It has been used in a few instances, e.g. cystic fibrosis and adenosine deaminase deficiency.
>
> ➤ Genetic screening allows intrauterine diagnosis of diseases such as Down's syndrome. Combination with in vitro techniques enables screening for affected fetuses and subsequent development allowed only for a normal baby.
>
> ➤ Ethical issues are very prominent for genetic screening e.g. prevention of disease through abortion.

the development of disease is not understood. Manipulation of the genome to eradicate disease is controversial in terms of understanding all the potential effects and on ethical grounds; however, even if it were ethical, social-decision making would still remain very difficult.

Surgical techniques and technologies

Surgeons develop new techniques as new devices and material become available. The development of new biomaterials some years ago made hip replacement feasible for the first time. The operation is undertaken to improve the quality of life for elderly people by relieving the pain and immobility caused by osteoarthritis of the hips. More than 90% of people still benefit 10 to 15 years after the operation and the reduced need for support services suggest a return of 400% on the cost of the operation.

The clinical picture in other diseases is often not so clear cut. In 1967, the first implantation of a graft to bypass a restriction in the coronary artery was carried out in a human subject. Major randomised controlled trails of coronary artery bypass grafting (CABG) have yielded evidence that CABG improves survival in high-risk patients with disease of the three main coronary arteries. It was introduced as a treatment for coronary heart disease of a life-threatening nature. However, once implemented it came to be applied to many different kinds of patient.

Ten years later, the further development of polymeric materials led to the practice of dilation of coronary arteries via catheterisation under visual control using X-rays; the technique of percutaneus transluminal coronary angioplasty (PTCA) was born. PTCA offers advantages over CABG in that the operation is much less invasive. Research work has suggested that it may improve myocardial ischaemia and restore functional capacity more satisfactorily than CABG but with an increased mortality rate. PTCA may also need to be repeated relatively frequently, which introduces considerations of relative cost effectiveness over time.

Endoscopy

More recently there has been widespread implementation of endoscopic techniques and keyhole surgery. Fibre-optic endoscopes initially proved their worth as diagnostic tools and then were employed for biopsies. The endoscope allows less invasive procedures to be carried out in the repair of inguinal hernias, joint surgery, cholecystectomy and a number of other techniques. This increases the proportion of surgery that can be undertaken on a day-care basis, accelerating the shift from hospital to home care. Endoscopes can also incorporate lasers, which can be used, for example, to fragment stones in the ureter. This combination of endoscope plus laser therapy opens up endless possibilities for surgery of the respiratory, urinary or gastrointestinal tracts as well as for re-canalisation of blood vessels.

Medical technologies

Medical technologies are often very interrelated with drugs, equipment and care requirements all involved. The intensive care unit (ICU) is an example of medical technology at its most complex. Judgements of what constitutes an appropriate number of ICU beds vary markedly between the UK and the USA. In the USA, ICU beds comprise about 15% of total beds, whereas in the UK they comprise only 1%. This is responsible for half the total difference in cost of hospital activity. The effectiveness of intensive care is good for cardiac surgery and coronary care, intermediate for head injury and relatively poor for chronic respiratory disease, hepatic disease or multisystem organ failure.

Kidney dialysis

There is no marked difference in the incidence of renal failure between the USA and the UK. Kidney dialysis and transplantation are effective but expensive technologies. In the USA in 1972 it was decided that Medicare would fund all patients requiring treatment, with the consequence that 5% of the health-care budget is now spent on 0.2% of patients. The UK rate of dialysis and transplantation shows a wide variation between regions. The rate in the UK is in the lowest quarter of 21 developed countries and is only half the rate in the USA.

When patients are not dialysed it is usually not because of a lack of kidney machines but because clinical judgements are made that the degree of likely benefit does not justify the treatment. Ten-year survival is less than 20% for these people. If patients over 50 years of age are excluded (the UK accepts fewer patients over 50 than most countries) and those with associated disease, then 10-year survival exceeds 50%. Diabetes worsens outcome, although evidence from small samples demonstrated that 60% of people who were blind because of diabetes were alive 5 years after starting dialysis.

Medical imaging

The first prototype computerised tomographic head scanner was tested in London in 1971, and in 1973 the Department of Health funded a head scanner for regional neurological centres. It deferred the funding of body scanners until evaluation had been undertaken, but the combined forces of the CT scanner manufacturers, the public, radiologists and charitable endowments led to a very rapid diffusion of the technology, as shown in Figure 25.1.

In 1978 a report by the Nuffield Foundation pointed out the problems of the rapid expansion of different types of high technology before they have been prop-

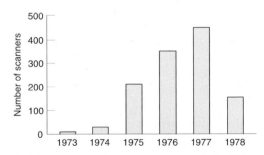

Fig. 25.1 Cumulative number of CT scanners installed in 1973–8 in the UK. (Hemmingway 1991)

erly evaluated. Despite this, the advent of magnetic resonance imaging (MRI) in 1981 was followed by a very similar diffusion of the machines without evaluation. In 1981, there were only three centres in the UK concerned with clinical applications of MRI but in the mid-1990s there are of the order of 100 fixed MRI units. The major application of MRI imaging is for the investigation of disorders affecting the brain and spinal cord and for examination of a wide range of musculoskeletal problems. It has a major advantage over CT scanning in that patients are not exposed to ionising radiation but it is much more expensive.

Both technologies and the even newer positron emission tomography (PET) make use of digital data. Approximately 20% of diagnostic imaging is now undertaken using digital data rather than X-ray film. These data are much easier to store and handle than film. They are also possible to transmit to remote sites using telecommunications, which will further revolutionise the current configuration of the delivery of diagnostic imaging services.

Neuroimaging techniques provide data for two uses: elucidation of the pathophysiology of conditions (i.e. a research output) and clinical assessment of the patient's condition as treatment (a medical outcome). With the emphasis on cost-containment, it is necessary to decide why imaging is undertaken and what clinical utility the findings will have.

Other medical technologies

A full review of medical technologies is beyond the scope of this chapter, but other well-recognised areas are:

- implantable sensory aids for vision and speech
- prostheses (including their microprocessor control)
- implantable reservoirs of drugs for diabetes, blood disorders and cancers.

Information on new technology

There are seemingly limitless possibilities of information technology (IT) applied to health care, either through information databases or computer-assisted diagnosis. Part 3 examines the availability of information and how to access it.

Technology assessment

Knowledge of the effectiveness of a new technology under ideal or test conditions is important but there is another activity that is largely overlooked and which

---

> **New medical and surgical technologies**
>
> ➤ New biomaterials enables replacement of damaged 'parts' in the body, e.g. hip replacements.
>
> ➤ Endoscopy and keyhole surgical techniques assist diagnosis, are used for biopsies and allow less invasive surgical procedures. In turn, this reduces some operative risks and length of hospital stays, which has cost implications.
>
> ➤ Medical technologies include intensive care methods, kidney dialysis and implant reservoirs for slow drug release.
>
> ➤ The effectiveness of new techniques such as nueroimaging has to be balanced against costs and clinical value.

---

is equally essential. The aim of this is to be as scientific about how new technology is used in the care of individuals and populations as about how it works, i.e. its effectiveness under less than ideal conditions. Once a technology has been adopted, questions are seldom asked about the appropriateness of its use. Drugs and devices and instrumentation are licensed as such and clinicians have freedom to choose the problems, patients and situations to which they should be applied. However, these judgements of appropriateness and extent of use are often more important than the quality of the technology itself. Technology assessment is a process, as outlined in Figure 25.2.

Identification

In the USA, the Food and Drug Administration (FDA) gathers information on drugs and devices that are being developed and the National Institutes of Health (NIH) support clinical trials. They are now required to provide the National Centre for Health Care Technology with lists of emerging technologies. Priority for evaluation is then given to technologies

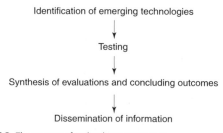

Fig. 25.2 The process of technology assessment.

suspected of being useless, dangerous, expensive or likely to be very widely used.

Testing

A major problem associated with testing is the stage of development that a technology has reached at the time of testing. During development, new clinical applications may emerge and risks and costs may change. For example, if mammography for breast cancer screening had been fully evaluated at an early stage of development when the X-ray doses and associated risks were high compared to current levels, and costs were also higher, then current screening programmes might never have emerged with their now known benefits. In addition, testing should be under optional conditions to measure effectiveness but insufficient account may be taken of how effectiveness may vary when translated into an average clinical setting. For example, keyhole surgery is effective and confers great benefit provided a skilled and trained surgeon practises it. However, its practice by untrained enthusiasts has been shown to be disastrous.

Problems of technology assessment

The most important problems of technology assessment are decisions about the level of use and identification of the appropriate kinds of patient to benefit from the technology.

- What proportion of total beds should be devoted to a particular form of care?
- Which subgroups of patients will most benefit from that care?
- Should all age, sex groups have the service available?
- Should patients with other diseases be excluded?

Those sorts of question can be asked of any medical technology. Who should supply the answers? These questions will become more pressing and strident with the development and implementation of genetic technologies.

The National Institute of Health in the USA has created a mechanism to consider the collective opinion of those professionally concerned with technology. The first consensus development conference dealing with breast cancer detection, particularly mammography, was held in 1977 and since then others have followed in different areas. Medical specialties have also recognised the problem and set up guidelines of good practice for their own field. In the UK, the Royal College of Radiologists began a programme in 1979 that has resulted in the development and implementation of guidelines for referral of patients for X-ray examinations and the appropriate use of X-rays in a particular instance.

There is a danger that technologists, specialists and scientists can become so excited by the possibilities of the activity in which they are engaged that they forget ethical considerations. Richard Feynman, the Nobel Prize winning physicist whose early years and work were concentrated on the development of the atomic bomb, has left a memorable statement of this danger. He described how the minds of the scientists working on the project were occupied with the 'technical sweetness' of their ideas and research. They hardly considered the end-point of their research and in fact partied at Los Alamos on the night the bomb was first dropped, happy at the success of their work! It is, therefore, very important that a representative group of society oversee the ethical, effectiveness and cost assessments of new technology.

Dissemination of information

Dissemination of information is recognised as still being of poor quality in developed countries but tentative steps have been made to put this right. The National Centre for Health Technology has a mandate to coordinate the dissemination of relevant information. More generally a cooperative attitude of mind towards the practice of evidence-based medicine is appearing in the medical community and certain initiatives such as the Cochrane Collaborative Centre in the UK will prove their mettle in this area as time progresses.

An individual cannot be comprehensively knowledgeable on new technology or its assessment, but the important thing is to know where to find the available evidence and how to assess it scientifically.

Information

➤ Information databases allow access to information on all aspects of medicine for health-care personnel regardless of their geographic location.

➤ Computer-assisted diagnosis is being developed in some fields.

➤ Technology assessment requires testing of new technologies, collection of results and analysis of the value of the technique and to which subgroups of patients it should be applied. This information must then be available to a wide audience.

Components of health care

International health

Christopher Potter

This chapter covers three aspects of international health:

- the health problems of developing countries
- the way Western medicine is delivered and practised
- the different models of health care used in some of the countries of Western Europe.

Developing countries

In most parts of the world, Western medicine is still a dream. It is seen as one of the great benefits of Western civilisation and is highly desired by developing countries. Much human effort and money goes into attempting to provide such care in developing countries, so it is useful to reflect on some of the features relevant to the provision of care.

The major improvements in health in developed countries do not result from health services but are the result of being richer, presumably through better housing, better nutrition and education. It is also said that immunisation, health education and surveillance are highly cost effective for improving patient outcomes compared with one-to-one treatment. Hospitals are increasingly seen as the equivalent of black holes absorbing money, which would be spent better elsewhere. Aid agencies and planners discourage the development of hospitals and emphasise public health and primary health care in developing countries with their growing populations and painfully low resource availability.

This emphasis is reasonable as far as it goes, but there comes a time when patients do need a Caesarean section delivery, a hiatus hernia repaired or an appendicectomy. If there is no functioning hospital, it can lead to a significant lack of faith in the whole system of Western medicine. Consequently, in more recent years it has become recognised that primary health care alone cannot meet the needs of the third world.

Dr H. Mahler, then Director General of WHO, indicated a change in attitude in 1981: 'A health system based on primary health care cannot, and I repeat cannot be realised, cannot be developed, cannot function, and simply cannot exist without a network of hospitals...'. He went on to say that hospitals in the Western image had to change their ways, for their primary function was to support the community and primary health care services.

Health systems in developing countries tend to be cash starved. A small percentage of the money available to a country may be spent on health, but even where the proportion is relatively high it needs to be remembered that the amount of money available is, in the first place, low. Typically care is provided free at the point of use, but often this means nothing.

Abel-Smith entitled a study of Tanzanian hospitals *Can the Poor Afford Free Medicine*? and came to the conclusion that they cannot! Without enough money in the system, there are no consumables, no maintenance, no drugs and in effect no services provided. Frequently there are many hidden charges for the patient. Sometimes this is because officials have not been paid or, more often, as a supplement to their earnings patients are expected to pay fees to various members of staff. They often have to buy drugs and equipment in the local market.

Western health care in developing countries tends to be uncoordinated. Ministries of Health have only weak or non-existent regulatory powers to monitor and control the private sector, or decentralised public provision. There are usually both vertical and horizontal health programmes. 'Vertical' programmes are discreet, self-contained programmes aimed at eradicating a single disease or problem, for example, river blindness, guinea worm or, in the past, smallpox. 'Horizontal' programmes attempt to deal with a wide range of health problems. In countries where there are a number of vertical programmes running, there will be duplication of staff, and poor communications.

Another characteristic of health-care delivery systems in developing countries is the lack of the supporting systems that we often take for granted.

- electricity is often available for only a few hours a day
- diesel generators are often expensive to run and yet hospital services require regular power supplies
- water for hygiene and drinking purposes can be scarce or non-existent; it is amazing how many hospitals have been built that have no water supply
- communication systems such as telephones and radio may not be available, with the consequent deleterious effect on referral systems and on resource coordination
- information systems are rudimentary, often with too little money to provide stationery for even the simple medical records systems that are the bedrock of all management information systems
- maintenance know-how and the money for spare parts and tools are usually problematic.

There are many staffing problems. The professions of the West have been copied whether or not these are appropriate for the country in question. Having invested significant amounts of public money in training health-care professionals, they have to be found jobs and it is not unusual to find that most government health-care spending goes on staffing. In Pakistan, for example, over 90% of public health-care money spending goes on the staff budget, and of that over 80% goes on doctors' salaries.

Educated health professionals prefer to be near centres of population, and the overall national figures showing doctors per head of population, or nurses per head of population are misleading because so many of them are grouped at very few centres in a country. In rural areas the numbers can be very low indeed and it would certainly be a mistake to believe that the quality of health staff from area to area is homogeneous.

Finally, Western health care in developing countries is characterised by poor quality. Because of poor information systems and because of the dominance of the system by professionals there is a lack of review and audit. In countries where the hierarchy or loss of face is important, discussing someone else's clinical practice can be even more difficult than in the West. Professional management is usually missing, and where it exists the managers are in a much weaker political position than the professionals.

However, professional cultures also have little con-

Developing countries

- ➤ Aspire to Western medicine.
- ➤ Need to have a balance of hospital- and community-based care.
- ➤ Often have problems with the basic infrastructure, e.g. water, power.
- ➤ Often have problems with the proper allocation of health-care professionals.

trol over individual members. The economic power of the public, their low literacy and education, and their inability to mobilise community support are typically such that they are in a very weak position with regard to the professional providers of health care. There is little effort to involve the community in health-care decisions, and even where health centres or other facilities are given this is often a manifestation of central paternalism that may be misunderstood or mistrusted by the community concerned.

Developed countries

Westernised medicine is practised in countries such as UK, USA, Western Europe, Japan, Australia, New Zealand and Canada. It is also the dominant form of medicine taught in what were the Soviet block countries, although Western doctors and health workers may find some of the practices unusual. It is the form of medicine taught in medical schools and practised in hospitals in developing countries. It is thought of as scientific. It is based on the medical model and embraces a wide range of technologies for diagnosis and treatment.

Most people living in the West take their form of medicine for granted, despite the rise of alternative therapies. Although many traditional practices can be shown to do more harm than good, it is arrogant to assume that all traditional approaches are worthless and only Western medicine can be helpful. Our own pharmacology is based on herbalism, and much healing occurs through psychological and placebo effects. Many people have spoken of modern hospitals as temples to the God of science, its priests and acolytes wearing the ritual white coats, stethoscope talisman worn like a pectoral cross, and the invocation of science forming its vocabulary.

However, there are many reasons for doubting how scientific Western medicine is. The application of the various sciences and technologies that are needed in this endeavour needs to be practised and creatively performed. Despite all of the emphasis on clinical audit, guidelines and standardised procedures, individual doctors vary considerably in the way they treat the same conditions. There are marked regional and national differences in such matters as:

- prescribing habits
- frequency of interventions
- diagnostic techniques preferred
- admission rate to hospitals.

This is surprising because most Western doctors take the same international journals and consult the same pool of medical textbooks. However, evidence from several sources, which we have quoted through this book, show that there is, in practice, a surprising variation. On an international level, researchers have shown, for example, that 20% of the population of Hamburg were diagnosed as suffering from a cardiac complaint because their blood pressure was so low. The same blood pressure readings in the UK, USA and France would be seen as an indicator of good health. In France, an analysis of the prescribed drugs showed that a tonic was the most widely prescribed drug and a number of other tonics were in the top 20. There were no general antibiotics in the list. By contrast, there were no tonics in the top 20 British drugs, a list which was headed by a general antibiotic, and other antibiotics also appeared on the list. The researchers showed that even among a small pool of Western countries what is considered as an illness varies, what is an appropriate treatment varies, and the use of drugs and technologies varies.

The same pattern is shown if we look at a health data file for length of stay in hospital for diseases in developed countries (Table 26.1). The mean length of stay for cancers, for example, varies from 10.5 in the USA to 51.7 days in Japan. The length of stay for mental disorders in Japan is a staggering 333.3 days compared with 11.6 in the USA. It might be argued that there are such cultural differences between Japan and the USA, and definitions of, for example, mental disorders, that this is not so surprising. If we compare Canada and the USA the variations are more surprising in that 80% of the population of Canada lives within 100 kilometres of the USA border. The mean length of stay for diseases of the blood is 11.1 days in Canada compared with 7.2 in the USA.

We see a different picture for reported admission rates. Table 26.2 shows the reported admission rates for tonsillectomies in Canada were 89 per 100 000 population compared with 205 in the USA. Admission rates for hysterectomies per 100 000 population were 405 in Australia, 479 in Canada and 557 in the USA. There might be cultural patterns at work for an operation often carried out for unclear reasons. It is less easy to explain why admission rates for appendectomies should be 143 in Canada and 340 in Australia for example, or 245 in Ireland and 131 in the UK and why Norway and Switzerland show rates of 64 and 74, respectively. Again with inguinal hernia repairs, Japan's 67 may be reflecting major cultural differences in attitudes towards hernias, but why would there be 145 in Australia and 219 in Canada?

Why have we emphasised this point? One can neither support overintervention (i.e. surgery, drug therapy, radiation therapy and so on), where it is not necessary nor the withholding of such treatment where it is necessary. With all of the variation, it is obvious that many people are not receiving the best service. Where there is excessive treatment, it is costing them or their governments (ultimately the same thing) too much money. It is because of these variations that so

Table 26.1 Mean length of stay in hospital (days) for disease categories by Country (OECD Health Data File, 1989) (World Bank 1993)

	UK	USA	Canada	Japan
Neoplasms	12.2	10.5	16.2	51.7
Mental disorders	50.3	11.6	24.7	333.3
Infections and parasitic diseases	9.6	6.9	10.5	117.6
Diseases of the blood	12.6	7.2	11.1	41.7

Table 26.2 Examples of reported admission rates (per 100 000 population) for selected procedures in 1980 (taken from OECD Health Data File, 1989) (World Bank 1993)

	UK	USA	Canada	Japan	Norway	Switzerland	Australia
Tonsillectomy	26	205	89	61	45	51	115
Coronary bypass	6	61	26	1	13	Not known	32
Appendicectomy	131	130	143	244	64	74	340
Hysterectomy	250	557	479	90	Not known	Not known	405
Inguinal hernia repair	154	238	224	67	78	116	202

much effort has been taken in recent years to try and standardise requirements, through the use of clinical protocols and clinical audit and feeding back information on length of stay to individual physicians.

UK data

Researchers have compared the Northern and Yorkshire regions of England with Scotland. As with Canada and Australia, it was felt that the populations living either side of a land border, of roughly the same size, and sharing similar cultural and socioeconomic features should have similar patterns of health service usage. This was not so. Considerably more money is being spent in Scotland per head than in England and Wales. However this is not reflected in better health for the Scots. Overall their health is worse than in England and Wales.

In this welter of comparisons between countries, we often think that the NHS is worse than it actually is. The average time of waiting to see a GP in parts of the USA in the 1980s was recorded as 3 weeks; an unacceptably long time in UK. The public perception is that there are no waiting lists in the USA, but data are not collected. It is clear that there is no single best way of providing health care, and that believing that better health care is a matter of more resources is highly simplistic. Political and cultural factors are at least as important in the way resources are used as are the scientific data on the medical techniques.

Governments and health care

Governments have three main rôles in the provision of health care:

● regulation
● planning
● provision.

Developed countries

➤ There are still wide variations in the frequency of use of many medical procedures in different locations.

➤ Prescribing habits, frequency of intervention, diagnostic techniques and hospital admissions/stays vary widely not only between countries but between regions within one country.

Regulation

Governments typically become involved in the regulation of:

● health-care practitioners
● institutions
● drugs, equipment and procedure
● financial affairs
● quality
● access and equity.

There is little argument about the responsibility for modern governments to regulate health care. The extent of that regulation varies. Doctors and nurses are obviously in a position of considerable power over patients. Medical technologies, such as radiation, drugs, and surgery can be harmful as well as good. There has, therefore, been an increase over the years in the laws that govern the medical professions and the use of drugs and technologies.

In most Western countries, there are detailed rules about who may practice medicine; safety standards on drugs, equipment and procedures; accreditation frameworks covering institutions; and so on. In the UK, the British Medical Association, UKCC (covering the various nursing professions including midwifery and health visiting), the Council for the Profession Supplementary to Medicine, the British Dental Association all license their members to practice. Non-members are not allowed to describe themselves as members, and there are regulations describing what members can do.

Not everyone accepts that professions should be protected in this way. In some Canadian and American states there have been calls for deregulation, and there has also been recently more blurring of the boundaries between Western medical practices and various alternative therapies. Not everyone accepts the unmitigated merits of domination of the health services by professionals. George Bernard Shaw described professions as a 'conspiracy against the laity' and others have argued that the approach makes people dependent – doctor knows best – and creates its own problems.

Another aspect of regulation is how far the government should try to regulate access to services. Within the UK, there is a general feeling that the government should take an interest in reducing waiting lists, whereas in USA nearly 40 million citizens do not appear on any sort of waiting list because they are not covered by health insurance at all. We have to decide if access includes providing financial assistance to poorer patients so they can afford to buy services. These are essentially political questions and different countries will have different answers.

The role of government in regulating the financial affairs of the health sector is even more controversial.

- Should governments cap the cost of drugs?
- Should it seek to regulate the cost of private surgery (assuming that it allows such a thing)? Should it only be interested in the public sector or try to control prices in the private sector as well?
- Is it right that in the UK there is an agreement controlling the cost of drugs supplied by manufacturers?
- Is it right that government make regulations restricting the ability of NHS health providers (trusts) to cross-subsidise services? A commercial approach would allow different providers within the NHS to set up services to give a particular provider some sort of commercial advantage, but within the UK they are not allowed to do this.

Regulating quality

There are a number of question marks against aspects of quality regulation.

- Is it acceptable in the UK for a private non-governmental agency, the King's Fund College, to develop an accreditation system?
- Is it acceptable that in the USA the non-governmental Joint Commission on the Accreditation of Health Organisations (JCAHO) is the main accreditation agency?
- Is it right that such quality systems tend to be input and process orientated, without looking at outcomes?
- Is it acceptable, for example, that in Britain (as in most countries) there is no simple way of knowing what postoperative embolism rates or postoperative infection rates are for different hospitals, specialties and surgeons?

Planning

Governments will inevitably become involved in planning health services, if only to try to stimulate provision in isolated areas (which can include social isolation, such as inner city areas) or during unsocial hours. There are various approaches to health-care planning, and each of the main structural reorganisations of the NHS has been characterised by a different approach.

There are essentially four types of planning:

- capital planning

- service planning
- business planning
- health needs/health gains.

Capital planning

Modern hospitals and their equipment are expensive. They are usually one-off investments described as capital expenditure, as opposed to revenue or on-going costs. Because of their expense, there is a tendency to try to ensure that they are in the right place. In the early 1980s there was one CT scanner in Wales, one in the whole of Western Australia and one in Saskatchewan. In Minneapolis, St Paul there were 22 scanners on 19 hospital sites, serving a population not much bigger than that of Bristol. Needless to say, the patients ended up paying for these expensive toys. There was obviously no central planning in St Paul.

Service planning

Service planning looks at the characteristics of the population being served, including:

- epidemiological needs, e.g. those diseases that are common
- demographic profile, e.g. whether the area in question is young or old; whether there are many people from the ethnic minorities
- environment, e.g. town or country, pollution or overcrowding risks.

On this basis planners can calculate the number of medical or other interventions that are likely to be needed year by year. Some areas may need more ENT provision than others, some may require more community psychiatric nurse interventions. It is a technical approach, which in theory is scientific rather than based on wants, either the wants of the population or the wants of the most powerful medical group in the area.

Business planning

The term business planning implies that the planning process concerns the economic viability of a service, with an emphasis on the local managers and clinicians managing the service according to the budget available. This forces managers to consider resources available and alternative ways of using those resources. There is constant pressure to persuade the government to take back these powers, for the managers and the nurses are much happier to blame the government than to have to try to work out a solution themselves.

Clinical quality may be jeopardised by business planning if we cannot save money. In addition the complexity of the internal market's contracting arrangements can make the whole process overly mechanistic and time consuming.

Health needs, health care planning

In this form of planning an attempt is made to prioritise the way that the service is run by giving greatest priority to those areas where most health gain can be taken. The approach concentrates on using effective treatment for relatively common diseases to gain the maximum effect on the population. The central point of planning in relation to health needs is that groups of people with common diseases effectively treated have priority over those who do not. This can sometimes pose problems with the general public when resources are scarce.

Provision

There are three strong arguments for public, as distinct from private, provision of some health services.

● Where the particular service is of public good or benefit to all yet there is no incentive for private provision. The classic example would be mosquito control, where it would be pointless for one householder to spray his or her house and garden if neighbours did not follow suit. To be effective, vaccination needs herd immunity, and there is an obvious argument for public provision of vaccinations. It can be argued that there are individual benefits and, therefore, people should pay for care where they can. If this were not the case, the comparatively well off, who can afford to pay, benefit from government funds that might be best targeted at the poorest in society.
● Where the public provision of health services is clearly more cost effective and alleviates poverty, there is an argument for not wasting resources on private provision.
● Where there is uncertainty, or the possibility of the health insurance market failing, it is sensible for the government to provide health care so that system does not collapse. In other words, the government plays the role of last resort, because there is always the risk that an unexpected epidemic, disaster or mismanagement could overwhelm the private or insurance system.

Funding for health services

Health services are funded from four sources:

● fees for service
● general taxation
● insurance: voluntary or compulsory
● third party, e.g. employer, usually through an insurance company.

There is a story that in ancient China physicians were paid by their patients while they were well but received nothing while the patient was sick. Although this appears to be a rational approach, it is not one that the authors have seen in any of the countries in which they have worked. Even where traditional healers dominate there is an expectation that gifts and fees will be given. Payment of such fees is the simplest approach and requires those patients, or their families, to find money for the health professional at the time they are ill. However, it has an obvious flaw. For most people sickness reduces their ability to work and, therefore, their access to money. In non-industrialised societies it is not uncommon for poor patients to have to beg and borrow funds from their extended family to pay for health services, and illness can often be the start of long periods of economic hardship.

The service providers are not especially happy with this approach either for they much prefer patients to pay when they are well off. It is of no advantage to a health provider to ask for money from people who are impoverished, ill or dead. They much prefer a system where they receive regular payment at a time when potential patients can afford it.

Methods of funding health services

Table 26.3 shows the different forms of funding health services that are found in different parts of the world. It can be seen that there are marked differences between the different categories of country in the amount they spend and the way that services are provided.

Taxation

In the UK, the state mainly uses taxes to fund the health services. Everybody who pays tax contributes to the system, and health care is available when they need it, typically for most people their main use is in the last 2 years of their life. The taxpayers pay the government, which foots the bill. This seems fair but raises other questions. Most people would accept that chronically sick or disabled persons should receive treatment. Not everyone would accept that the general

Table 26.3 Clinical health systems by income group (World Bank 1993)

Category of country (1990 per capita income in dollars)	Health expenditure in 1990		Main characteristics	Examples
	As share of GNP (%)	Dollars per capita		
Low income (100–600)	2–7	2–40	High private spending for traditional medicine and for drugs Public services financed from general revenues Little insurance	Bangladesh, India, Pakistan, most sub-Saharan African countries
Middle income (600–7900); private insurance	2–7	20–350	Government services for middle- and low-income groups financed from general revenues Private insurance and private provision for affluent (less than 10% of population)	South Africa, Zimbabwe
Social insurance	3–7	20–400	Public health and clinical care for low-income groups financed from general revenues Social insurance for wage labour force, with mixed provision	Costa Rica, Republic of Korea, Turkey
Formerly socialist economies of Europe (650–6000)	3–6	30–200	Public services (which are low in quality or collapsing) financed from general revenues Large underground market in privately provided services	Czech Republic, Poland, Slovak Republic, republics of former USSR
Established market economies, excluding, USA (5000–34 000)	6–10	400–2500	Universal or near-universal coverage through general revenue financing or compulsory social insurance Use of capped third-party payments and global budgets	Social insurance: France, Germany, Japan General tax revenues: Norway, Sweden, UK
USA (22 000)	12	2800	Combination of private voluntary insurance and use of general revenue from taxes Unregulated and openended free-for-service compensation High administrative costs associated with health provision and insurance	USA

public should obtain free services that add to a patient's quality of life but are not in the same league as, for instance, treating someone who is severely injured. There has to be some line drawn for what is a health service and what is not. Examples of services that may or may not be considered legitimate parts of a health service are:

- infertility treatment
- breast reductions or enhancements
- tattoo removals
- stress counselling.

UK health service patients were expected to pay for replacement of their spectacles or false teeth if these were broken from carelessness, from its inception. There has always been a moralising argument that some people did not deserve to have all of their care free at the point of receiving it.

The insurance approach obviously spreads the risk around the population. In the UK, because of the limited capacity of the private sector, the health insurance market has grown quite slowly. People see private insurance as a useful way of jumping queues where there are waiting lists, and for getting private beds with a wider choice of food, TV and privacy. Its benefit in the UK for most people is questionable.

Voluntary insurance

The USA has remained more reliant than any other Western country on what may be termed an optional system of health care. People can buy health insurance with different degrees of cover, many of which are attached to the perks that they get from their employment. The government of the USA defends this approach by saying that if a large number of insurers are paying for care the task of making sure that the service is giving good value for money falls to the private insurers. Their argument is that this will keep the doctors and nurses on their toes to give a high-quality service.

Even the USA uses taxes to fund services for poor people, elderly people or government employees, e.g. through Medicare and Medicaid. They are also used to fund services provided by the Veterans Administration (for military and ex-military personnel), for end-stage renal failure services and for some catastrophic or emergency services. For those not in these categories the costs of falling ill may be covered by the use of health insurance. Such health insurance is voluntary in the USA and some people fall between the two stools of not being poor enough to qualify for Medicare or Medicaid while not being rich enough to keep up with the very expensive insurance premiums required through the health insurance system. In some states, up to 15% of people are not sufficiently covered for health care.

The quality is high, in so far as the service intervenes much more than in most health services. With such close scrutiny by the health insurers and the tendency of the US public to sue if anything goes wrong, the professionals tend to use a 'belt and braces' approach to treatment and care. There is a tendency for the service to do something rather than wait and see. This is one reason for the expense of the system.

Compulsory insurance

Germany was the main pioneer of a third method of paying for its health care. It has been said that Bismarck built up this system in order to win over the workers to the conservative cause. In this system of 'compulsory insurance', workers and employees are obliged to make payments to designated health funds, which pay the treatment costs of their members. People pay a predetermined percentage of their income to these funds, the employers pay an equal amount, at present about 12%. When Bismarck introduced a nationalised insurance system to cover the health of Prussian miners, his lead was later followed by Lloyd George in the UK prior to the advent of the NHS.

One of the ironies of health-care history is that the fairly right-wing state of Queensland in Australia was one of the first to introduce a totally state-funded health service.

Specific countries

Germany

In Germany in the 1990s the compulsory insurance

funds make contracts with different care providers, for instance the associations that represent the GPs. There are more than 1000 insurance funds that people can pay into. Membership of a fund covers a worker and his or her family. Those not working have a different fund, so that virtually everyone is covered for health care. Another feature of the German system is an absolute separation between institutional care and other forms of care. As a result, the GPs dominate, for instance, all day and out-patient care.

There have been talks in Germany for over 20 years on keeping down the costs of the health-care system. One reason for the difficulty in reaching agreement has been differences between the different states in the federation. Doctors dominate the health service and have an important say in the insurance funds themselves, so these cannot exert pressure on the medical profession.

Variations on the insurance-based theme have been set up in other European countries, notably Belgium, France, the Netherlands and Greece. The German system remains the flagship of this type of care, with the biggest health care system in Europe.

France

In France, the main characteristic of the system is that patients have free choice, with no restrictions on their access to a GP or specialist. They may even go to hospital without seeing either. There is also equal opportunity in care. The private sector is very powerful with two-thirds of all doctors working in the private sector. Patients pay their doctors and are then reimbursed by the insurance system. About three-quarters of the cost is reimbursed. In hospital, the system pays the hospital directly.

A sickness insurance scheme or a social aid scheme guarantees health care for people who do not pay their social security insurance. The system is very expensive, probably because professionals feel the need to overtreat as patients have the freedom to go elsewhere. The government attempts to control costs by regulating the number of professionals, especially doctors and pharmacists. Despite this they still have twice as many doctors per head as in the UK. Social security insurance comes from three different branches; sickness at work, old age and family. All three are separately funded.

The chairman of the board of a hospital is the mayor of the local commune and the local authorities are very involved in the management of the hospital. It is, therefore, virtually impossible to reduce the number of hospitals.

Sweden

The system in Sweden has traditionally depended on financing health care through general taxation and, like the UK, it is experimenting in the 1990s with an internal market model. The Swedish health service is more decentralised than that in the UK, being run by the equivalent of the county councils. The system has been predominantly public, as in the UK, though in contrast to the UK the finances for the service have come from local not central taxation. Each county of 200 000 to 400 000 has one main and a number of smaller hospitals. The system is very hospital based despite numerous efforts since the 1970s to strengthen primary care. They have recently set up a primary care system similar to that in the UK. Sweden has actually succeeded in reducing its spending on health care in the 1990s.

The internal market model that they have been setting up in parallel to the UK is different in detail from county to county. Ten units have been set up as purchasers and these hold the government finance. The hospitals are paid according to the diagnoses of the patients (DRGs, see Chapter 22) in their care. Each patient, therefore, has a clearly defined 'price tag' and it appears that professionals are becoming more aware of this and responding by spending less.

The Swedes are discussing moving to an insurance-based system but this is unlikely to happen, given that this would undermine the power of the counties and reduce the government's control over costs.

Tax-based versus insurance-based systems

Table 26.4 lists the advantages of tax-based and insurance-based schemes.

Table 26.4 Tax-based versus insurance-based health schemes

Advantages of a tax-based system	Advantages of an insurance-based system
Usually cheaper overall	Patients can choose insurers
100% coverage	Patients can choose not to pay for health care
Less bureaucratic	People can pay for extras on the margins of health care
Less pressure to overtreat	Insurers help to ensure quality of care
Less likely to give 'two-tier' care	Less government interference

Health services

➤ Governments have three major roles in health care: regulation, planning and provision.

➤ Health services are funded from fees, general taxation, insurance and a third party (e.g. an employer through an insurance company).

➤ Tax-based health systems give 100% coverage and are usually cheaper to run than insurance-based systems. They tend to be less bureaucratic and are less likely to overtreat or give two-tiered care.

➤ Insurance-based health systems give more choice to patients on what they pay for; there is less government interference and quality of care is overseen by insurers.

The National Health Service in the UK

Christopher Potter

In this chapter the health provision in the UK is described:

- the setting up of the NHS
- the internal market in the NHS
- general practice budgets
- funding.

Introduction

The debate about what form the UK health service should take has continued since at least the 1920s. The debate continues and because there are no technically correct solutions to deciding what are really political issues it will no doubt continue into the future.

The setting up of the NHS owed little to the Labour Party or the Socialists in its early days. Left-wing thinking during the 1920s '30s and '40s, was that health was not a priority. Their argument was that if matters such as wage rates, housing, nutrition, education and so on were dealt with, sickness and illness would look after itself. It is certainly true that the biggest health gains during the last century have come through improved housing and sanitation, but it was fanciful to believe that health could be ignored.

The Dawson committee in the 1920s, the BMA and various other commissions and writers had seen the need to address the ramshackle patchwork of services which had grown up in the UK by the time of the Second World War. In particular, there were two hospital services that were always on the edge of bankruptcy. The war itself added to the pressures on the health services and showed up their inadequacies, though it did improve the financial state of the hospitals temporarily as people injured in the fighting or as a result of bombing were paid for from taxation.

A committee under Lord Beverage, a Liberal peer, during the Second World War set up a blueprint for a welfare state in the UK in 1942. After much talk, the 1946 National Health Service Act was introduced on 1 April, 1948. Probably the most important feature of the Act are the opening words in which the Secretary of State is made responsible for providing a comprehensive health service. The word 'comprehensive' is defined in terms that cover the whole population and included 'all necessary forms of health services'. There are no restrictions. In consequence, if a patient or health professional can make a claim that their health is being adversely effected and that a treatment or intervention is available to avoid this situation, it must be given.

This comprehensiveness is remarkable and singles the NHS out from all other forms of social services and welfare provision made in the UK. In education and transport there is a clear appreciation that not everyone can have all they want. Since 1948, there has been an ever-increasing accumulation of different services that politicians have been reluctant to challenge. Every health-care professional has a career to nurture and he or she can make a case for their particular service or specialty interest needing to be funded. Sufferers of any condition will raise a hue and cry if their services are not available.

Purchasers and providers

Mrs Thatcher's government set up an NHS Review in 1989, which led to the NHS and Community Care Act, 1990. The central core of the NHS part of the act was to set up an **internal market** within the health service with purchasers and providers, in the belief that where there is a choice of services market pressures will improve the cost and quality of those providing the choice. The Labour government in 1997 decided to keep purchasers and providers but to get rid of the internal market.

Purchasers

At a local level, the health authorities are the purchasers. As protectors of the health of the people, they are responsible for purchasing services from trusts, who are the providers. The intention is that the money to pay for services follows the patients. For many years, the efficiency trap had been recognised, where more efficient hospitals with shorter length of stay would see more patients but would also run out of money.

Providers

The providers consist of:

- hospital trusts
- community service trusts
- ambulance trusts
- specialist groups, e.g. radiotherapy, dental hospitals.

In theory, private hospitals, voluntary organisations and charitable organisations are also providers of services. All health authorities purchase some of their services from such groups, but the proportion of the services bought in this way is tiny.

Boards of executive and non-executive directors run the trusts. Trusts own their own buildings and employ their own staff. They:

- enter into service agreements as providers with GP commissioners (see later), health authorities and other trusts
- undertake research
- undertake training
- work jointly with one another
- take in fee-paying patients, but not to the detriment of NHS contracts
- generate income but have no automatic right to retain that income.

Rationale for the purchaser–provider split

With the purchaser–provider split, the intention was that more efficient units providing better-quality services would attract more patients from the health authorities and commissioning GPs and would flourish. In practice, health authorities tend to look after and use their local hospitals. Restrictions are placed on trusts in their ability to provide subsidised services or cross-subsidise between services, which would let them compete unfairly with other trusts. The purchaser–provider split might, if purchasers had been aggressive about not using expensive or poor-quality services, have resulted in hospitals that were not well managed becoming bankrupt. However, with a few exceptions, such an occurrence is so embarrassing to the government that they do not let it happen.

The health authorities are given a sum of money by the government each year based on their population and needs, including a measure of the poverty of the population (measured by a formula). The health authorities then set up agreements with their provider trusts to treat and care for the population within that health authority boundary. The agreements may be quite detailed or very simple. For some services, such as an A&E department, the authority simply wants the service to be available for whoever turns up at all times of day and night. The agreement can, therefore, be quite simple and is known as a block contract. The exception might be the quality standards, where it might stipulate that all patients should be seen within a short period of arriving at the department.

General practitioner fundholding and Primary Care Groups

GP budgets were also introduced in the 1990 Act with GP-estimated, prescribing budgets. This was a new departure for before this GPs were not restricted on the cost of their prescribed medicines. As part of the act, GPs were also given the option of becoming **fundholders**. GPs who opted to become fundholding practices had to have a list size of at least 5000 patients. GPs with 3000 patients or more could opt to hold the budget for out-patient and community care only.

Fundholding practices could purchase secondary services, i.e. hospital or community nursing services. They were given a budget from the health authority allocation to cover the cost of non-emergency in-patient and out-patient care. These were originally the services that were best known for their long waiting lists. Early suspicions were that the government was trying to off load the blame for long waiting lists onto the GPs. The money transferred from the health authority also covered the cost of their prescribed drugs and the staffing costs of the practice. The GPs then needed to draw up agreements with the hospital or community trusts specifying the cost of the service and its quality.

GP fundholders have been until recently purchasing increasingly large proportions of the health service budget. In 1996, about half of the population were registered with fundholding practices. Practices were increasingly being encouraged to opt for a series of different approaches for providing their services. A wide range of experiments was tried, including total fundholding, where the GPs, in groups, purchase the emergency as well as the non-emergency care. Other approaches include GPs working for NHS trusts as salaried employees and groups of 'multifunds' where non-fundholding GPs work with the health authority to organise the contracts for their patients.

The Labour government in 1998 stopped the fund-holding scheme. In its place, all GPs have been invited to take part in commissioning services with the health authority. These groups are known as Primary Care Groups. Purchasing services by the four main models (Local Health Groups in Wales). They will consist of 10–15 people with an executive board of five people. The groups will be subcommittees of the Health Authority. They will commence in April 1999 and will totally replace GP fundholding at that time. Each Primary Care Group will purchase services for a population of about 150 000 people.

The **stage one model** is one where the Primary Care Group will assist the Health Authority to purchase the services it wants. The Primary Care Group will act mainly in an advisory capacity. The Primary Care Groups will also oversee the GPs in the area, checking on the quality of their services and ensuring that the GP practices remain within their budgets. The groups will consist of representatives of all of the GPs in an area together with representatives from the Health Authority, the Local Authority and other primary care groups, such as nurses. The groups will also have representatives of the public and voluntary organisations.

The **stage two model** for the groups will be when they purchase some services for themselves, bearing in mind the needs of the local population. The groups will obviously need assistance from the Health Authority finance team for this. The sort of services purchased this way include patients who require non-emergency surgery or medicine. These are often services that have waiting lists. Part of the aim of the purchasers will be to try to reduce these lists as far as possible.

The **third stage** of development of the Primary Care Groups will be for them to purchase the great majority of services, including the emergency services for an area. These day-to-day emergency services that are usually needed at short notice, often without the general practitioner seeing the patient. Examples of such patients are those admitted to accident and emergency departments and those with emergency surgical or medical conditions, such as appendicitis or a heart attack. Some total purchasing practices already work with populations of about 50 000 people at this sort of stage.

The **fourth stage** will be for the Primary Care Groups to form what are known as Primary Care Trusts. These appear to be Primary Care Groups, which will purchase virtually all services and be integrated into the other primary care services in an area, but the model is not yet completely clear.

In Scotland the new groups will go straight to this stage. In England and Wales it is expected that all of the groups will start at stage one and work up to the later stages.

Purchasing all of the services in an area for a population of 150 000 will be difficult for some services. The rarity and expense of some, so called, regional services means that a small number of extra cases could completely upset the budgeting of the Primary Care Group. There are a number of conditions that fall into these categories, for example people who need renal and cardiac transplantation, those mentally ill people who need regional secure accommodation and children with rare genetic disorders. The population base for such services has, in the past, generally been about two million people, though this will, of course, vary with the condition. The government appear to be aiming to get around these problems by setting aside money for them at the beginning of a pay round. This is known as 'top slicing'.

Strengths and weakness of the purchaser–provider approach

Strengths for purchasers

- Can specify what they buy in as much or as little detail as they wish. There are some limits including giving the provider 6 months warning about proposed major changes proposed in the service. The Department of Health has also issued general strictures not to undermine the viability of trusts. There is a new emphasis to be placed on long-term agreements, over 3 or more years, rather than new agreements to be drawn up annually as at present.

- In practice, purchasers have been responsible about their demands on providers. After all, only a few years back they were colleagues in the same organisation. Many people, especially in management, move from the one side of the service to the other.

- All areas and providers have their black spots. These black spots may be a specialty, a service or an individual, which are known to give a poor service. The purchaser–provider split does not solve all of these problems, but it does allow the purchasers to have the ultimate sanction if things are not improving. That sanction is to remove the contract from one provider and give it to another. The Primary Care Group purchasers will be able to ask for services which match closely with the needs of their local population.

Strengths for providers

- More freedom to develop and try to sell new ideas. The boards of the trusts have a greater stake in their work for, if a trust fails, the executives will be out of a job.
- There is greater pressure for hospitals and community units to keep within their budgets than before the development of the split.
- Trusts have to be aware of what they do well and to concentrate on that, rather than trying to do a wide range of tasks, some badly.
- In practice this aspect of the market has been disappointing. Some trusts have been fast to develop new, exciting approaches to the delivery of services, but these are a minority. Generally the trusts have been on the defensive, worrying about their budgets and trying to keep their heads down.

Weaknesses

- Built in competition between providers so that collaboration between them is difficult.
- There are also problems, especially for Primary Care Groups, of buying in rare services. The need to make overt choices when purchasing one of two alternatives, a central point of the purchaser–provider split, can also be seen as a weakness. This is the case if the choice is not explained to the public promptly and clearly.
- Trusts that lose services they have provided for some years tend to cry foul to the press. Sometimes the decision not to give a service, even at the individual patient level can hit the headlines.
- This is only a weakness of the service if the purchaser or provider in question is unable to give coherent reasons for their decisions.
- Unfortunately there is no tradition within the health service for doing this, so patients often get a distorted view of the service.
- There is a new overt emphasis on costing. This emphasis upon money appears to make the service appear less altruistic than it has in the past. There has been a long tradition in medicine, from the days of the voluntary hospitals, of giving free treatment and the National Health Service inherited some of this ethos so that until recently there has been only sporadic talk about the cost of effective care.

Conclusion

Mrs. Thatcher's favourite image of the market was of a group of costermongers vying with each other about the price and quality of their goods to sell their wares. In this the price is not something one mentions as an afterthought, it is shouted as part of the marketing. The internal market she set up in the health service was different from such a free approach. It had to keep within budget and to provide a full range of medical care free at the point of use. It is hard to envisage a group of costermongers developing a market under such constraints. It might just do so under heavy threat from the local spivs. It is interesting to surmise who has that role in the health service.

The Labour government, which came to power in 1997, has abolished the internal market, but is keeping purchasers and providers. They have put a great deal of emphasis upon collaboration between purchasers and providers instead of confrontation. The system did not involve a great deal of outward confrontation but there are inevitable tensions when all providers want more money and the purchaser is unable to satisfy all of these demands. The amount of money provided by governments has increased only minimally under the Labour government so these tensions are not likely to disappear.

Is the NHS underfunded?

In the UK where the bulk of the health-care sector is paid for from general taxation, it is frequently argued that the NHS is underfunded. There is a belief that the UK spends less than comparable countries on health care. This common perception, with widespread complaints from health professionals, gives rise to the idea that there is underfunding of the NHS and it naturally leads to the view that the UK should spend more on the NHS and reinforces the possibility of rationing care to certain core services.

The reality is that in nearly all developed countries of the world, government spending on health-care provision falls within a band of about 6.5 to 8% of GDP. The UK spends more than the average on publicly funded health care and is only unusual in that the general public puts so little of their own money into the system. The only country that comes close to spending double the UK's percentage of GDP on health care is the USA, which has developed a system demonstrating the futility of throwing money at a problem like health care:

- a quarter of its expenditure goes on administration
- 37 million people are uninsured (30% of Hispanic males)

- prices for common surgical procedures are far higher than in its neighbour, Canada.

As for the professionals complaining that they want more money, that is a problem in every country in the world.

One cannot draw the conclusion that the UK government should spend more money on the NHS because:

- it is already spending more than most on *publicly funded health* services
- all expenditure does not inevitably lead to quality
- there is no evidence that all current expenditure in the NHS is justified.

In fact it is clear that underfunding means nothing without defining what needs to be funded. It is at least as logical to say that too much is expected from the funds available. However, most people in the health service have a vested interest in taking the former position.

There are a number of reasons for the clamour for more resources:

- governments do not like to look bad by seeming miserly
- opposition leaders and the media like to show government in a bad light
- health professionals want higher salaries, more freedom and newer technologies
- managers find it easier to say that they need more money than to take unpopular decisions. An example of this was the fate of the Chief Executive of a local hospital trust, who tried to make three consultants redundant. The rest of the consultants passed a motion of no confidence in him and his board fired him.

Other people have been keen to control the demand for health services, to raise the threshold at which people come for treatment. The argument is that if there is no immediate cost to a person he or she is more likely to look for care. The other side of the argument is that any restrictions form a barrier, which will probably hurt those who are most in need. There is evidence, for instance, that increases in charges for dental and ophthalmic services have led to a fall in demand. It seems likely that a nation brought up to believe that health care should be provided free is reluctant to put money aside for health-care expenditure, even if they have employment and the means to put money aside.

The NHS provides a very wide range of high-quality health services very cost effectively. However, there is still waste, and resources could clearly be better used to improve health in many areas.

Areas where waste could be reduced are:

- reducing *ineffective* care, such as D&Cs (dilatation and curettage) in women with menorrhagia under 40 years of age
- reducing *unnecessary* care, such as recalling patients to out-patient appointments several times routinely instead of moving their care to their GP
- reducing *wastage* by avoiding using highly skilled, highly paid people for tasks that do not require their expertise; an example would be using untrained staff rather than nurses for giving patients their food and washing them
- reducing *costs* by using, for instance, unbranded (generic) medicines.

Inevitably the NHS is a subject for political debate. Unfortunately that debate is frequently based on sentiment and ignorance. Even more unfortunately, it is often based on self-serving positions adopted by health professionals, and equally self-serving hysteria by the media and politicians, who ignore the effects on lives and health caused by their point scoring. We feel that the public ought to have more say in the range and choice of treatments available to them, with less arrogance on the part of the professions and politicians and more assertiveness on the part of patients.

The NHS

➤ The act setting up the NHS required a comprehensive health service covering the whole population and all necessary forms of health service.

➤ The NHS review in 1990 set up an internal market with purchasers – the health authorities and GPs – and providers – hospital, community service and ambulance trusts and special groups.

➤ GP budgets for prescribing drugs were introduced and GPs could become fund holders, having a budget they could use to purchase services.

➤ The question of whether the NHS is underfunded or uses funding poorly is complex and has political implications. A move to payment for services is thought to be most likely to hurt those most in need.

Preventative health care, health promotion and screening

28

In this chapter methods of promoting health are examined:

- disease prevention strategies
- health education and lifestyle changes
- screening.

Disease-prevention strategies

General methods of disease prevention can be considered as:

- environmental
- personal
- medical.

Environmental strategies

A number of preventative strategies can be considered as environmental and these often involve legislation. They include:

- water purity and treatment, e.g. the chlorination of water to reduce bacteria and fluoridation to reduce caries in teeth
- air purity
- noise legislation
- housing quality, including provision of sewerage
- factory regulations, health and safety at work legislation
- food regulations, including the prevention of the contamination of meat and other products and exclusion of food handlers with certain diseases or carrying certain disease.

The importance of food regulations has been underlined by severe outbreaks of a strain of *E. coli* in Scotland in 1997–8.

Personal strategies

Some strategies that affect personal behaviour may also have legislation attached to them, such as:

- pre-employment examination of bus and train drivers and pilots
- exclusion of people with epilepsy who have had fits in the past 12 months from driving (unless fits were exclusively while sleeping)
- wearing seat belts in cars, helmets on motor cycles.

Others are not related to legislation except to exclude young people from taking part:

- smoking cigarettes
- drinking alcoholic drinks.

Others are related to advice without legislation:

- diet
- exercise.

Medical strategies

Prevention can equally apply to the work that doctors do:

- avoidance of iatrogenic disease from, for example, inappropriate use of medicines; avoiding making available large quantities of dangerous drugs to people who are depressed
- inappropriate labelling of people as ill when they are not, especially by screening for disease with poor screening tools.

The most effective form of prevention of disease is **immunisation** and **vaccination**, against infectious disease. We perceive these diseases, since vaccination became so widespread, as less important than they were formerly.

Health promotion

Health promotion is the process of helping people to take control over their lives so that they can choose options that are health giving rather than those which are health risky.

There has been an increased emphasis upon health promotion within primary health care teams. The government has encouraged this by offering special funding for health education and promotion clinics in primary care. They have recently promised to ban cigarette advertising. Health authorities have to set out their priorities for health promotion. Examples are:

- support for smoking cessation
- promotion of school no-smoking policies
- smoking advice for pregnant women
- helping primary health-care teams give healthy eating advice
- helping schools with healthy eating projects
- promotion of advice on emergency contraception
- peer group education projects for adolescents about contraception
- training of primary health-care teams in brief interventions for abusers of alcohol
- training youth workers to educate young people about healthy alcohol drinking.

Generally media campaigns seem to be as effective as group work, though smoking cessation is still best brought about by the patient's doctor telling them to stop.

Health promotion is about much more than setting up campaigns. It is about getting full community participation in promoting healthy approaches to life generally. It is about removing the blocks to taking healthy choices when a choice is offered. There are a number of components of such community development:

- creation of a sense of social cohesion on a neighbourhood basis and strengthening group inter-relationships
- encouragement and stimulation of self-help, through the initiative of individuals in the community
- stimulation by outside agencies when initiative for self-help is lacking
- persuading people to change through their own efforts
- identification and development of local leaders
- development of civic consciousness and acceptance of civic responsibility
- use of professionals to support the efforts of the people in the community

- coordinating services in the area for local needs
- training in democratic procedures.

The list, if read carefully, suggests some of the problems perceived with health promotion. On the one hand, individuals may need help and advice with their health about what services do and how to get hold of them. On the other, there is a paternalism about the list that suggests that 'we' will show 'you' what you need. There is a danger that, with this model, health and the pursuit of greater health will come to dominate the reasons for people taking part in activities such as sport, dancing or music. Given a chance, health issues can even come to dominate the relationships between two people. There is a danger of turning 'good health' into a religious activity.

Having said this, there is a need for a greater understanding by the population of health and disease and the extent to which the health services can help. This is much more limited than appears to be generally believed, possibly because of images of medical practice and research presented in different public media.

Lifestyles

Much of the work of health promotion is aimed at altering people's lifestyles. The traditional areas of interest include:

- smoking
- diet
- alcohol
- physical activity.

These have important impacts on health, being implicated in a number of major health problems. Smoking cigarettes is a cause of a large number of diseases, the most important of which are ischaemic heart disease, cerebrovascular disease, chronic bronchitis and lung cancer. Researchers have added high-fat, low-fibre diets as causes of ischaemic heart disease, bowel cancer and diabetes. Alcohol misuse is associated with motor vehicle accidents and violence generally. Physical activity appears to promote bone strength and may help to reduce the likelihood of other diseases.

The great majority of people who have one or other unhealthy lifestyle habits know that they do. Altering their lifestyle is, therefore, more complex than simply pointing out to them the risks that they are taking. The chances are that they will already know. Resistance to change occurs because of:

- family behaviour
- past experience

- peer pressures
- advertising media
- lacking the skills to break the habit
- healthy eating and exercise may have significant time and financial costs.

Social class and lifestyle

Social class is an important determinant of morbidity and mortality. It is, therefore, not surprising to find that lifestyles between the different social classes are different. Figure 28.1 shows the percentage of people who smoked daily in Cardiff and the Vale of Glamorgan by manual and non-manual occupations of the main wage earner. We can see that considerably more people with manual occupations smoke than with non-manual. The occupational class difference is greater in women than men. This is exacerbated by the fact that women where the main wage earner in the household is in a manual occupation are continuing to increase their rates of smoking. The other groups are all reducing their smoking habit.

Dietary factors also differ between the occupational classes. Figure 28.2 shows the percentage of people eating fresh fruit at least four times a week by occupational class. Again the distinction is marked. In this

> ### Disease prevention
>
> ➤ Disease-prevention strategies are aimed at stopping people becoming ill and can be environmental, personal or medical. Most effective are immunisation and vaccination.
>
> ➤ Health promotion is educating the population on healthy options and helping them to chose and implement these.
>
> ➤ Lifestyles are associated with social class for several health risk factors, e.g. smoking and diet.

case, however, all four groups were eating more fresh fruit than they had been 5 years before.

Some behaviour does not appear to be related to occupational class, especially drinking alcohol and taking exercise.

Screening

Prevention is qualitative so that there is no sharp boundary between prevention and treatment. People relate screening to prevention, but prevention, as we have seen is much more than simply using screening. Professionals aim most screening done in the health service at early treatment, rather than the total avoidance of disease. Prevention generally is about stopping well people from becoming ill. The medical input in prevention is, therefore, quite restricted, often being carried out by educationists.

Screening for asymptomatic disease

A screening test, by definition is not diagnostic. The screening test is usually a single test. It is simpler and much cheaper than a full diagnostic work-up. Relatively unskilled people can often carry it out, reducing its cost still further. People with positive findings on the screening test are referred for full assessment and treatment. This type of screening may be a simple procedure, but because the screeners carry it out on large numbers of asymptomatic people it can be very expensive overall. The general public tend to be keen to introduce screening for a large number of rare diseases, but this can clash with health authorities who are aware of the cost consequences. Table 28.1 shows some of the screening tests that have been proposed. More are constantly being added.

Decisions must be made about two main issues before asymptomatic screening can be shown to be a

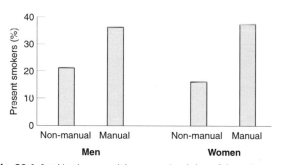

Fig. 28.1 Smoking by sex and the occupational class of the main wage earner in a household, in 1990. (OPCS 1997)

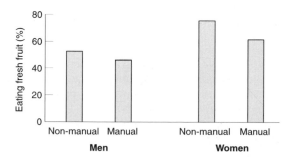

Fig. 28.2 The percentage eating fresh fruit four or more times a week by sex and the occupational class of the main wage earner. (OPCS 1997)

Table 28.1 Some areas of asymptomatic screening

National service	Provided in places	Suggested
Breast cancer	Apgar score (babies)	Cystic fibrosis
Cervical cancer	Congen ht disease (infants)	Galactosaemia
Phenylketonuria	Chromosomal abnormalities (fetal)	Endocrine disorders
Dental	Prostate cancer	Learning disabilities
Congenital hip dislocation	Cholesterol	Bacteriuria
Venereal disease (pregnancy)	Anaemia	Abdominal aneurysm
Childhood milestones	Lead poisoning (some industries)	Rheumatic heart disease
Deafness (infants)	Colour blindness (some industries)	Sex chromosome abnormalities
Sight (infants)	Tuberculosis	HIV
Height & weight (infants)		Inguinal hernia
Examination 3 yearly (middle aged)		
Examination yearly (over 65)		

reasonable approach: the disease and the test. The **disease** being screened for should be:

- serious or potentially so
- treatable or controllable
- early diagnosis must lead to a better prognosis than late diagnosis
- it must be reasonably prevalent in the population studied
- screening costs must compare favourably with the costs of not screening, i.e. lives saved or disabilities avoided must be in line with costs for other diseases.

The test should be:

- acceptable: the test must not be excessively painful, embarrassing or potentially dangerous; some tests that require fetal venous blood may fall into the last category
- reliable: the test must be carried out with an instrument of proven accuracy, the inter- and intraobserver variation must be low and variations between subjects must be small; the reason for the latter is that if we try to separate a measure into two groups – those likely to and those not likely to have the disease – marked variations in the normal range will mean that we will classify many people into the wrong group
- valid: the test must be confirmed by a 'gold standard' and have high sensitivity and specificity.

Table 28.2 is the fourfold table (discussed in Chapter 3), which illustrates the concepts of sensitivity and specificity. Sensitivity for a screening test is the accuracy of the test in identifying all the diseased subjects. Specificity is the accuracy of the test in identifying those without the disease. False positives are those found to be positive by the test but who do not have

Table 28.2 Selection of a screening test with good sensitivity and specificity

| Test | Disease | |
	Present	Absent
Positive	Agreement (a)	Overreferral (b)
Negative	Underreferral (c)	Agreement (d)

Sensitivity = a/(a+c)
Specificity = d/(b+d)

False-positive rate of the test $= \dfrac{b}{a+b}$

False-negative rate of the test $= \dfrac{c}{c+d}$

the disease. False negatives are those who are negative by the test but who do have the disease.

The reader will remember from Chapter 00 the importance of prevalence when measuring these entities. When screening for asymptomatic disease, the prevalence of the disease in the population being screened will inevitably be low, leading to large numbers of people in cells (b) and (d). We will need to test fully those in cell (b), also known as the false positive group, to ensure that they are disease free. The cost of caring for these people will be a result of the screening process. This is an additional cost, which would not have arisen if we had not set up the screen. This group will also be very anxious about their result, so it is important that we should follow them up as soon as possible. The group in (d) will have been told that they do not have a disease that they had not thought they might have had until they were screened.

For a given test, improving sensitivity generally reduces specificity and vice versa. For serious diseases with effective treatment, there is a temptation to go for high sensitivity at the cost of specificity. This produces high referral rates. An example is breast self-examination where the sensitivity is only 67%. People have improved on this by mammography, but the overreferral rate goes up to 76%. More importantly breast self-examination alone does not catch the cancer early enough in its progress to alter the prognosis. It is no longer recommended on its own. The national breast screening campaign screens all women between the ages of 45 and 65 in the country for breast cancer by mammography.

Sometimes specificity may be more important, where the consequences of not receiving therapy are less important, e.g. a test for hepatic function before taking the contraceptive pill. It would not be crucial if the screening test for hepatotoxicity had a low sensitivity as long as the test had a high specificity. In this situation, all of the cases would be caught but some without the problem could be advised not to take the pill. This is a better option when there are other good methods of contraception available.

Screening in particular diseases

Screening in cancer of the breast

A number of randomised controlled trials have shown that breast cancer screening through the use of mammography can be effective in identifying women with early breast cancer. The trials also suggested that the screening reduced the mortality rate from breast cancer. As a result, the national breast screening campaign was set up in the UK. It is early to say whether, at a nationally organised level, it is effective in terms of mortality. Detecting cases earlier means that screened patients will live longer than those with symptomatic tumours simply because they were diagnosed at an earlier stage of the disease. In the national campaign, the rate of detection has been higher than was anticipated, especially so in Wales. Early therapy in *symptomatic* disease seems to make little difference, for the outcome is still poor.

Screening for cancer of the lung

Although 6-monthly X-ray examinations increase the early detection of lung cancer, there is no good evidence that this increases the 5-year survival rate. Such an approach has not, therefore, been suggested as a screening method. The results of early treatment remain so bad that there does not appear to be much point in screening by any method and certainly not by a method that has intrinsic hazards (Chapter 21).

Screening for cancer of the cervix

The Papanicolaou smear test has a sensitivity of 66% for carcinoma in situ. There is a high overreferral rate because of the rarity of cervical cancer. There is little evidence that carcinoma in situ progresses to the full disease. The pressures to continue screening are largely political, spurred on by women's groups. New methods of screening using direct visual approaches, DNA testing and other methods are being developed. In future it may be that the screening system may concentrate on high-risk women, especially in low-income families.

Screening for cancer of the large bowel

Cancer of the large bowel is a treatable form of cancer. No good screening test is employed routinely in asymptomatic individuals in this country. It has been suggested that a two-tier screening test, with fecal occult blood testing followed by sigmoidoscopy where the first test is positive should be used. Using sigmoidoscopy would be unpleasant and potentially liable to side effects in large numbers of healthy people. A preliminary screen to produce an 'at-risk' population makes sense in tests of this nature.

Screening

➤ Screening is aimed at detecting early treatable disease.

➤ Diseases are worth screening for if they are treatable or controllable, more easily treated with early diagnosis and reasonably prevalent.

➤ Screening tests must not be excessively painful or dangerous, must be reliable and must be valid (high sensitivity and specificity).

➤ Sensitivity is the accuracy of the test in identifying all diseased subjects. It is important for serious diseases with effective treatment.

➤ Specificity is the accuracy of the test in identifying those without the disease; it becomes important when the consequences of false positives are serious.

➤ Screening for specific diseases varies from the routine highly effective tests (e.g. for phenylketonuria) to more controversial areas (e.g. for cancer of the bowel).

Antenatal screening

Antenatal screening is carried out in many countries. The most effective method of reducing the incidence of disease in the population by screening is for neural tube defects, where the birth prevalence has fallen by 95% between 1970 and 1990. Screening for high concentrations of alpha-fetoprotein at 16 to 18 weeks gestation detects about 75% of pregnancies where the fetus has spinal bifida. Routine ultrasound at 18–20 weeks can detect a similar proportion. The serum test gives a 10:1 overreferral rate. The diagnostic test is to carry out an amniocentesis, which carries a risk of aborting a normal fetus of 1 in 1000. The 'treatment' for an affected fetus is abortion at a fairly late stage. Most effort at present is going into trying to detect abnormalities earlier in pregnancy.

For Down's syndrome, maternal age and antenatal serum screening are used together to isolate a group of people at high risk of having a baby with Down's syndrome. Current research is concentrating on the use of other markers and ultrasound to improve diagnostic accuracy. Isolating the abnormal chromosomes from the fetus is also progressing. There are also efforts to diagnose abnormalities in the first trimester. Screening tests for other chromosomal abnormalities such as trisomy 18 (Edward's syndrome) are being developed.

Primary health care

In this chapter aspects of primary health care in the UK are described:

- the primary care team
- types of practice
- funding.

Introduction

Primary care was defined by Starfield as 'first contact, continuous, comprehensive, and co-ordinated care provided to populations undifferentiated by gender, disease or organ system'. This describes the ideal service.

In the UK GPs provide primary health care, the initial contact of individuals and families with the health service. There are 30 000 GPs in the UK; these take up about 9% of the NHS spending for their service costs and another 10% for their prescribing costs. On these figures they are a formidable part of the health-care spectrum.

Within the practices are **practice nurses**. In the community, based in local clinics, but increasingly working directly with general practitioners, are the **community health services**. The latter services include district nurses, health visitors, domiciliary midwives, physiotherapists, occupational and speech therapists and chiropodists.

Other points of first contact between patients and the health service are:

- accident and emergency departments
- genitourinary departments
- child health services
- community mental health teams
- family planning and well women clinics
- occupational health programmes.
- the national breast cancer screening programme is a special case; it calls women between the ages of 45 and 65 to be screened.

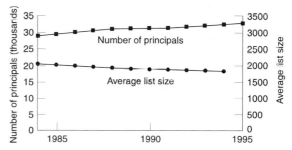

Fig. 29.1 GP list sizes and the number of practice principals in the UK. (OHF 1997)

The UK is unusual in providing health care where access to hospital services is mainly controlled by GPs. The GPs look after a defined list of patients of all ages and have continuous responsibility for their care. People consider that this initial filtering of patients by the GPs has contributed to the relatively low cost of the hospital services in the UK health service. Figure 29.1 shows the number and list size of GPs since 1981. The number of GPs has increased steadily throughout the 1980s and the average list size has fallen.

In the UK, 97% of the population is registered with a GP and only a small proportion change practices, usually when they move to another area. In any one day GPs see around 650 000 patients in their surgeries and visit a further 100 000 in the community. The number of GP home visits has remained unchanged despite falling list sizes.

The number of consultations per patient per year has increased slightly as can be seen in Figure 29.2. All the age groups have increased their contact with GPs to some extent over the 15 years shown on the figure. This has been greatest for infants, possibly because of increased numbers of contacts as GPs have taken over the immunisation programme over the past few years from the community services. Young women and recently retired men have also most markedly increased their contact with GPs. This may because of

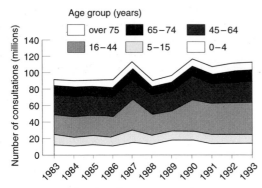

Fig. 29.2 Estimated number of GP consultations by patient age group in the UK. (OHE 1997)

the need for contact during pregnancy in the former group, as GPs have been taking over obstetric care from the hospitals. Newly retired men attend for routine check-ups as part of the GP's contract.

The primary care team

The definition of the term 'primary care team' has been the subject of considerable discussion. One suggestion has been:

A multidisciplinary team with a common purpose and responsibility for the health care of patients at their first point of contact.

The core team consist of:

● doctors
● practice nurses
● attached health visitors, community nurses
● practice administrators, receptionists and secretaries.

In some practices, particularly those in health centres, midwives and other attached health professionals and even social workers, paid for by the local authority rather than the health authority, work from the building. In others they are based outside the practice. GPs may extend the team in some instances by the inclusion of community psychiatric nurses, counsellors or dieticians. Some practices employ phlebotomists to take blood and may have some laboratory facilities.

Primary health care teams were promoted by the Harding Report as long ago as 1981, but while some have developed according to the definition we have suggested, mostly they have not. Team approaches to primary care were expected to develop as health centres were created in the 1970s. However, there has been virtually no growth in the proportion of GPs working from health centres in the 1980s and 1990s. Cumberlege has pointed out that primary health-care teams rarely work because they have few established protocols or aims. These would encourage discussion and help them to monitor their successes and failures. The move from health centres has had more to do with financial incentives for GPs to set up in their own premises.

The WHO approach to primary health care emphasises the role of community participation and health promotion. Although some general practices have formed their own patient participation groups, the numbers are small and a considerable number have failed to survive. This is often because they lacked a clear role or depended on the activities of a few enthusiasts. Reviewing the very limited development of patient participation, Tudor Hart, a renowned GP in South Wales, proposed that special interest groups aimed at particular problems (e.g. hypertension, diabetes or asthma) might be more productive.

The new development by health authorities of commissioning services using primary care groups gives an opportunity for involving the community along with voluntary organisations, and primary care professionals to shape local schemes. Primary health care refers to that care which is given when the patient first seeks help. In the UK, specialists give secondary health care. Patients virtually always have to go through the primary system to be referred on to the specialists. Table 29.1 lists the professionals who offer unselected and on-going care for patients. Medical professionals in the community include public health doctors dealing with child health in schools. Speech therapists and occupational therapists can complement the efforts of pharmacists, midwives and physiotherapists.

Table 29.1 Primary care: potential members of the team

Area	Potential team member	The core primary care team
Medical	GP	GP
	School medical officer	
	Community geriatrician	
	Community psychiatrist	
	Dentist	
Paramedical	Community nurse	Community nurse
	Midwife	
	Physiotherapist	Physiotherapist
	Pharmacist	
Administrative	Practice assistant	Practice assistant
Social	Social worker	Social worker
	Phycologist	
	Domiciliary aid	

Primary care is oriented to the local community, and local circumstances dictate who will be suitable partners in the team. In an inner-city area, social and community psychiatric workers may be essential members, whereas the GP in an isolated rural community is more likely to favour community nurses. All the disciplines listed in Table 29.1 may be found in various combinations in different places.

Origins of the team

The idea of the primary care team as distinct from the new Primary Care Commissioning Groups has been taken up most vigorously in countries with a strong primary care orientation: Canada, the Netherlands, Scandinavia and the UK. An important reason for their development has been the shift from cure to care. Teamwork allows delegation of tasks and the role of nurses, practice assistants and midwives can be seen in this light. This delegation is not just a way of being more efficient with facilities. For some things other workers can do better than the GP: physiotherapists in rehabilitation, the practice assistant in organising prevention, and so on.

Table 29.2 shows the sort of work that involves various members of the team.

Group practices

Group practices are partnerships of three or more GPs working from the same building. The UK has a long tradition of GPs working in partnerships. Group practices are more efficient than single-handed practices at providing continuity of care and are able to employ more staff for management and administration. Group practice also brings together practitioners who formerly worked in isolation, with a resulting peer review of their patient care.

Table 29.2 lists the most important areas of work for the primary care team. A good example is terminal care. Terminal care provided in the intimate environment of the patient's home, in close relation to the patient's family and friends benefits greatly from a multidisciplinary approach. It is important that those giving the care are clear about its objectives and the place of professional support compared with that provided by relatives and friends.

Another area in which primary care has recently expanded has been prevention. Many people may be screened but abnormal findings need to be pursued; chronic diseases are diagnosed but in the long term not adequately treated. About 80% of the younger people in the community will consult a GP at least once every 3 years, and these visits offer good opportunities for health promotion and prevention. The practice assistant is important in exploiting this potential, by combining an individual primary care approach and administrative support. This strategy greatly improves follow-up care in screening and in chronic diseases. We should say that, in common with much of the work in primary care, the effectiveness of such approaches has not been proved.

One hazard of the team approach is that it reflects a 'professionals know best' attitude, making the patient feel alienated. Some say that it is the patient, rather than the professionals, who should be responsible for continuity of care and who decides where to turn for help. Experiments with patients as the budget holders of their own care underline that this approach is feasible. In this way patients would gain real influence on the running of the primary care team.

Table 29.2 General practice care, with primary care team involvement	
Topic	Disciplines involved
Health surveillance	
Perinatal, early childhood, elderly,	
screening	Health visitor
	Midwife
	School medical officer
	Practice assistant
Management of chronic diseases	
Asthma	Pharmacist
Diabetes mellitus	Practice assistant
Hypertension	
Terminal care	Community nurse
	Physiotherapist
	Pharmacist
	Social worker
Psychosocial impact of illness	Social worker
	Physiotherapist
	Community
	psychiatric services
	Psychologist

A primary care led health service?

Countries with more highly developed systems of primary care tend to have lower health-care costs. Policies designed to shift the balance from secondary to primary care have, therefore, been popular with governments, often leading to health service reforms. But saving money is not the only reason. The other side of the coin is that a health service dominated by secondary, tertiary and emergency, mainly hospital-based, care will tend to be fragmented, discontinuous, uncoordinated and costly.

In the UK, some procedures are being transferred from hospital to community settings. For example, triage systems and hospital-at-home schemes are being set up to avoid hospital admissions and allow for early discharge. Attempts are being made to reduce the number of patients referred to specialist services by developing referral guidelines. GPs and community nurses are being encouraged to develop new skills and new practice-based facilities. Shared care schemes are being introduced for chronic disease management, paediatrics, mental health and maternity care. Some GPs and specialists are experimenting with direct booking to surgical waiting lists, avoiding the need for specialist out-patient consultations.

There are some problems. Hard pressed primary care staff do not usually welcome more work unless there is more money to pay for it. If we take money from the hospital service for primary care the new primary care services will have to substitute for secondary care by looking after more ill patients. The difficult part is moving the money from one service to another without damaging patient care while this is happening.

In recent years GPs in the UK have been encouraged to do more and more things that have traditionally been done in hospital. One example is minor operations. The hope has been that, by removing this workload from the hospital, this would reduce waiting times for both minor and major operations. Evaluating this policy has so far shown no reduction in demand for hospital-based minor surgery. GPs' willingness to do these operations seems to have encouraged patients to come forward for treatment who would not otherwise have done so. The increased availability of equipment for near patient diagnostic testing in general practices has had a similarly disappointing impact on demand for hospital services. One researcher found that after practice-based equipment for two biological and four biochemical tests were introduced in 12 practices the overall rates of investigation went up and costs increased. GPs seemed to be using the practice equipment as an addition to, rather than a substitute for, hospital laboratory investigation.

Financing general practice

The vast majority of GPs are independent contractors with the health authority. The contract is set at a national level according to a schedule (the red book) for a basic payment, the number of patients on the GP's list and separate fees for some services, such as immunisation. The patients on the list attract fees

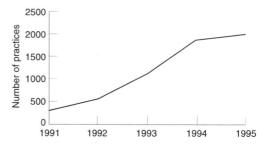

Fig. 29.3 The number of fundholding general practices in England. (Mechanic 1995)

according to a weighted capitation formula, which gives the general practitioner more for some groups of patients thought to need intensive care, such as elderly people. The health authorities have other finances for the development of general practices, for extra staff or equipment.

GP fundholding

Figure 29.3 shows the number of GP fundholders over time. Over 3000 GPs applied in 1996 in over 1200 practices, to make over half of all the GPs in the country fundholders. In that round, the maximum list size for standard fundholding was reduced to 5000. The scheme was extended to cover virtually all elective surgery, out-patients and specialist nursing services. The Labour government halted the extension of the fundholding scheme in 1997 and discontinued it in favour of Primary Care Groups.

Effectiveness of fundholding

Prescribing costs

It was hoped that general practitioner fundholding, with its emphasis upon GPs paying for their drugs, would reduce prescribing costs. Traditionally, UK GPs are conservative prescribers. Those who are fundholding took over the drugs' budget and the power to reinvest any savings that they could make in other services for their patients. At the same time an indicative prescribing scheme for GPs who were not fundholders was set up to help them to control their costs. This means that GPs have a theoretical budget for their drug costs. The health authority sets a financial target for each practice based on their previous prescribing costs, together with an estimate for inflation. No penalties were imposed on practices that fail to meet their targets. They receive information on their prescribing pattern compared with the pattern in other practices. It seems likely that all GPs will be expected to keep within a drugs budget in future under the supervision of the Primary Care Groups.

A group of researchers set up a study to look at the prescribing patterns of the practices taking part in the Oxford region fundholding groups. In the fundholding and non-fundholding practices the cost of drugs and the number of items prescribed rose steadily over the 3 years of the study. This study discovered that the group of non-dispensing fundholding practices had the highest costs at the end of the study. Paradoxically this was the group who had the greatest incentive to keep its costs low. In the initial stages of the study, a year after fundholding started, fundholding GPs seemed to have been more effective than non-fundholders in controlling their costs. Three years later, however, the pattern reversed and the difference between the types of practice reduced.

Inflationary influences on prescribing costs caused both groups to increase their costs despite the cost-control measures. Heavy marketing of some new anti-depressants and other drugs led to an increase in their prescribing although they were no more effective than those already available. This pressure from the drug companies appears to have been more powerful than government policy. This is not really surprising for pharmaceutical companies put very large budgets into persuading GPs to buy their goods. This publicity grows increasingly sophisticated and is very effective.

Referral to hospital

The fundholding scheme was intended to cut down the number of referrals GPs made to hospital by giving fundholders the non-urgent hospital in- and out-patient budget for their patients. There is some suggestion from research that GP fundholders are, because of their fundholding, becoming more critical in their decision to send patients to different surgeons. GPs mentioned that when choosing a surgeon to refer patients to they were most influenced by their confidence in the consultant's ability, short waiting times and informative response from the providers. The costs of the treatment and the convenience to patients were less important. Fundholders send the majority of referrals locally. Another study suggested that referral patterns to hospital were not different for fundholders and non-fundholders. Primary Care Groups at the second stage will take over such purchasing.

Patient care

Another detailed before and after study suggested that, after becoming fundholders, GPs were less good at giving time to people with subtle sociomedical problems. They were more effective at treating the traditional medical problems seen in general practice. This group examined the way fundholders and non-fundholders managed people with joint pain and found that the fundholders were maintaining their times for consultation with patients at much the same level as before becoming fundholders. They were, however, less likely to refer patients for investigations or to hospital. Patients showed less satisfaction latterly than formerly with their care. There is no evidence about whether they were more or less successfully treated.

Evaluating fundholding generally

A National Audit Office survey has looked at the effect of GP fundholding. The report suggested that many fundholding practices have improved communication with hospital services, with open access to pathology and radiology. They also had practice-based services for many groups including those needing physiotherapy, dietetics, chiropody, psychiatric nursing and psychology. The fundholders spent less on drugs than non-fundholders.

However, fundholders, as purchasers of hospital services, had not bought services according to the best evidence of effectiveness. They have not taken the opportunity to use or develop guidelines for the best treatment of complicated diseases. Very few tried to assess the needs of their practice population before purchasing services. The survey, a simple comparison between fundholders and non-fundholders, cannot separate the effects of fundholding from those general changes that were happening in general practice.

The general practice fundholding scheme was an attempt to shift the balance of power, and hence

---

Primary health care

➤ In the UK the GP is the usual first point of contact for the general population with the health service.

➤ The primary care team consists of doctors, practice nurses, attached health visitors, community nurses and administrators.

➤ General practice has moved towards group practices and a large number of larger practises have become fundholders, controlling drug budgets, hospital referrals and wider aspects of patient care.

money, into primary care. The new Primary Care Groups, working with the health authorities, may maintain that momentum. It seems unlikely that a committee of GPs and other primary care workers advising the health authority will have as much enthusiasm for its task as the fundholders working for themselves, but the Groups will have the benefit of overseeing a complete area.

Perhaps the gatekeeper role of UK GPs already delivers the nearest thing to an optimal balance. Healthcare systems that allow patients direct access to specialists generally have higher rates of intervention and higher costs. A study in North Carolina found that patients with back pain who consulted orthopaedic surgeons or chiropractors incurred much greater costs than those who consulted a primary care practitioner. The outcomes of treatment in terms of functional recovery and return to work were similar in the three groups.

Secondary health care

30

In this chapter secondary care in hospitals is discussed:

- what events result in referrals
- admission levels and policies
- the effectiveness of hospital treatment.

Introduction

Secondary care is that care which is given as a result of a referral from the primary care provider. Most commonly this is a specialist service referred to by a GP, but there are a number of other primary care professionals. We may think of nurses who often uncover problems that they refer working in community-based clinics or schools. The most costly part of the health services is the hospital service.

Development of hospitals

The centre point of most health services in the UK these days is the district general hospital. These developed in the mid-1960s as a response to the euphoria and relative prosperity of the country after the war. The new district general hospitals usually replaced groups of smaller hospitals. There have been a number of attempts to reduce the power that hospitals exert over the health services. These have usually been seen as a move to reduce the power of hospital-based specialists. It has, therefore, been greatly resisted. At the same time as the development of the district general hospitals, the government published a plan suggesting the development of large health centres for GPs. The government intended this to boost the development of the GP-based services. The primary health-care teams in these health centres would, it was hoped, develop more preventative services and reduce the pressure on casualty and out-patient departments in district general hospitals.

The enthusiasm for health centres was partially triggered by an enthusiasm for polyclinics developed in the Eastern bloc countries and in parts of Scandinavia. In those countries, the great majority of the health care needed by a local population was carried out in such places. This could include minor surgery and some specialist out-patient facilities. These plans never really came to fruition in the UK, but interestingly GPs are now increasingly being advised to follow this approach.

The cost of hospitals

Hospitals are the most costly part of any health service. The cost of hospitals and other institutional care have been rising very rapidly in all developed countries. Figure 30.1 shows the costs of a health authority in relation to the functions carried out. It can be seen that the hospital services dominate. Figure 30.2 shows the costs of health care for in-patients since 1970 by different OECD countries. All the countries showed a marked rise in the price of their health costs. Interestingly New Zealand, with one of the most extreme rises in costs, has felt driven to make rapid

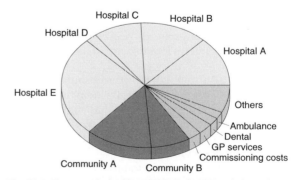

Fig. 30.1 The costs of a health authority in the UK in relation to its functions.

227

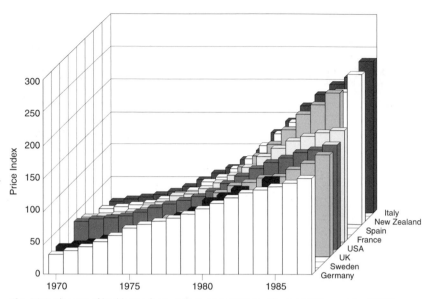

Fig. 30.2 The cost of health care for in-patients since 1970 by different OECD countries. 1980 is taken as the index year with a value of 100 to adjust for changing money values. (World Bank 1993)

and extensive changes to the administrative structure of its health service in a similar manner to the UK. It has split the service into two groups: purchasers who plan the service and providers who provide the care for patients.

The increase in the price of health care is not confined to hospitals. Figure 30.3 shows the changes in prices for ambulatory medical care. There are three aspects to such care. First, the primary care services that patients go to first when they have a problem, mainly GPs and a small number of others such as chiropodists. The second group of services is the out-patients' services provided by specialists or secondary care givers and usually based in hospital. The third group are the community services, which traditionally give their care in patients' homes and comprise mainly district nurses, community psychiatric nurses, health visitors, chiropodists and, in some areas, therapists. More specialist groups are also developing in the community, such as nurses looking after diabetes or stoma care.

Figure 30.3 on ambulatory services shows that they have increased, if anything, slightly more than the hospital services. Italy, in particular, has made a heavy investment in ambulatory services. For all of these increases in prices, the UK has remained low on the list of price increases on health care.

There is a huge range in the overall amount spent on health care in different countries, with Switzerland spending nearly five times as much per head as Greece

or Portugal. Countries that spend more or less than others on health services tend to spend it on both in-patient and ambulatory care. However there are some differences. Spain spends less than a fifth of its total on ambulatory care, whereas Luxembourg spends almost two-thirds. In other words, Luxembourg puts much more emphasis on GP, community-based services and out-patient services than Spain. Figure 30.4 shows the data for the proportion spent on ambulatory care in OECD countries compared with the wealth of the different countries. The figure shows that there is a trend for countries that are wealthier to spend a greater proportion of that wealth on ambulatory, rather than hospital care. There are a number of possible reasons for this. It may be that the poorer countries within the OECD group are keen to ensure that secondary services, based around the hospital, are in place before the full development of primary and out-patient services. There may be strong pressure from the population for governments to develop acute general medical and surgical services first. The pressures for the treatment of emergencies as the priority has been well described by Ivan Illich. He says that labelling a problem as an emergency is one way of ensuring that money will be spent on it, no matter how poor the country.

There will certainly be pressure from professional groups to do so, for most training, even today, is performed in hospital. This is despite the fact that the majority of doctors and many other professions in the

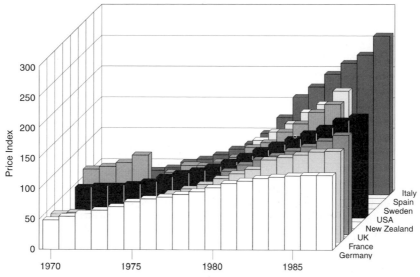

Fig. 30.3 The cost of ambulatory care, indexed to 100 as in Figure 30.2. (World Bank 1993)

medical field will spend their careers in community-based or primary care. It may be that pressures from urban, more politically aware populations, who will also be more likely to benefit from hospital services, may be strongest in poorer countries, where the rural population has little voice. It is interesting that this tendency completely cuts across the WHO policy of developing primary care services first.

Costs of hospital staffing in the UK

In the UK, the hospital sector continues to absorb about two-thirds of the money put into health care annually. This has been changing over the years. Figure 30.5 shows the percentage increase in spending on the hospital and GP sectors of the health service decade by decade since the NHS began. The figure shows that the heyday of expansion for the hospital sector was in the 1960s, as the district general hospitals were developing. Nearly a million people work in NHS hospitals in the UK. This has increased by more than three times since the founding of the health service. The number of beds for each staff member and the number of patients discharged per member of staff in hospitals fell steadily from the 1950s until the 1980s when they rose a little. In other words, the service became more labour intensive until the 1980s. This, of course, will have increased the costs of hospitals, for staffing makes up at least 70% of the cost of the NHS.

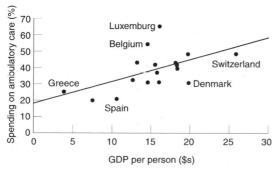

Fig. 30.4 The proportion spent on ambulatory care in OECD countries compared with wealth. (World Bank 1993)

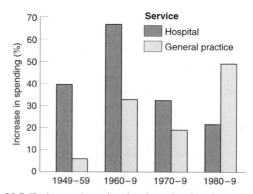

Fig. 30.5 The increased spending decade on decade on hospital and GP services (adjusted to inflation). (OHE 1997)

Admission to hospital

It is an astonishing fact, given the cost of hospital admission, that, where researchers have measured their need for admission against standard criteria, the majority of people going into hospital do not need to. Indeed their admission and stay has, more often than not, been shown to be unnecessary and inappropriate. The criteria used in these studies have not assumed that new services are available, or that any change needs to take place to accommodate these people elsewhere. Clinicians running the local services in their existing state drew up the criteria for these studies.

A number of studies have compared the attitudes of the patients to their services in different settings. The most relevant to this book compared hospital-based and non-hospital-based care. One study looked at day surgery based in a large teaching hospital in Northern California. The researchers compared this with a free-standing surgical unit. This approach is especially interesting because it shows that people can perform surgery outside what we would normally define as a hospital. The facility is attached to a large general practice. It consists of an operating room, a three-bedded recovery unit, a minor procedure room, waiting and reception areas and a changing room for patients.

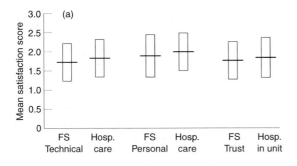

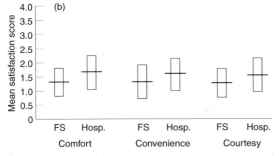

Fig. 30.6 Comparison of patients' response to two types of surgical care: (a) technical aspects of care; (b) social aspects of care. FS, Free-standing day hospital; Hosp., hospital-based day hospital. (Pica-Furey 1993)

In order to compare like with like patients assessed were restricted to those who had had one procedure, a cataract extraction. Ninety-eight patients had been to the free standing day hospital and 95 had been to the hospital-based day hospital. The effectiveness of the procedures was measured in terms of the physical and mental state of patients. It was similar for both groups. The success of the facility, therefore, revolved around the preference of the patients for one or other of the day units. The groups were not randomised but the patients appeared to be very similar for age, sex and severity of the disease before being treated. There was no difference in the degree of satisfaction with technical aspects of the care. The way that the operation was performed, the personal relationships with staff and the degree to which patients trusted the staff were similar (Fig 30.6a). The free-standing day unit scored better on all scores but this difference was not great enough to rule out a chance finding.

When less technical aspects were examined, the patients in the free-standing day hospital scored much more highly and were significantly more satisfied (Fig. 30.6b). Things that pleased them especially were:

- the comfort of the surroundings
- the convenience of getting to the unit
- the courtesy of staff
- the speed and seriousness with which complaints were handled.

This was quite a small study and was not methodologically entirely satisfactory. It was not, for instance, a randomised trial. It is possible that the patients going to one facility or the other had important differences in their attitudes to care before they went into surgery. However the study did show, over a range of measures, that good results can be obtained for surgery in units that are peripherally based rather than being in a central hospital complex. Patients preferred these. In other words secondary care in this instance was not tied to hospital care.

Variations in admission rate

We have mentioned several times that there is a great variation in the use of hospitals for what appears to be the same cause in different places. This suggests that there is a great deal of waste in the system as it stands. We have mentioned the American figures, which suggest that in the treatment of children there are 18-fold differences in the rate of admission to hospital for gastroenteritis and 15-fold differences for respiratory disease. We have also mentioned a study comparing only teaching hospitals, which still showed five-fold differences for respiratory tract infection .

Referral to hospital

Referrals to hospital come from a number of sources. Figure 30.7 shows the way that different groups of patients arrived in hospital from different sources in a UK hospital. Rates of referral by GPs vary greatly from GP to GP. The central reason for some GPs referring more than others appears to lie with the personality of the individual doctor. However, there are some patterns within this variation, for we have discussed above the fact that the rate of referral of patients is related to the unemployment rate in different areas.

Who should be treated in hospital?

In principle, it seems reasonable to avoid admission to hospital whenever possible for all age groups. As far back as 1959, the Platt Committee recommended the extension of community nursing services so that the hospital admission of young children could be avoided wherever possible. There was little obvious response to this recommendation at the time. The treatment of children in hospital, especially visiting rights for parents, continued to be rudimentary. The Court Report 17 years later re-emphasised the need to avoid admission to hospital, mainly by the strengthening of the community paediatrics services.

These early recommendations were, again, not taken up. The central idea was the development of GP paediatricians who were to be unusual in the UK as primary care workers with a specialty interest. This would have mixed secondary care with primary, something people have been very resistant to in the UK. Following this report, a few consultants in community paediatric medicine were appointed. From the 1950s until the 1980s a few areas paved the way, showing that paediatric care could be provided largely at home, but this did not start to expand rapidly until the

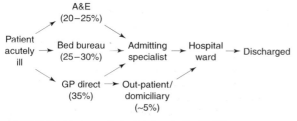

Fig. 30.7 Emergency medical admissions in Cardiff, UK.

late 1980s and is still not universally provided at the end of the 1990s.

Measuring the effect of hospital

A study of patients aged 65 and over discharged from NHS hospitals in Wales showed that one-fifth of all patients died during the year following their admission to hospital. Not surprisingly, this was highest in the over 85s where a third died in the year. The highest death rates were amongst those originally treated for cancers, stroke, coronary heart disease and those admitted for social reasons. About three-quarters of those who died in the year following their admission died of the same thing with which they went in.

The researchers measured the patients' disability after discharge. One-fifth of the patients were worse compared with their state before admission, 1 in 20 had improved. The rest were no different. A year after leaving hospital, a third was more disabled than when they went into hospital, a fifth was less disabled. Curiously older patients did not fare any worse, in terms of their disability rates, than younger. If someone has an illness serious enough to send them to hospital the older ones have a greater chance of dying from it, but if not their likelihood of being disabled is the same as those who are younger.

Changes in disability were related to the patients' diagnoses. Three months after leaving hospital, patients who had arthritis (who were admitted mainly for hip replacements) showed the greatest improvement in disability, while stroke patients and those with fractured hips showed the most marked deterioration. Cancer and ischaemic heart disease patients occupied an intermediate position between these two extremes. A year after going into hospital, patients admitted originally with a stroke continued to deteriorate, while patients with coronary heart disease showed, on average, a modest improvement in disability. Patients treated for surgical repairs such as cataract operations or hernia repairs showed few changes in disability after discharge, but they were, by and large, a fit group of people before they started.

Overall, a substantial fraction of patients were more disabled after discharge than before admission to hospital. The effect of hospital on disability for these patients was that short-term elective stays, which are increasingly these days being given as day care, reduced the subsequent level of disability. Acute illnesses, requiring emergency admission, were disabling and the hospital stay made little impact on that degree of disability. This sort of information needs to be borne in mind before one advocates widespread hospital care.

Dangers of hospitals

Hospitals can do harm. The significant burden of nosocomal infections has already been mentioned. Several studies, notably a follow-up of stroke patients treated in hospital, have suggested that the loss of the routine of the ward combined with an overprotective attitude by relatives and carers may well lead to an increase in disability after discharge from hospital. This may be a more important effect for patients treated in intensive care. People have suggested that relatives are more afraid of a condition when patients get home if they have been treated in a special unit. As a result, the family, fearing for the safety of their relative, tend to inhibit that patient's rehabilitation in case they have a recurrence of their acute episode. This tendency is increasingly being overcome by complicated regimes to ensure the rehabilitation of patients. Some people have suggested that psychological support may help in the rehabilitation of patients, especially those who have had heart attacks. The evidence for the effectiveness of these approaches is conflicting.

Hospitals do not appear to be greatly effective for the treatment of people with acute very disabling or chronic disease. The deaths and disability suffered by patients in hospital in the studies mentioned were heavily dependent upon the age of patients, their initial disability and their medical condition. These are things which are not possible to change by treatment in hospital or elsewhere.

The place of hospitals

There are several indications that hospitals may not be the ideal place to treat patients:

- many people in hospital do not need to be there
- given the choice, patients prefer to be treated in a community-based unit rather than a large hospital
- the main reason for this preference is the better communications in the peripheral units
- there are great variations in the proportion of patients admitted to hospital in different places
- research suggests that children and old people are especially vulnerable if treated in hospital.

Secondary health care

➤ Ambulatory care includes community-based services and out-patients: the proportion of health-care costs spent in this area tends to be higher in wealthier countries.

➤ Countries with a higher proportion of community care tend to have less expensive health services.

➤ The hospital budget uses two-thirds of the health-care budget in the UK; it employs nearly a million people. Staff costs make up 70% of the cost of the NHS.

➤ Hospitals are sources of infection in themselves (nosocomical) and there is evidence that hospitalisation in itself may lead to subsequent disability.

The move to community care

31

In this chapter the move from hospital to community care is examined:

- the extent of the change
- why the change is occurring
- what advantages community care offers
- how it works and how it is funded.

The aim of this chapter is to describe the origins, implementation and problems with the move towards community care.

Introduction

There has been an increasing interest in providing services in the community, rather than in institutions for a number of years. These changes have also been controversial, partly because of the opposition of the vested interests controlling hospitals and other institutions, partly because such moves result in the closure of large high-profile units to be replaced by small, less-obvious means of treating people.

The public became aware of the move to community care with the implementation of the community care part of the NHS and Community Care Act 1990 in April 1993. Since then, although the changes affected the care of elderly people most directly, there has been much media attention on the care of mentally ill people. The media have highlighted a number of cases where mentally ill patients have murdered people or put themselves in danger. The media have accompanied such news with comments about the failure of community care to prevent these tragedies. In fact mentally ill people cause a very small proportion of violence to others. People who are mentally ill carry out one serious assault for every 600. On other occasions, mentally ill people have been hurt, one notable case being a patient who climbed into a lion's cage and was mauled. The media comments have strongly suggested that such people should be locked up for their own and other people's safety. In fact the Mental Health Act 1983 is very specific about who may or may not be locked up in mental institutions. The working of the Act is more closely watched and monitored than any of the other areas in which health services work.

The move to community care

Reduction in hospital beds

The number of hospital beds in this country has been diminishing for a long time in virtually all specialties. Figure 31.1 shows the number of hospital beds in the UK since 1951. It shows that since the early 1970s there has been a rapid reduction in the numbers. The figure also shows the number of discharges and deaths from hospital at the same time. The figure presents the conundrum that if present trends continue the last hospital bed will close in 2014, at which time it will look after about 12 million patients. It is obvious that much of the decrease in the number of beds has been made possible by improvements in techniques and policies that allow patients to be treated in a much shorter time than previously. Other changes have been the increased use of day surgery for many of the common surgical complaints and the reduced length of stay for acute medical cases. Since the early 1970s, the expected length of stay for a patient with an acute myocardial infarction, the commonest single diagnosis for hospital in-patients, has fallen from 6 weeks to less than a week, often 2 days in uncomplicated cases.

Patient and client groups

Community care has been increasingly important for all patient groups. The government in the UK has earmarked some money since the 1970s in some specialties to increase the extent of the care given in the

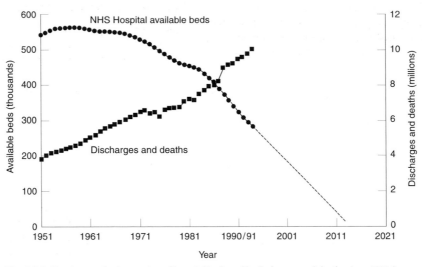

Fig. 31.1 The changes in the number of hospital beds and in discharges and deaths since 1951 in the UK. (OPCS 1997)

community and to reduce the amount given from an institutional base. These specialties are outlined in Table 31.1, together with the time over which the policy has been in force. We can see that, for some groups, policies for moving people into the community considerably pre-date the Community Care Act. Changes have been obvious for much longer than this. Figure 31.2 shows the number of mental illness beds available for mentally ill people in the UK and USA over the past 100 years. We can also see that the number of hospital places in England and Wales began to fall in the 1940s, in the USA in the 1950s.

Reasons for the move to community care

There are a number of reasons for the move from hospital into the community for all specialties:

● *demographic:* The ageing of the population, community care is safer for old people

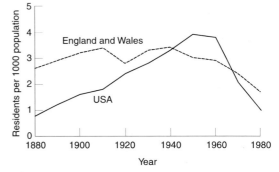

Fig. 31.2 Residents in psychiatric hospitals in England and Wales and the USA. (Mechanic 1997)

● *economic*
  — value for money
  — flexibility of community services
  — lack of fixed costs

● *technological*
  — more can be done at home
  — more can be done by the GP
  — community nurses can do more

● *consumer choice:* liked because it is user friendly.

We will discuss these reasons in more detail.

Demography: the ageing of the population

There is a general feeling that the increased longevity of people in this country will result in a greater use of hospital beds by elderly people in the future. This is not

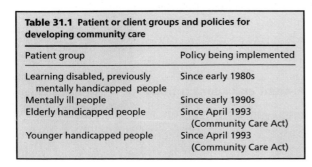

Table 31.1 Patient or client groups and policies for developing community care

Patient group	Policy being implemented
Learning disabled, previously mentally handicapped people	Since early 1980s
Mentally ill people	Since early 1990s
Elderly handicapped people	Since April 1993 (Community Care Act)
Younger handicapped people	Since April 1993 (Community Care Act)

at all certain. Some important studies have looked at the idea of healthy life expectancy or life expectancy without disability, instead of simply looking at survival. Using these ideas to study populations of elderly people over time, researchers in the USA showed that 85-year-old people in 1989 required considerably less assistance to go about their normal lives than they did in 1982. These researchers also found that community-based programmes for caring for elderly people over the long term had greater benefits for both the elderly person and their family. They were more expensive than hospital-based approaches. Peter Laslett, among others, has made a strong plea for us to try to be more flexible when discussing age. In particular he has suggested the ideas of the third and fourth age.

The third age, represents the great majority of older people, who are reasonably fit and who, in medical terms, are treated as any other middle-aged people. The fourth age requires a different medical approach. The essential thing to remember is that the difference between the third and fourth age or indeed between either of them and any other age is not a matter of chronology. There is no age at which one automatically becomes the other.

In the third age people are living longer and are probably fitter than they used to be; therefore, they do not require as much hospital care. In the fourth age, it is likely that hospital will be irrelevant to the needs of these people and probably dangerous when comparing the risks of being there with the benefits obtained.

Flexibility of community services

Community services are flexible. They may be provided in the patient's own home or in a local clinic or in the GPs' premises. They can easily move, for instance to provide a child-care clinic on a new housing estate where a new sudden demand for the service arises. Similarly in an era where the population is ageing, child clinics can move out again.

Lack of fixed costs

As we saw in Chapter 30, in the UK the hospital sector continues to absorb about two-thirds of the money put into health care annually. Hospitals are built to last a long time. Many UK hospitals are over 70 years old. The cost of these buildings, especially heating and lighting them and often caring for their extensive grounds, is a fixed cost on the health service. This means that no matter how many patients are cared for, whether 10 or 100, the costs of upkeep on the building remain an albatross around the neck of the service.

More can now be done at home

The medical professions have taken up several advances in technology for the development of home and community-based care. Developments in office and management methods are as useful to the health service as an important industry as for any manufacturing company. Telecommunications and computer technology are good examples of this. Many of the new technologies will help with the development of a less institutionalised health service.

Technological developments for people living at home have been emerging over the last few years. Sometimes they are obviously effective, but there needs to be as much scrutiny of these as of any other new approach. The following shows a list of just some of these technologies, which will lessen the need for in-patient services over the next decade or so.

- diagnostic kits and analysers
- assessment of symptoms using personal computers
- vaccines
- computer-controlled prostheses
- automatic drug delivery and treatment systems.

Diagnostic kits particularly those using monoclonal antibodies are discussed in Chapter 25. These kits will be especially useful in reducing the need for in-patient care because the kits can be used in clinics or at home with little expertise required. They give diagnostic information quickly and may allow patients to remain at home or shorten their stay in hospital.

The most common uses for such kits at present are for diagnosing pregnancy or ovulation, with the kit being used to detect the presence of certain hormones. They can also be used for deciding upon the cause of respiratory infections, the presence of some bacteria, (such as streptococci) and for sexually transmitted diseases. Manufacturers may eventually offer tests for a number of diseases on sale to the public, including screening tests for cancer of the cervix or prostate. They may use a wide variety of other kits to diagnose skin diseases, tooth disease and eye problems. Some companies plan to develop and market tests for common diseases with a part genetic cause, such as diabetes. The kits, together with new analysers, allow reliable diagnostic testing virtually anywhere.

A number of new technological developments assist in maintaining people who would normally depend on their family or their health providers. Treatments include artificial sphincters and electrical stimulators for the prevention of urinary incontinence to relieve problems caused by poor bladder function. In future, devices may be developed to replace parts of the nervous system. These will stimulate nerve fibres or nerve cells electrically and restore functions that are lost because of disease or injury. One type of device that has been used in the mid-1990s is cochleal implants for improving hearing. Other devices are likely to follow for speech and even smell. These devices work by electrically stimulating nerves, or parts of the spinal cord, or areas within the brain. They attempt to stimulate the normal signals given off by those organs and improve senses, which may have been damaged. The aim of these advances is to make dependent people more independent and to keep them out of hospitals and other institutions.

More can be done by the GP and community nurse

Some new technology can be used within the community by the GP or community nurse. Diagnostic kits have already been discussed in this context. As a high proportion of in-patient stays is for confirmation of diagnosis, any technology that enables sophisticated diagnostic methods to be used in the primary care area will reduce the need for hospital stays. A good example of this is for gastrointestinal disease. This is an area where medicine, surgery and radiology overlap, so that any move towards community care also will involve a blurring of the traditional divisions within medicine. A study has examined varied approaches using gastro-intestinal endoscopy to confirm the diagnosis.

There are three possible options for the treatment path for duodenal ulcer. (i) The first one where a GP refers patients directly to a hospital-based consultant who confirms the presence of a duodenal ulcer by endoscopy and monitors the treatment given. (ii) In the second case the GP again refers to hospital where they carry out minimally invasive therapy. (iii) A third approach is totally community based, where the GP performs open-access endoscopy to confirm the diagnosis and initiates and monitors therapy.

The experts considered all three approaches to be satisfactory in terms of their safety and acceptability. However, the community approach was the most efficient and cost effective. In addition it was felt to be marginally safer, largely because of a reduced chance of cross-infection. They thought that most patients would prefer the community-based route though they suggested that for first attacks of duodenal ulcer symptoms patients did not need investigation. They felt that, in the future, all patients with uncomplicated duodenal ulcer would be treated in the community. This may require some extended GP training, but the use of hospital services would be restricted only to those patients who have poor initial results.

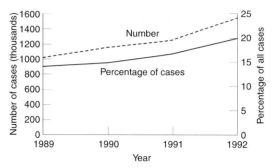

Fig. 31.3 The number of hospital-based day surgery cases and the proportion these form of total surgery cases in England. (OPCS 1997)

There have been rapid increases in the amount of hospital-based day surgery performed. Figure 31.3 shows the data since 1989.

The Royal College of Paediatricians has recommended that the care of children should be carried out at home or in the local community wherever possible. This is partly to avoid the adverse psychological and social effects of hospital care on children. The dangers of hospital care for elderly people have led to a new term **cascade iatrogenesis**, where inadvertent overtreatment of patients has led to more treatment to counterbalance the first.

A further interesting example is in obstetrics, where women have demanded home care despite the expert opinion that it may be harmful. Their persistence has paid off to such an extent that the experts have now measured the possible harm that home care might do and have found it preferable to hospital care.

Consumer choice

We showed earlier in this chapter that some patients had been moving towards community care since the 1960s. For mental illness, some therapeutic advances

---

Community care

➤ The shift to community care has occurred because of demographic change (ageing population), economic advantages, technological advances and because consumers prefer it.

➤ New technologies (e.g. diagnostic kits) enable diagnosis to be confirmed without an in-patient stay and may allow treatment outside the hospital setting.

➤ A move to community care led by consumer choice has occurred in areas such as obstetrics.

made this possible, especially developments in drug therapy. A more important influence was a change in emphasis on the way that mentally ill people were thought of by the public at large. As opposed to obstetric care, where the drive for change came from the direct consumer, mental illness treatment is an area where intense discussion has involved hospital-based professionals, community-based professionals and the general public.

A Canadian, W. Wolfsenberger, boosted the policies for these changes in mentally ill people in 1972 with his philosophy of 'normalisation'. This was initially about people with learning disabilities, then known as the mentally retarded, but was also developed for the care of mentally ill people. Part of this movement related to civil rights campaigns in the USA, with a belief that people should not be discriminated against simply because of their external characteristics. It was believed, rightly, that many of the problems suffered by learning disabled and mentally ill people were caused by people rejecting them and, more specifically, locking them up in institutions for life. There are still a few patients in hospital today who were incarcerated for the rest of their lives because of some minor legal infringement and a mild learning disability. We locked up some because they were deaf and believed to be learning disabled.

This feeling that everyone has a set of inalienable rights that we should protect developed into the move towards making it possible for these patients to be cared for in the community as far as possible. The changes were also brought about as a result of some professional battling between the medical profession and social workers. There is no doubt that the horrors of some institutions have tarred all the others with the same brush. Doctors were seen as supporting the institutional approach with an authoritarian drug-orientated approach to patients who found it difficult to adjust. Social workers and psychologists were seen as interested in social care and allowing patients out into the community. This was never really true. Many doctors were committed to community care and some social workers were, no doubt, advocates of the asylum rôle of the institutions, with patients protected from the outside world. Nevertheless there was, and is, some difference in emphasis between the professions.

The community has traditionally been of lower status than hospitals. Some people certainly saw moving the power base into the community as a way of getting back at medical consultants. Policies for the development of mental illness services continued to progress slowly in the UK. In 1975, there was a Royal Commission report *Better Services for the Mentally Ill*, pointing out some of the worst aspects of life in mental hospitals. There followed an expansion of social services within the mental illness service and the gradual localisation of the specialist services to cover geographical areas. There were calls for closer collaboration between the health and social services and more staff began to be appointed.

Despite much work, a Select Committee Report in 1985 in the UK was again critical of the services and suggested closer work and joint planning between health and social services. They also suggested bringing in the voluntary sector to help with treating patients. Some saw this as the government attempting to treat patients cheaply. Table 31.2 shows the main suggested changes between the old and new services.

Other countries, most notably Italy and the USA, made dramatic changes to their care of mentally ill people. In the UK some areas led the way. One, rather extreme, early experiment was in Torbay, where it is said that consultants were given offices with their multidisciplinary community teams and forbidden to go back into the hospitals. This caused considerable consternation and anger initially. Common sense prevailed shortly after this and a community-based service, based on teams covering geographical areas has been built up.

Each team contains community psychiatric nurses, psychiatric social workers, psychiatrists and psychologists, with some administrative staff. To ensure that the teams are, in fact, dealing with patients who would, in the old model, have been in hospital, the teams are expected to confine most of their work to patients with severe mental illness. This is important, for about a third of the patients seen by GPs have a mental illness component to them. If the teams took on a few of these patients, most of which have relatively mild anxiety or depression, they would become rapidly swamped.

Table 31.2 Suggested changes in the service for mentally ill people

Treatment area	Old service	New service
Acute care	In mental hospital	In district general hospital
Rehabilitation	In hospital or day hospital	In day hospital or social services day centre
Long-term care	In hospital	At home or in homely settings
Planning and management	Mainly by the health service	Joint

Paying for the changes

The changes towards care in the community can, to some extent, be paid for by the reduced costs brought about by the closure of the big institutions. Table 31.3 shows the marked differences in what is available for different patient or client groups. There is a marked difference between the ways that each approach to community care is paid for.

Implementing community care policy

Figure 31.4 shows the main changes in places used in the community for mentally ill people. However the reductions in the number of hospital places do not equal the increased number of community places; the figures do not add up. Some people seem to disappear when they leave the mental hospital. This study showed that the development of services in the community was slower than the rate at which patients were being discharged. This figure also shows the large number of different options that we must make available in order for community care to work.

Another factor, which has been important, has been the difference between different areas of the country in the amount of money given to community care. In the English regions the amount varies between £17 per person in Wessex to £28 in Merseyside. To some extent these differences may reflect differences in the number of people with severe mental illness in different places.

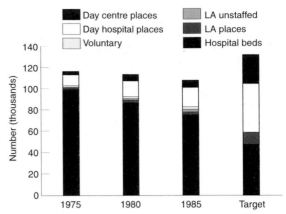

Fig. 31.4 The main changes in places in hospital and the community for mentally ill people (LA, local authority). (Mechanic 1997)

The numbers that are affected in the populations cannot possibly explain the extent of the difference in financing.

Community care, exemplified by the community mental health teams, requires a different approach from the traditional medical treatment approach. In the latter, the doctor makes the decisions. Other people, mainly nurses, carry these out. Community care has an important social element in which doctors are not skilled. There is, therefore, the need for a wide range of different skills. The usual means of dealing with this problem has been a team approach. There is, within the team, a blurring of professional rôles so that

Table 31.3 Paying for community care

Patient or client group	Resources available	Releasing resources	Who gets the money
Learning disabled people	Closure of old hospitals	Most money can be transferred but this takes time as places in the community are developed. A few places needed in small institutions for the very severely affected	Most money transfers to social services; small group of clients/patients
Mentally ill people	Closure of old hospitals	Some money can be transferred to community but acute wards still needed for some patients, usually these need to be built new in district general hospital or free standing	Some money transfers to social services but not much; large group of patients
Elderly handicapped people	Release of social security money previously used in private nursing homes	Money transferred from social security to social services. Health service can discharge patients from hospital to these services. Health service must keep some long-stay places for people with 'long-term medical need'. This has to be defined locally	Social services now manage all of this money, but budgets are under great pressure as they are competing with education etc. Large numbers of patients
Young handicapped people	Poor existing service. No money to be released	If they have a 'long-term medical need', the health service must care for them; very few facilities available. Otherwise social services may adapt home	No extra money; health or social services have to find extra

different professionals may overlap with others in what they do. Nurses may be involved in some social work. Social workers may help with what has been traditionally a therapeutic approach usually given by doctors.

The point of this change is to try to overcome one of the difficulties that have dogged the care of people with complex problems. Patients with complicated health and social needs, often for rehabilitation or for maintenance of someone who is not likely to improve, have, in the past, been assessed and treated separately by large numbers of personnel representing different professions, with little contact between them. I have heard elderly disabled people say 'I have had five comprehensive assessments over the past 3 months but still no one has fitted a rail to my bath so that I can get myself out'. In the team approach, the first person that sees the patient deals with the problem, whether this is a nurse, social worker, doctor or therapist. They carry out an agreed multiprofessional assessment. A plan, known as a 'care plan', is agreed with the patient. One of the team, usually the one with the skills most relevant to that patient's problems, acts as a 'key worker'. This means that he or she will keep in close contact, explaining to the patient and their family how the various bits of the care work and how they inter-relate. This whole process is known as case or, more recently, care management.

Effectiveness of teams

Case management arose in the USA in response to the dispersal of psychiatric and social care that followed the closure of large mental hospitals. The basic idea was that a designated person, the 'case manager', would take special responsibility for a 'client' in the community. The case manager would assess the client's needs and ensure, through a care plan, that suitable services were provided to meet them. They would also monitor the services the patients received and maintain contact with the client as key workers.

Case management has been bedevilled by a tendency to lump two different approaches under one name. The first is a low-intensity approach in which case managers offer an office-based service, buying in services from other agencies. The second approach is more intensive. It bears little resemblance to standard case management. People provide this approach using a dedicated multidisciplinary team of mental-health professionals that generally include a psychiatrist. The patient–staff ratio is low and the amount of contact with patients high. Team members work with patients as and when their particular skills are required. The team concentrates on avoiding hospital admission and developing patients' independent living skills. They make strenuous efforts to retain contact with patients. This can be difficult when severely mentally ill patients do not believe themselves to be ill.

There are at least 13 randomised controlled trials of this assertive community treatment in the world literature, 12 of which have found the approach beneficial when compared with routine management. There are at least nine randomised controlled trials and two well-designed non-randomised controlled studies, comparing non-assertive case management with the traditional approach where each professional acted separately on the patient's behalf; all but one of which have largely negative findings.

In the UK, social services care management rapidly increased after the publication of the Griffiths report on community care. This report recommended that case management (provided by social services) should be at the heart of community care for severely mentally ill people. Meanwhile, the case management idea was being imposed on the mental-health services as the 'care-programme approach'. This was intended to run in tandem with care management, though how or why this should happen has never been clarified. Originally it was reserved for the most severely ill patients. The mental-health services were required to appoint key workers, case managers by another name, for these patients. The patients were to receive an assessment of need, a written care plan and regular reviews organised by the key worker.

It is possible to see how, with proper funding and guidance, this approach might have evolved into an approximation to assertive community treatment. In practice, the care-programme approach has meant standard case management for all, through a combination of lack of funding, mushrooming paperwork and its extension to all psychiatric patients. No one has ever fully evaluated the care-programme approach but a partial evaluation in a recent randomised controlled trial produced disturbing findings: a doubling of hospital admission rates for the care-programme group. There is a simple explanation for case management's immunity to scientific analysis: in Britain it is no longer just an intervention but rather a government policy.

The patients' views of community care

There is no doubt that when asked and where it is a reasonable option patients prefer community care and do better using this approach. This has been well researched for mentally ill people. Patients have a

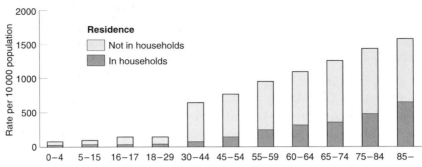

Fig. 31.5 The relationship between age and long-standing illness in Cardiff (from 1991 census).

better chance of having a more normal life. They are more likely to use shops and pubs, they have fewer behaviour problems, improved morale and better skills. This means, of course, that the general public is more likely than previously to meet people who behave oddly. Some people find this disturbing. There is a great deal of educational work to be done with the general public to stop them despising and being afraid of mentally ill people.

Bringing about community care: keeping records

We need to know what is going on in the community and yet information is hard to come by. In hospital, there are good computer systems so that one knows when a patient comes in and goes out and what was wrong with them. This is not so for the community. The patient may need to be cared for for the rest of their life with intermittent treatment. It is difficult to capture such data, for the patient may move or go to different people for treatment. The only central record system, which follows patients around in the community, is the GP's record. GPs often still keep these in 45-year-old envelopes.

Patient and client groups: elderly people

The needs of elderly people and their treatment in the community or elsewhere are dominated by the demographic structure of the age group and their dependency. Figure 31.5 shows the numbers of people in Cardiff by the proportion with long-standing disability. We took these data from the census in 1991 when there was such a question included as part of the census. It shows clearly the large number of severely disabled elderly people. Figure 31.6 shows the figures projected forward to 2001 for dependent elderly people. We can see that the numbers for the youngest

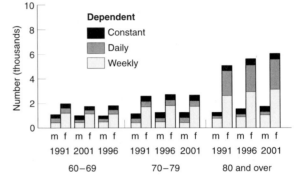

Fig. 31.6 Future dependency by age and sex: projected data from 1991 census (the figures used in Figure 31.5) to 2001.

groups will decrease slightly then increase markedly for the over 80s. A 65-year-old person with severe disability will have differences in their need for support when compared with an 85-year-old person. The severe disability is likely to be complicated by multiple problems, especially mental problems.

An important topic for the maintenance of community care is the impact of an elderly person on his or her family and friends. This is also an important component of their assessment, as is careful monitoring of any service which may be provided. Figure 31.7 shows the person upon whom older people (both men and women) are dependent in the over 70s.

Relatives and other carers are essential to the development of community care. One of the main functions of health services in future will be to maintain the help that these people give.

Community service development in different countries

The government in Denmark has tried to limit the financial costs of caring for elderly people by develop-

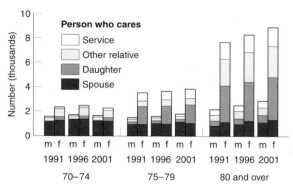

Fig. 31.7 Carers who elderly people rely on for help. Data from the 1991 census in Cardiff projected forward to 2001.

Community Care Act in the UK

Under the Community Care Act, social services are able to offer the money that might have been used to maintain an elderly person in a nursing home to maintain elderly, disabled or mentally ill people in their homes. Patients, especially those being discharged from hospital with some remaining disabilities, have more choice, they can be maintained at home or in a nursing home. In most areas about a third of patients who are eligible for private nursing home care choose to remain at home with extra support. Social services in the UK, unlike health services, are not free at the point of delivery. People who are poor and receiving income support from the government will get their social services free but only about two-thirds of disabled people are on income support.

ing community services. These services include home nurses and special housing for elderly people. It is suggested that it is cheaper to provide 30 hours a week of home care than to place an elderly person in an institution. The question remains about whether the care is equivalent.

In Germany they have made attempts to reduce the admission of people to hospital. They have provided home nursing and other assistance. Interestingly, it has proved difficult to bring about this change because people in Germany felt that they were entitled to a specific type of care. This probably reflects the insurance-based system that they have. The public wanted more for the money they pay. There have been similar problems in Belgium, France, the Netherlands and Greece. Change has been a little easier to implement in countries that pay for their health care out of taxes, as in Denmark, the UK, Italy and Sweden.

Community care for mental illness

➤ To care of the mentally ill is one of the major areas changed by the move to community care.

➤ The 'care plan' is an overall strategy to deal with a patient's needs; it is overseen by one member of a multiskilled professional team. Community mental health teams are effective only if properly funded.

➤ Patients with mental illness prefer community care but facilities have not kept up with the closure of hospital beds.

Managing waiting lists

Christopher Potter

Waiting lists are discussed in terms of:

- positive and negative aspects
- contributory factors
- management.

Introduction

Waiting lists are firmly fixed in the popular imagination as a bad thing, to be the subject of breast-beating by health-service staff and brow beating by the press and politicians. They are regularly deplored by the health-services' critics as a symbol of its poor management, and by the staff to win more resources. The following quotes from politicians indicates their use as a political weapon.

> The number of people who have waited more than a year for hospital treatment in England increased by 15.2% between March and June this year, according to a survey of health authorities by the Labour party … equivalent to an annual rise of 60.8% … more than one million people were on waiting lists in England in June.

> People waiting more than a year for treatment numbered 64 881. Change over the preceding three months ranged from an increase of 378.6% in Mersey to a reduction of 47.6% … for London's postgraduate teaching hospitals.

> … the minister … was not dismayed by the figures, noting that the number of patients waiting for more than a year had fallen from 119 000 since the NHS reform in 1991 … Half of all admissions to hospital are immediate. Of patients on waiting lists, half are admitted within five weeks, nearly 75% within three months, and 98% within a year.

These quotes also illustrates some other factors, such as the need to look closely at the particular region or specialty being referred to (there are great variations), and the time period under question. Two important points, usually overlooked in discussions about waiting lists, must be made before any detailed consideration of their management is made. First, waiting list records are only kept in a few parts of the world. Some health services simply do not keep the data. It is probable that the UK collect the data centrally only because it has been made a political issue and because it is reasonably easy to collect the data in this way. In a private health-care service, the data are often impossible to collect. Waiting lists are, therefore, to some extent, an artefact of publicly funded health systems, and it is usually impossible to find figures to compare with the UK's performance. On a recent visit to a German medical school, one of us was met by blank surprise when he asked about how long people waited for treatment. Not because there were no people waiting, but because there was no reason why the hospital should keep such records. American critics of the UK health service and its waiting lists ignore the uninsured in their own country who never even make it onto a waiting list.

Waiting lists exist only where there is a

- well-defined referral system controlling access to secondary and tertiary care
- there are relatively limited places where such care is offered
- there are administrative procedures and discipline to keep records
- where there is political and public debate about the matter.

Positive values of waiting lists

Waiting lists have a number of positive virtues. The debate about waiting lists rarely addresses the question of what would be a reasonable and even desirable length of waiting. A little thought demonstrates the importance of this. If health-service capacity (buildings, staff, etc.) was increased so that any condition needing treatment was able to be treated immediately, it would result in spare capacity for much of the time, in other words waste. Seasonal variations, for example, would require beds and other facilities to be available unnecessarily all year round.

If conditions do not lead to death, disability or excessive discomfort, some degree of waiting clearly reduces the cost of the NHS to the country quite significantly. The amount of waiting that is acceptable is impossible to define exactly by appeal to objective standards, so that the actual wait will be a subjective decision. In the 1990s, the NHS in the UK has become more sophisticated, but it still breaks waiting lists into 3-month and 12-month periods without separating the time waited from the severity of the condition. This is clearly pointless.

The Patients' Charter sets standards without any reference to need or severity except for a small number of conditions, especially those waiting for cardiac surgery. This was in response to special pleading on behalf of that group of patients, rather than an overview of the severity of the condition for all of those waiting. Excessive concern with numbers hides both the cost to the nation and the effect on the clinically more needy. We could do far more with the contracts between the purchasers and providers to set standards for reasonable waiting times for many specific conditions. At present, we often use broad categories such as urgent versus non-urgent. It would not be hard to indicate a target wait for, say, the 20% of conditions that probably account for 80% of our waiting list activity in each specialty.

Overcapacity also has an indirect impact on cost. For example, it reduces the pressure to use beds efficiently. It is a well-known rule that if beds are provided they will be filled. It has been suggested that much of the furore over the need for acute medical beds in hospital over the past few years has been an artefact, largely caused by a lack of overflow beds in other specialties and a recent tendency to increase the availability of acute medical beds. But waiting lists are not just beneficial from a financial point of view. They have one important clinical benefit, and two secondary benefits.

First, they limit unnecessary and overhasty intervention. It is commonly recognised that, because of its funding system, the USA enjoys overcapacity within the health-care sector. If the patient or their employer/insurer can pay, the treatment is available immediately. As a result there is overintervention. Not only are doctors tempted to react immediately but also

patients are not given time to find out if they prefer to live with the condition, or for natural remission of symptoms to occur.

It is not cynical to argue that time should be allowed for this, it is merely to challenge the ethos that if something can be done it is always in the patient's best interests to do it. Treatments do not always have the intended consequences. Excessive care carries with it excessive iatrogenic disease, and speedy intervention can simply lead to speedier distress.

For many conditions, there is an optimal time for intervening, especially surgically. Cataracts are a classic example. The reason may be that tissues change, or the extent of disease becomes clearer, or that the patient reaches the point where the discomfort of the condition, pain of treatment and risk of outcome reach some sort of threshold.

In a TV documentary, there was a scene in which a British cardiologist told his patient that his condition had reached the stage where they can and should operate. He reassured the patient that the operation has an 80% success rate, but the real blow as far as the programme maker is concerned, there was an 18-month waiting list. The incident was supposedly a genuine interview between a real cardiologist and a real patient.

It raises several questions, such as why the doctor could not have predicted the natural history of the disease and 'booked' a slot, on the possibility it would be needed, a year earlier. Or why he has to talk about waiting at all. Why not simply say to the patient, 'You will need an operation in 18 months, we will book it in now, and meanwhile here is how your GP and I will help you manage your care…'. It seems like strange ethics to worry a patient instead of reassuring him. But, what is most interesting is the idea that 80% success is reassuring; what of the one in five non-successes?

Causes of waiting lists

Given that waiting lists have been a cause of concern or embarrassment for decades, and various structural reforms, financial packages and research programmes have addressed the problem, they have remained remarkably resilient in the NHS. So much so that many have accepted the doctrine that the more capacity is provided in the NHS the greater the demand created. Just as building more roads seems to encourage more car use, so dealing with one level of health-care demand simply exposes more of the demand 'iceberg'. At a local level this is not true. We have several times come across a situation where a new senior registrar has decided to clear the waiting list for his or her boss and has done so quite quickly. The other common situation we have come across is when research into a subject is being done. A comparative study of day surgery versus in-patient care in Edinburgh rapidly removed the waiting lists for hernias and varicose veins. On a wider scale, however, these appear to be unusual occurrences.

We mentioned some of the benefits of waiting lists to put their management into a wider context than is normally considered. Despite this general benefit, there is no question that, because of the poor management of the lists, some people wait unnecessarily and for too long. John Yates has attacked NHS waiting lists for many years, illustrating how badly the service has sometimes served its patients. Internal markets, the Patients' Charter, and Waiting List Initiatives, in which special centres are set up to take on the waiting-list patients, have all tried to address the very real problem of bringing waiting lists under control.

Managing waiting lists requires some understanding of what causes them. There are at least five possible explanations:

- political: waiting lists reflect an imbalance between inputs and outputs, in other words there is too little money put into the NHS
- functional waiting lists have purposes or benefits that either by design or not have a function within the NHS or in the wider system
- managerial: waiting lists are caused by bad management
  — poor administration of facilities
  — poor clinical management of cases, including poor referral systems and poor admission procedures
- cynical: key players, particularly surgeons, have a vested interest in maintaining long waiting lists either for status reasons, boosting private earnings or both
- Multifactorial: waiting lists are the product of many small-scale professional, personal and managerial local decisions.

None of these explanations can fully account for the persistent size of waiting lists in the UK health service, though each can be justified as a partial explanation.

Political causes

This is the least easy argument to defend, although the commonest response to waiting lists is to suggest providing more money. We have already seen that it would be very expensive for the country to provide sufficient excess capacity to cope with complete removal of waiting lists. It may be reasonable to increase capacity to some extent, and increasing theatre lists, providing centres to focus on cataracts, hip replacement, etc. will have an impact. A great deal of money has been spent on 'blitzes', 'waiting list initiatives', overtime payments for extra sessions, etc., but lists do not respond in any 'straight line' way. Some impact does occur if extra resources are provided but the underlying issue is still, 'How big is a reasonable waiting list, and how much are we willing to spend'?

Functional causes

The possible positive benefits to the system from having waiting lists has been discussed above. As well as keeping down direct costs, it is obvious that maintaining a waiting list allows the system to use its finances flexibly, coping with emergencies yet allowing elective cases to be fitted into vacant slots. Expensive inputs (i.e. facilities, equipment and staff) are used to maximum effort. Spending on consumables can be spread over time. Seasonal variations can be accommodated. There can be some 'rationing' of demand, reflecting cultural values on what is important and what is not. (Not absolute rationing, i.e. denying access to services completely, but letting 'cosmetic' cases wait, or treating some groups as more deserving of quick responses than others.)

Waiting lists can be used deliberately to blur the rationing issue. Rather than be forced to either find treatments or exclude them from NHS provision, some cases can be postponed, to be dealt with as and when it is least inconvenient. This is harder under the new quality-monitoring systems such as the Patients' Charter, because they only allow a limited period of postponement. Similarly, they limit the final use of waiting lists as a humane way of treating 'no hopers', i.e. telling people for whom there is unlikely to be any amelioration of their condition that they are on the list. However, the ethics of this are questionable, and not everyone would accept that offering false hope is humane.

Poor management

Waiting lists are often said to be caused by poor management. In an organisation the size of the NHS, examples of errors and poor administration are easy to find:

- failure to ensure that patients are called in time
- failure to use operating theatres for longer hours,

perhaps carrying out more day surgery

- failure to ensure staff are available, causing operating lists to be cancelled
- failure to ensure equipment or facilities are operational
- failure to start clinics and operating lists on time
- failure of surgeons to mix their lists efficiently; failure to screen patients before admission
- failure of liaison between departments
- failure to discharge old patients and doctors consequently spending too long in out-patient departments
- failure to ensure patients can be discharged to their homes.

The list goes on and on and it is important for all NHS staff constantly to strive to identify failures and try to obviate them. We often are too prone to perpetuate old practices, and too complacent.

For clinicians, one important area of criticism concerns poor clinical case management. First, it is agreed that many treatments are unjustified and ineffective, or provided in the wrong way. Second, it is clear that there are great variations between countries, between regions and between individual clinicians in the rate of intervention, treatment regimes, length of stay and resources used. If there was more consistency around the average of the better performers and if unnecessary (i.e. not provably effective) treatments were excluded, there would be much more (usually estimated at 20%) capacity available for more justified cases. Third, in the UK, a 1% increase in GP referrals means 2.5 million additional hospital cases, so better clinical protocols and liaison with GPs could have a disproportionately positive impact.

Cynical view

The cynical view holds that waiting lists are the result of vested interests. Despite the rhetoric of the internal market, money has singularly failed to 'follow the patient'. Hospitals still fall into the 'efficiency trap', dealing with patients early in the financial year and finding themselves short of money to use their theatres and beds properly later in the year. Specially earmarked waiting-list allocations of money by the government have, in effect, rewarded the hospitals that have allowed lists to grow. It has helped to avoid the embarrassing possibility of some hospitals going bankrupt. Individual clinicians also benefit from long waiting lists. There is a perverse incentive under which the length of a list is deemed to reflect a consultant's importance and status. And obviously the

prospect of a long wait may encourage patients to go into private practice, often under the same consultant.

A waiting list can give clinicians bargaining power, for everything from a new facility, extra staff or upgrading their secretaries. It is a way of controlling demand on them. It gives them a chance to choose interesting cases for themselves, or for training purposes. Less cynically, it can be argued that waiting lists grow because the clinician psychologically prefers to take better care of existing patients or refuses to allow clinical priorities to be distorted by administrative criteria.

Multifactorial cause

The most convincing explanation for waiting lists is that they are actually the product of a great many local decisions and situations. Consequently, reducing them will need many sustained interactions, rather than finding one catch-all solution. The senior managers tackled various administrative aspects of a Swansea hospital's waiting lists and brought about a 22% reduction. They also carried out detailed interviews with consultants and concluded that 'the waiting list problem is not simply related to resources, but involved more profound issues of professional power and control'. This involved the relationship between hospital doctors and other hospital doctors, managers and GPs.

In discussing their findings, the authors made 24 specific recommendations for change, and discovered that the early cooperation with consultants evaporated! Although some proposals were administrative, others classified clinical and non-clinical issues in a way that threatened professional interests and led to the authors being threatened with legal action. They report that 'the application of qualitative research techniques to management problems proved to be a salutary lesson…'.

Another analysis in Swansea showed a 20-fold variation in referral rates between GPs. A GP who referred excessively in one specialty did not necessarily do so for another.

GP referral is a function of his or her confidence, which in turn can be affected by:

- proper referral protocols
- doctor education
- patient expectation
- specialists, attitudes locally
- access to diagnostic facilities
- the financing system
- their knowledge of existing waiting lists.

Patients fail to turn up for operations, even where special clinics or lists have been arranged for them. One of the authors once investigated an 'urgent' case who had been on an ophthalmology list for over 2 years, and who became a *cause celebre*. Looking more closely it was found that he was a seaman who had been given a number of appointments to match his home leave, but who chose to put it off each time. But the card index of waiting cases just showed him as a persistently waiting urgent case.

Out-patient waiting lists

Factors that can cause long waiting lists in out-patient departments include:

- a widespread failure to define consultants' rôles

Waiting lists

➤ Waiting lists only exist where there is a well-defined referral system, limited places where the referral care is offered, the procedures to keep records and political and public urge to debate the issue.

➤ Positive values of waiting lists include avoiding overcapacity and waste and avoiding overhasty intervention.

➤ Waiting lists are caused by inefficient funds, poor management, vested interests within the medical profession and a composite of many local decisions at different levels of management.

---

vis-à-vis those referring to them, so that cases are not referred back to GPs for management
- automatic follow-up of all postoperative patients in out-patient departments, when they and / or the GP / community nurse could be advised of how to manage postoperatively
- consultants preferring a personal referral rather than accepting a 'pool' referral
- junior staff automatically giving old cases a follow-up appointment (usually 6 months ahead so their successor can take on the case)
- GPs and patients referring cases as 'emergencies' to jump the queue, thereby distorting the referral patterns
- individual variation amongst specialists about how they prioritise their lists – or even letting their secretaries do the prioritisation
- failure to 'cull' lists: it is commonly found that 20–30% of patients have been admitted as emergencies, been tested privately, moved, died, or decided to live with the condition.

Managing waiting lists

It will be obvious that there are many causes and, therefore, many possible options for managing waiting lists. Figure 32.1 shows examples of guidance for good practice and Table 32.1 shows ways of reducing waiting lists. The following are all approaches that have been used with some measure of success to reduce waiting lists.

The use of severity indices. These have been developed to categorise patients more precisely than the traditional 'urgent/non-urgent' classification used by

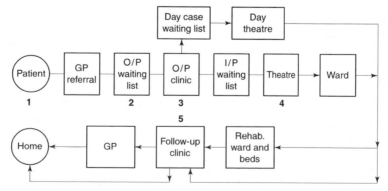

Fig. 32.1 Patient flow and opportunities for reducing waiting lists: 1, agreed referral protocols; 2, structured waiting list by condition; 3, clinics run according to capacity and pressures; 4, flexible operating lists; 5, using protocols for follow-up. o/p, out-patient; I/P, in-patient; Rehab, rehabilitation.

Table 32.1 Ways of reducing waiting lists

Key elements	Minimum	Good practice	Best practice
Publish clear waiting time priorities	List waiting time issues by specialty	Prioritise issues by specialty	Prioritise issues by condition/procedure
Generate options to respond to priorities	Analyse waiting list/time problems and generate options to tackle them	Analyse problems: generate options and prioritise on specialty basis	Analysis and generation of options appraised on cost–benefit basis
Agree and set waiting list/time targets	Set target based on in-patient, out-patient, day-case and emergency/elective mix	Set target as minimum with reference to historical referral patterns	Set target as good practice together with prospective analysis of case mix
Incorporate targets within service contract	Agree and prioritise specialty-based targets	Agree and prioritise targets linked to investment	Agree and prioritise condition/procedure targets. Link to investment in specific schemes
Identify and implement actions	Actions supported by outline project plan	Actions supported by project plan and risk factors identified	Actions supported by risk analysis and contingency planning
Put monitoring systems in place	Compare monthly actual versus target activity by specialty	Compare monthly actual versus target activity on procedure/condition basis	As good practice, with referral, rare and prospective case mix analysis added
Take follow-up action	Agree contingency action: purchaser and provider	Agree contingency action linked to activity and waiting list/time projections	As good practice linked to agreed/planned variation in contract: cost and activity
GP referral	Referral letter format agreed by consultant	Referral letter to state urgency, reason and provisional diagnosis	Referral protocols agreed between GP and consultants
Categorisation and prioritisation of patients	Categorise patients according to urgency	Categorise patients according to urgency and condition	As good practice and link to condition clinics
New out-patients appointments	Ensure appropriate mix of new and return patients	Organise specific clinics for most common conditions	Offer booked admission date
In-patient treatment	Ensure efficient use of capacity to minimise turnover interval	As minimum, with, in addition, development of discharge procedures	Develop in-patient protocols, length of stay and discharge procedures by condition
Day theatre use	Dedicated day theatre available	Day theatre linked to preoperative assessment clinics	Develop day case protocols: identify patient groups for day surgery
Return out-patient appointments	Monitor return-to-new out-patient ratio	Develop clear criteria for discharge to GP	Develop out-patient protocols: number of and reason for return visits
Theatre management	Emergency theatre available	Identify sessions available to be booked by consultant or specialities	Introduce three session working theatre to be utilised over 12 hours
Structure waiting list by priority	Prioritise waiting list by urgent (1), semi-urgent (2) and routine (3)	As level 1 and by age group	Identify average, maximum and minimum waiting time by priority
Structure waiting list by condition/procedure	Identify five most common conditions: structure list according to numbers in five areas	Structure list as minimum and by priority within each condition	Structure list by diagnoses/intended management of patient
Link structuring of list to out-patient resources	Link out-patient booking systems to list prioritisation	Introduce condition-specific clinics	Introduce out-patient booking systems linked to condition/procedure and priority
Link structuring of list to in-patient resources	Allocate in-patient beds according to waiting list priorities	Link waiting list structure to categorisation of in-patient beds: emergency high/low dependency	As good practice and link to introduction of discharge procedures
Link structuring of list to programme of investigations	Ensure out-patient investigations programmed according to priority	Ensure out-patient and in-patient investigations programmed and linked to waiting list priorities	Link protocols of programmed investigation unit to waiting list priorities and conditions

GPs. More work could be developed in this area, with greater use of clinical protocols and guidelines by GPs and specialists.

Validation of waiting lists. This involves checking whether all patients still want treatment, are alive, have been treated as emergencies or have been treated privately. Those not still requiring treatment are removed from the list. Whether patients offered appointments and not showing up should be culled is a controversial issue.

Management. Improved management systems for out-patient department, theatres, admissions department, etc., including better liaison, instituted to reduce unnecessary waits.

Waiting list managers. These have been used to improve coordination and use of resources and to develop procedures and protocols to use facilities to maximum capacity.

Use spare capacity. Using theatres for longer hours, using capacity elsewhere, or even using the private sector, has increased flow through the system.

Booking systems. A forward booking system has been tried; this could run perhaps much further in advance to anticipate need – unnecessary bookings can always be filled. Such cases could legitimately be described not as 'waiting' but as being under managed care.

More use of referral protocols. These give clear clin-ical guidelines, using clinical audit to identify non-compliance with agreed procedures, better definition of consultant rôle and guidance for junior staff.

Use of 'treatment centres'. Centres specialising in the commonest cases, perhaps using semi-retired or part-time staff have been used successfully to deal with cataracts.

'Blitzes'. These have been used to try to clear backlogs. They could use specifically allocated resources or concentrate on certain cases.

Clearer protocols for junior staff. These concerned follow-up procedures; improved community and GP liaison was also used to alleviate hospital visits for some postoperative or chronic cases.

Reducing waiting lists

➤ Use agreed referral protocols: severity indices ensure list only carries patients still requiring treatment.

➤ Structure waiting lists by conditions; treat some conditions in separate treatment centres.

➤ Use spare capacity and flexible operating lists to ensure maximal flow through the system.

➤ Use protocols for follow-up, allowing some to occur in the primary-care sector.

References for figures and tables

Alberti K G 1993 Problems related to definitions and epidemiology of type 2 non-insulin dependent diabetes mellitus: studies throughout the world. Diabetologia 36:978–84

Anonymous 1973 Oral contraceptives and venous thromboembolic disease, surgically confirmed gallbladder disease, and breast tumours. Report from the Boston Collaborative Drug Surveillance Programme. Lancet 1:1399–404

Anspaugh L R, Catlin R J, Goldman M 1988 The global impact of the Chernobyl reactor accident. Science 242:1513–9

Anto J M, Sunyer J, Rodriguez-Roisin R, Suarez-Cervera M, Vazquez L 1989 Community outbreaks of asthma associated with inhalation of soybean dust. Toxicoepidemiological committee. New England Journal of Medicine 320:1097–102

Benhamou E, Benhamou S, Auquier A, Flamant R 1989 Changes in patterns of cigarette smoking and lung cancer risk: results of a case-control study. British Journal of Cancer 60:601–4

Bithell J F, Dutton S J, Draper G J, Neary N M 1994 Distribution of childhood leukaemias and non-Hodgkin's lymphomas near nuclear installations in England and Wales. BMJ 309:501–5

Cartier A 1998 Occupational asthma: what have we learned. Journal of Allergy & Clinical Immunology 102:S90–5

Citterio A, Azan G, Bergamaschi R, Ernetta A, Cosi V 1989 Multiple sclerosis: disability and mortality in a cohort of clinically diagnosed patients. Neuroepidemiology 8:249–53

deDombal F T 1975 Computer-aided diagnosis and decision-making in the acute abdomen. Journal of the Royal College of Physicians of London 9:211–8

Editorial 1989 Radiation Exposure. Practitioner 233:1631–2

Ennals S 1991 Industrial injuries benefits. BMJ 302:400–1

Evans J G, Seagroat V, Goldacre M J 1997 Secular trends in proximal femoral fracture, Oxford record linkage study area and England 1968–86. Journal of Epidemiology and Community Health 51:424–9

Gale R P 1984 Progress in acute myelogenous leukemia. Annals of Internal Medicine 101:702–5

Griffith D E, Levin J L 1989 Respiratory effects of outdoor air pollution. Postgraduate Medicine 86:111–6

Hartnett B J, Marlin G E 1976 Doxycycline in serum and bronchial secretions. Thorax 31:144–8

Hemingway A P 1991 25 years of imaging. Hospital Medicine 46:235–7

Illing H P 1989 Assessment of toxicity for major hazards: some concepts and problems. Human Toxicology 8:369

Ions G K, Stevens J 1987 Prediction of survival in patients with femoral neck fractures. Journal of Bone & Joint Surgery (British Volume) 69:384–7

Kabat G C 1998 Aspects of the epidemiology of lung cancer in smokers and non-smokers in the United States. Lung Cancer 15:1–20

Kannel W B 1990 CHD risk factors: a Farmingham study update. Hospital Practice 25:119–27

Keighley M R, Buchman P, Minervini S, Arabi Y, Alexander-Williams J 1979 Prospective trials of minor surgical procedures and high fibre diet for haemorrhoids. British Medical Journal 2:967–9

Khaw K T, Rose G 1989 Cholesterol screening programmes: how much potential benefit. British Medical Journal 299:606–7

Lowe C R 1973 Congenital malformations among infants born to epileptic women. Lancet 1:9–10

Lowe J E, Gall S A Jr. 1997 Correlates of survival in patients with postinfarction ventricular septal defect. Annals of Thoracic Surgery 63:1508–9

Malmgren W B, Warlow C, Bamford J, Sandercock P 1987 Geographical and secular trends in stroke incidence. Lancet 20:1196–200

McCulloch P 1996 Gastric cancer. Postgraduate Medical Journal. 72:450–7

McKeown T 1979 The role of medicine. Blackwell Ltd, Oxford

McPherson K, Wennberg J E, Hovind O B, Clifford P 1982 Small-area variations in the use of common surgical procedures: an international comparison of New England, England and Norway. New England Journal of Medicine 307:1310–4

Mechanic D 1995 The Americanization of the British National Health Service. Health Affairs 14:51–67

Mechanic D, McAlpine D D, Olfson M 1997 Changing patterns of psychiatric inpatient care in the United States, 1988–1994. Archives of General Psychiatry 55:785–91

Mosser M 1989 Suppositions and speculations—their possible effects on treatment decisions in the management of hypertension. American Heart Journal 118:1362–9

Mossman B T, Gee J B 1989 Asbestos-related diseases. New England Journal of Medicine 320:1721–30

Morrow R H, Bryant J H 1995 Health policy approaches to measuring and valuing human life: conceptual and ethical issues [see comments]. American Journal of Public Health 85:1356–60

OHE Compendium of Health Statistics, 10th edition 1997

OPCS 1997 General Household Survey. HMSO

OPCS Rates of incapacity for work. Cause 1970–1993 HMSO

OPCS 1997 Bed use statistics for the United Kingdom. 1950–1997 DoH, OPCS

Open University Press 1984 The Health of Nations. The Open University Press, Milton Keynes

Orszulak T A, Schaff H V, Chesebro J H, Holmes D R Jr 1986 Initial experience with sequential internal mammary artery bypass grafts to the left anterior descending diagonal coronary arteries. 1986 Mayo Clinic Proceedings 61:3–8

Paling J, Paling S 1993 Up to your armpits in alligators. The Environmental Institute, Gainsville, Florida

PHLS Communicable Disease Surveillance Centre 1994 Quarterly communicable disease review October to December 1993. Journal of Public Health Medicine 16:235–41

Pica-Furey W 1993 Ambulatory surgery—hospital based versus freestanding. A comparative study of patient satisfaction. AORN Journal 57:1119–27

Reingold A L, Hargett N T, Shands K N et al 1982 Toxic shock syndrome surveillance in the United States, 1980 to 1981. Annals of Internal Medicine 96:875–80

Sadovnick A D, Ebers G C Wilson R W, Paty D W 1992 Life expectancy in patients attending multiple sclerosis clinics. Neurology 42:991–4

SIGN (Scottish Intercollegiate Guidelines Network) Report of Findings. 1997 Royal College of Physicians of Edinburgh, Edinburgh

Smith D C 1986 A historical overview of the recognition of appendicitis—Part 1. New York State Journal of Medicine 86:571–83

Stykowski P A, Kannel W B, D'Agostino R B 1990 Changes in risk factors and the decline in mortality from cardiovascular disease. The Farmingham Heart Study. New England Journal of Medicine 322:1635–41

Tokuhata G 1981 1980 Mortality Figures. News Release. Pennsylvania Department of Health

Vessy M P, Doll R, Sutton P M 1972 Oral contraceptives and breast neoplasia: a retrospective study. British Medical Journal 829:719–24

Weston C, Donelly P 1995 Management of cardiac arrest by ambulance technicians and paramedics. Studying only admissions is a source of potential bias [letter; comment]. British Medical Journal 311:509

Wolf P A, D'Agnostino R B, Kannel W B, Bonita R, Belanger A J 1988 Cigarette smoking as a risk factor for stroke. The Farmingham Study. Journal of the American Medical Association 259:1025–9

World Bank 1993 Investing in health. World development report 1993. Oxford University Press, Oxford

Index